Leprosy and Empire

An innovative, interdisciplinary study of why leprosy, a disease with a very low level of infection, has repeatedly provoked revulsion and fear. Rod Edmond explores, in particular, how these reactions were re-fashioned in the modern colonial period. Beginning as a medical history, the book broadens into an examination of how Britain and its colonies responded to the believed spread of leprosy. Across the empire this involved isolating victims of the disease in 'colonies', often on offshore islands. Discussion of the segregation of lepers is then extended to analogous examples of this practice, which, it is argued, has been an essential part of the repertoire of colonialism in the modern period. The book also examines literary representations of leprosy in Romantic, Victorian and twentieth-century writing, and concludes with a discussion of traveller-writers such as R. L. Stevenson and Graham Greene who described and fictionalized their experience of staying in a leper colony.

ROD EDMOND is Professor of Modern Literature and Cultural History at the University of Kent. His previous publications include *Representing the South Pacific: Colonial Discourse from Cook to Gauguin* (1997) and, as co-editor with Vanessa Smith, *Islands in History and Representation* (2003).

Cambridge Social and Cultural Histories

Series editors:
Margot C. Finn, *University of Warwick*
Colin Jones, *University of Warwick*
Keith Wrightson, *Yale University*

New cultural histories have recently expanded the parameters (and enriched the methodologies) of social history. Cambridge Social and Cultural Histories recognises the plurality of current approaches to social and cultural history as distinctive points of entry into a common explanatory project. Open to innovative and interdisciplinary work, regardless of its chronological or geographical location, the series encompasses a broad range of histories of social relationships and of the cultures that inform them and lend them meaning. Historical anthropology, historical sociology, comparative history, gender history and historicist literary studies – among other subjects – all fall within the remit of Cambridge Social and Cultural Histories.

Titles in the series include:

Leprosy and Empire

A Medical and Cultural History

Rod Edmond

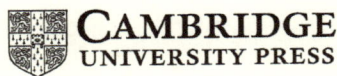
CAMBRIDGE
UNIVERSITY PRESS

CAMBRIDGE UNIVERSITY PRESS
Cambridge, New York, Melbourne, Madrid, Cape Town, Singapore,
São Paulo, Delhi, Dubai, Tokyo

Cambridge University Press
The Edinburgh Building, Cambridge CB2 8RU, UK

Published in the United States of America by Cambridge University Press, New York

www.cambridge.org
Information on this title: www.cambridge.org/9780521123129

First published 2006
This digitally printed version 2009

A catalogue record for this publication is available from the British Library

ISBN 978-0-521-86584-5 Hardback
ISBN 978-0-521-12312-9 Paperback

'Whan he was in his lusti age,
The leper cawhte in his visage
And so forth overall aboute,
That he ne mihte ryden oute.'

(John Gower)

'A distemper so noisome, that it might well pass for the utmost corruption of
the human body, on this side of the grave.' (Anonymous seventeenth-century
traveller)

'It is in truth a distemper corrupting the whole mass of the blood, and therefore
considered by Paul of Aegina as an universal ulcer.' (William Jones)

'There is hardly anything on earth, or between it and heaven, which has not been
regarded as the cause of leprosy.' (Arneur Hansen)

'The ugly troubles and weakens man, it reminds him of deterioration and
impotence.' (Friedrich Nietzsche)

'Death is the most contagious plague and we've all got it; it moulds its features
upon the features of the living.' (Robin Hyde)

'Wonderful! To study history as if it were a body!' (Michael Ondaatje)

Contents

Illustrations

Acknowledgements

Grateful acknowledgement is made to the Wellcome Trust for a research leave fellowship that allowed me to do much of the research for this book. Particular thanks are due to Michael Worboys for his advice and guidance as I began the project, and for his support as I pursued it.

I also wish to thank librarians at the Wellcome Institute; the British Library; the Mission Houses Museum Library, Honolulu; the Hamilton library at the University of Hawaii, Manoa; and at my home institution, the University of Kent.

Colleagues in my own department, especially those in the Centre for Postcolonial Studies – Abdulrazak Gurnah, Lyn Innes and Caroline Rooney – have provided an unfailingly supportive context in which to write and teach. Colleagues in Kent's History Department – Ulf Schmidt and Charlotte Sleigh – have offered a new and welcome context in which to pursue my research.

Elsewhere, it is a pleasure to thank Sara Salih and Vanessa Smith for their friendship, emails and support.

Bits and pieces of this book have been aired at several conferences and research seminars, and I am grateful to audiences at the 'Reconfiguring the British' seminar at the Institute of Historical Research, London; the Wellcome Unit for the History of Medicine, Oxford; the Centre for the History of Science, Technology and Medicine, and the Wellcome Unit at the University of Manchester; the History of Medicine Centre at the University of Warwick; and the University of Sussex for their suggestions and criticisms.

I have previously published some of the material in chapter 3 in 'Returning fears: tropical disease and the metropolis', in Felix Driver and Luciana Martins (eds.), *Tropical Visions in an Age of Empire* (Chicago and London: Chicago University Press, 2005), and in ' "Without the camp": leprosy and nineteenth-century writing', *Victorian Literature and Culture* 29:2 (2001). A shorter version of chapter 4 was published as 'Abject bodies/abject sites: leper islands in the high imperial era', in Rod Edmond and Vanessa Smith (eds.), *Islands in History and Representation*

(London: Routledge, 2003). I am grateful to the publishers of this material for permission to republish it.

Many individuals have helped in many ways, often by pointing me in the direction of new sources and references. These include (I'm sure the list isn't exhaustive): Tim Armstrong, Henry Bernstein, Jo Collins, Cilla Corlett, Hugh Cunningham, Harriet Deacon, Ursula Deith, Brian Dillon, Felix Driver, Marion Edmond, Murray Edmond, Catherine Hall, Mark Harrison, Colin Jones, Jonathan Lamb, Andrew Lincoln, Allan Mitchell, Jan Montefiore, Nancy and Al Morris, Dave Murray, Emily Nash, Maria Nugent, Felicity Nussbaum, Evelyn O'Callaghan, Marion O'Connor, Bill Purcell, Nigel Rigby, Jo Robertson, Stephanie Rudgard-Redsell, Martin Scofield, Lynette Shum, Tony Skillen, Amy Smith, Murray Smith, Scarlett Thomas, Marina Warner, Val Wilmer.

As before, thanks to Sarah, Cassius, Daisy and Jo, and for the first time, Ed and Molly; Claudia, Louis and Otto.

Introduction

Revulsion and fear have been the most common responses to leprosy since biblical times, yet there is slight medical basis for the recurring stigmatisation of a disease with such a very low level of infection. Leprosy, it seems, has had extraordinary potential for becoming more than itself. The reasons for this, the myths that accrued around the disease, and particularly the manner in which these were refashioned in the modern colonial period, is the subject of this book.

Carlo Ginzburg has described the panic in early fourteenth-century France around an alleged conspiracy of lepers to kill the healthy by poisoning the fountains and wells. As alarm spread, the rumoured conspiracy grew to include the Jews (there was an ancient tradition that among the ancestors of the Jews was a group of lepers driven out of Egypt), and then, somewhat improbably, the Muslim king of Granada. Ginzburg argues that lepers and Jews were pariah groups because of their ambiguous borderline status. Lepers were unclean, but loving them was, as Francis of Assisi had shown, a sign of sanctity. Jews were the deicide race but also those to whom God had chosen to reveal himself. Muslims were the threat from without, the menacing world beyond Christendom, conspiring with those groups within whose marginality made them susceptible to promises of wealth and power, as well as potential targets of social purification. Ginzburg also sketches a wider social context for this outbreak of victimisation. Tensions provoked by the establishment of a monetary economy were finding expression in anti-Semitic hatred, behind which lay the determination of an aggressive mercantile class to sweep away the competition of the money-lenders. The role of the lepers in this is more obscure, but there were large revenues to be derived from the administration of the many leper asylums.[1]

In the cold war Hollywood movie *Big Jim McLain* (1952), John Wayne plays an investigator for the Un-American Activities Committee sent to Hawaii to root out communism in the islands. As his plane approaches

---

[1] Carlo Ginzburg, *Ecstasies: Deciphering the Witches' Sabbath* (Harmondsworth: Penguin, 1992), part 1.

Honolulu the film zooms in on the famous leper colony on the adjacent island of Molokai, providing a focal point for the hero's mission to protect these beautiful islands from the modern infection of communism. If the 'ancient leper colony of Kalaupapa' as the film has it (in fact it was established in 1865) is the islands' traditional worm in the bud, communism threatens to be its modern equivalent. When Big Jim visits Pearl Harbor we are reminded of the threat from without, but more disturbing is the new insidious threat from within. Just as the arrival of Chinese indentured labourers in the mid-nineteenth century had brought leprosy to Hawaii and threatened the good health and stability of this United States colony-in-the-making, communism now presents an analogous danger. The communists plan to cripple Hawaii in two ways. Union action will stop exports, while a sinister bacteriologist will infect the people. Communism, like leprosy, is a contagion, and both are definitely un-American. This identification is associative rather than precise, but the narrative implication is clear; communism, like leprosy, is infective, deforming and horrifying.

Both episodes demonstrate how leprosy readily becomes a focus for almost anything that Judeo-Christian cultures have found particularly troubling. The origins of this are biblical. When Big Jim McLain climbs nervously out of the light aircraft that has flown him to Molokai in his quest for communist subversion, he recalls his childhood revulsion at Bible stories of lepers read to him by his mother. The biblical figure of the leper is, in fact, a deeply ambivalent one. In the Old Testament the leper is to be sent 'without the camp', as the Book of Leviticus has it. Out of this grew the tradition of proclaiming the rites of death over the still living body of the leper, and of regarding leprosy as a moral as well as a physical disease: as an emblem of sin. In the New Testament, however, the leper becomes more a figure of pity, and leprosy a metaphor of divine salvation, with the emphasis on treatment and cure rather than on diagnosis and segregation. Francis of Assisi exemplified this by cherishing the pariah of the Old Testament. Something of this ambivalence can be seen in the lepers' squint, that feature of church architecture which allowed the leper to see into the church but not to enter and partake: in other words to be simultaneously present and absent.

Chapter 14 of the Book of Leviticus concludes: 'To teach when it is unclean, and when it is clean: this is the law of leprosy.' Chapters 13 and 14 are preoccupied with the difficulty of interpreting and applying this law, as the following examples from chapter 13 show:

38. If a man also or a woman have in the skin of their flesh bright spots, *even* white bright spots;
39. Then the priest shall look: and, behold, *if* the bright spots in the skin of their flesh *be* darkish white; it *is* a freckled spot *that* groweth in the skin; he *is* clean.
40. And the man whose hair is fallen off his head, he *is* bald; *yet is* he clean.

42. And if there be in the bald head, or bald forehead, a white reddish sore; it *is* a leprosy sprung up in his bald head, or his bald forehead.

43. Then the priest shall look upon it: and, behold, *if* the rising of the sore *be* white reddish in his bald head, or in his bald forehead, as the leprosy appeareth in the skin of the flesh;

44. He is a leprous man, he *is* unclean: the priest shall pronounce him utterly unclean; his plague *is* in his head.

46. All the days wherein the plague *shall be* in him he shall be defiled; he *is* unclean: he shall dwell alone; without the camp *shall* his habitation *be.*

If Leviticus is regarded as a handbook for priests to help them diagnose leprosy and distinguish it from less serious skin afflictions, these verses illustrate how difficult this was. They circle and return obsessively to the spot, blemish or sore in question in the attempt to decide whether it is clean or unclean.

Why was leprosy one of the abominations of Leviticus? Mary Douglas has suggested a general answer to this question: 'Those species are unclean which are imperfect members of their class, or whose class itself confounds the general scheme of the world'.[2] Allied to this was the idea of the human body as an expression of wholeness and completeness, the 'perfect container'.[3] Wholeness is a metaphor for holiness, and involves definition, discrimination and order: 'Holiness means keeping distinct the categories of creation'.[4] Although there is no specific discussion of leprosy in *Purity and Danger*, Douglas opens up an approach to my question. Leprosy undermines the integrity of the body and its significance as an expression of cherished distinctions and categories. Most vividly the leprous body challenges the fundamental distinction between life and death, putrefying and decomposing while alive and still able to reproduce. This, in turn, suggests Julia Kristeva's concept of abjection, which partly derives from *Purity and Danger*. In *Powers of Horror*, Kristeva argues that the human corpse, which is almost universally surrounded by rituals and taboos to prevent contamination of the living, is the most horrifying manifestation of the impossibility of a clear distinction between the clean and unclean, and thus between order and disorder. The leprous body, even more than Kristeva's example of the corpse, is a mordant instance of what she means by abjection: 'a border that has encroached upon everything ... death infecting life ... something rejected from which one does not part'.[5] If, in

[2] Mary Douglas, *Purity and Danger: An Analysis of Concepts of Pollution and Taboo* (Harmondsworth: Penguin, 1970), p. 70.

[3] *Ibid.*, p. 65.   [4] *Ibid.*, p. 67.

[5] Julia Kristeva, *Powers of Horror: An Essay on Abjection* (New York: Columbia University Press, 1982), pp. 3–4.

Douglas's words, '(h)ybrids and other confusions are abominated', then the leper becomes the most disquieting hybrid of all.[6]

In *Leviticus as Literature* Mary Douglas has elaborated and modified her earlier study. Importantly she reminds us that Leviticus was composed and edited during a long period of continuing political upheaval.[7] Leprosy's tendency to become more than itself has frequently been heightened at moments of social or political disturbance. Douglas also demonstrates the correlative literary style of Leviticus and the way in which this works through analogies. Most, if not all, literary treatments of leprosy seem to share this characteristic: testament to the extraordinary signifying power of the disease. Douglas reads chapters 12–15 of Leviticus as constructing from the human body prone to sickness a microcosm of the sanctuary in danger of defilement.[8] Chapter 12 is concerned with the blood impurity of a woman menstruating or giving birth; chapters 13 and 14 with leprosy; and chapter 15 with genital discharges from men or women. These exposed and risk-prone conditions are sources of impurity, and in terms of the body logic of Leviticus, constitute a threat to the integrity of the living being: 'The breach of the body's containing walls evidenced by an escape of vital fluids and the failure of its skin cover are vulnerable states which go counter to God's creative action when he set up separating boundaries in the beginning.'[9]

The two chapters specifically concerned with leprosy extend outwards from the diseased body to the garments clothing that body, and then to the house that encloses both. Each is given the same diagnostic treatment and the cleansed house as well as the cleansed body receives atonement.[10] These three analogies of leprosy – the pustulating body, the garment and the house – are a cover for the person inside, each enclosed by a further cover and leading to the tabernacle 'where the series of spoilt covers converges'.[11] The laws of leprosy, like those of bodily discharges, expound the meaning of bodily impurity and its relation to the sacred as expressed in the body of the tabernacle. Contact with the polluted thing will transmit that pollution on and on until it impinges on the sacred body of the tabernacle.[12] Leprosy, therefore, is a form of 'sacred contagion': not a consequence of the maleficent power of demons but a result of the action of God for some breach of his covenant. Ritual impurity, such as that represented by the leprous body and its enforced removal from the camp, is a way of reimposing God's order on his creation. For the Leviticus writer, 'unclean' is not primarily a term of psychological horror and disgust but a

---

[6] Douglas, *Purity and Danger*, p. 67.
[7] Mary Douglas, *Leviticus as Literature* (Oxford: Oxford University Press, 2000), p. 7.
[8] *Ibid.*, p. 176.   [9] *Ibid.*, p. 190.   [10] *Ibid.*, p. 177.   [11] *Ibid.*, p. 191.   [12] *Ibid.*, p. 187.

way of demonstrating the comprehensive nature of God's care and control.[13]

Already there are problems with my discussion. Does the leprosy of Leviticus, of fourteenth-century France and twentieth-century Hawaii describe the same clinical entity? And does the concern of the Leviticus writer, the panic of late medieval southern French society, and the fear of the anti-communist investigator derive from some common trans-historical Judeo-Christian revulsion at the disease, or does each of these instances have a historical specificity that makes it misleading to run them together in the way that I have so far been doing? The simple answer to the first of these questions is almost certainly not. Even within the Bible, the symptoms of leprosy in Leviticus are different, for example, from those described by Aaron in Numbers. The Leviticus writer is concerned with blemishes of the skin, and there is no equivalent of the account in Numbers, which describes it as a condition in which the flesh is 'half consumed' (12: 12). Mary Douglas argues that Leviticus's description suggests not one but various skin diseases, including skin cancer, psoriasis, tropical ulcers, yaws, and major infectious diseases such as smallpox or measles.[14] In medieval and early modern Europe leprosy was very often a generic term for a wide range of skin diseases and, clinically speaking, it is only in the early nineteenth century that a sustained attempt was begun to distinguish leprosy from other skin disorders, and to distinguish between different types of leprosy itself. That said, the Leviticus writer is obsessively concerned with establishing 'true leprosy' and with distinguishing it from other superficially similar diseases. And for all that leprosy continued to be run together with other skin diseases, it was also imperative to differentiate a disease that was believed to be highly contagious and whose consequences for the sufferer were so serious. Accurate diagnosis was, on the one hand, impossible, and on the other, essential. Versions of this dilemma haunted the disease until well into the twentieth century.

Does a constant set of causes underlie the apparent continuity of response to leprosy since biblical times? For a medical scientist such as Olaf K. Skinsnes, leprosy is a disease with a unique medical pathology that produces a unique social response; a constant set of causes results in an identical stigma wherever the disease appears.[15] And a literary critic like Nathaniel Brady also sees the resurfacing of fears about leprosy in Europe in the nineteenth century, after centuries during which the disease had virtually disappeared, as testimony to its constant power as an emblem of

---

[13] *Ibid.*, pp. 149–51, 188.   [14] *Ibid.*, pp. 183–4.
[15] Zachary Gussow, *Leprosy, Racism, and Public Health: Social Policy in Chronic Disease Control* (Boulder, Colo.: Westview Press, 1989), p. 8.

sin and moral decay.[16] For Zachary Gussow, however, to regard the reaction to leprosy as a psychological and cultural constant is to augment the very process being described and to endorse the idea of the long unchanging history of leprosy's taint; '[h]umanity's dread is termed a natural response', and leprosy becomes perpetually identified with stigma. Biblical tradition and the literary imagination, he suggests, have been particularly important in sustaining this account of the history of the disease.[17]

Gussow himself denies the universality of both the response and its causes, arguing that leprosy was 'retainted' in the modern colonial period; around the turn of the twentieth century it was transformed from 'a feared clinical entity' into 'a stigmatised phenomenon'.[18] He sees a number of interlocking reasons for this: the discovery of the leprosy bacillus in 1874 which offered scientific support for those who argued the disease was contagious rather than hereditary; the belief that leprosy was racially selective, and had become a tropical rather than a European disease; the movement of indentured labour around the world following the abolition of slavery, and consequent fear of the disease spreading; and the organised involvement of Western missionaries in leprosy work in the wake of the expansion of European empires.[19] This approach is clearly more satisfactory than trans-historical and trans-cultural explanations that see the fear of leprosy as constant and unchanging. The idea of 'retainting' also fits the sequence proposed by Foucault in which leprosy disappeared from the Western world at the end of the Middle Ages, with criminals and the insane taking the part previously played by the leper.[20] Gussow builds on some of the possibilities opened up by Foucault's argument.[21]

There are, however, significant differences between the two. Gussow treats modern leprosy almost as if it were a new disease, although he declines to be drawn into the question of the continuity or otherwise of biblical and medieval leprosy with its modern forms.[22] In terms of its stigmatisation he insistently emphasises discontinuity: 'It is unnecessary to search the human psyche deeply or to reach far back into history to account for modern lepraphobia. A close look at the expanding Western world during the late nineteenth and early twentieth centuries suffices.'[23]

---

[16] *Ibid.*, p. 12.   [17] *Ibid.*, p. 4.

[18] Zachary Gussow and George S. Tracy, 'Stigma and the Leprosy Phenomenon: The Social History of a Disease in the Nineteenth and Twentieth Centuries', *Bulletin of the History of Medicine*, 44 (1970), 440.

[19] Gussow, *Leprosy, Racism, and Public Health*, pp. 201–9.

[20] Michel Foucault, *Madness and Civilisation: A History of Insanity in the Age of Reason* (London: Tavistock Publications, 1979), ch. 1.

[21] Gussow, *Leprosy, Racism, and Public Health*, p. 18.   [22] *Ibid.*, p. 6.   [23] *Ibid.*, p. 23.

For Foucault, however, the structures of exclusion built around the figure of the leper persisted, even if the disease disappeared.[24] Foucault also bypasses the question as to whether modern, medieval and biblical leprosy describe the same disease. For him the important point is that Judeo-Christian societies at different historical moments have used the label as if it did describe a constant condition. Although many of the causes underlying the prominence often given to leprosy have undoubtedly changed, the need for a disease that provided a physical basis upon which to exclude certain groups persisted. Or, more precisely, this need became urgent at particular periods. Within the smaller, more circumscribed cultures of Europe in the Middle Ages the question of who did and did not belong must often have been pressing. Large-scale movements of people, such as the Crusades, were particularly disturbing. Disease spread, new diseases were introduced, and other kinds of imagined contamination followed. Similarly in the modern colonial period, the mass movement of indentured labourers from India, China and Japan across the Caribbean, Indian and Pacific oceans brought heightened fears of the spread of disease, which in turn offered a language with which to stigmatise and denigrate these migrants.

So although Gussow is surely right to insist that the meanings attributed to leprosy have always been historically fashioned, this is not to deny the persistence of certain causes of both a social and psychological kind. The disease might or might not have been the same, the specific social groups which leprosy has been used to stigmatise have varied, but the suitability of leprosy for the purpose of stigmatisation has been remarkably persistent. There might have been periods when the stigma that leprosy attracts was less intense, but it has remained more constant than Gussow allows. His determination to destigmatise the condition by insisting on the historical specificity of late nineteenth- and early twentieth-century lepraphobia leads him to understate the persistent tradition of stigmatising the disease that has characterised European cultures. My concern is to try and read the stigma through time and to understand better the varying historical conditions in which it has been produced.

Foucault, however, overstates the case when he claims that leprosy disappeared from Europe in the sixteenth and seventeenth centuries. It lingered in parts of Europe, particularly in Spain and Norway, and during the first half of the nineteenth century there was growing awareness of its persistence and its possible return to other parts of Europe. The prevalence of leprosy among sections of the Norwegian peasantry was confirmed by

---

[24] Foucault, *Madness and Civilization*, p. 7.

leprosy surveys and censuses in the 1830s and 40s and resulted in a national leprosy register in Norway by 1856.[25] This began to cause anxiety in Britain, especially in Scotland where it was believed that leprosy had persisted longest before its eventual disappearance. The possible recrudescence of the disease sparked a revival of interest in its history and aetiology. During the 1840s and 50s the *Edinburgh Medical Journal* carried a series of articles on whether or not present-day leprosy was identical to that in Britain and Europe during the Middle Ages,[26] on its 'probable reappearance on our shores', and on why it had 'disappeared' in the first place.[27] Alexander Fiddes, who had first-hand experience of the disease from Jamaica, wrote: 'It seems not unreasonable to suppose, that in the same manner as the scourge declined spontaneously in the sixteenth and seventeenth centuries, so it may resume its activity at a future time, should the external causes which favour its development ever regain their ancient ascendancy.'[28] The unexplained disappearance of leprosy from many parts of Europe in the early modern period contributed directly to fears of its return in the nineteenth.

Foucault's claim that leprosy disappeared is therefore as misleading as Gussow's that it was reinvented. The disease never entirely went away, and so it did not need to be reinvented. Instead, the persistence of leprosy in parts of Europe, and an enduring tradition of stigmatisation, intersected with a rapidly changing imperial world from around the turn of the nineteenth century to produce a modern version of the disease that drew heavily on biblical and medieval ways of understanding it. This process whereby a Judeo-Christian discourse on leprosy was inflected by the modern history of colonialism to reconstruct leprosy and the figure of the leper was extremely complex. Neither Foucault nor Gussow take sufficient account of the profound ambivalence that was intrinsic to Judeo-Christian responses to the disease. Foucault swings from medieval horror of the disease to its disappearance in the post-medieval world. Gussow is preoccupied with the peculiarly modern stigmatisation of the disease and the ways of overcoming this in the contemporary world, locating the most intense reactions to it in the era of high imperialism. Horror and pity have, to varying degrees, always co-existed in tension with each other, one requiring the leper to be removed 'without the camp', the other prompting those who are clean to go and live with and tend the

---

[25] Gussow, *Leprosy, Racism, and Public Health*, p. 69.

[26] James Y. Simpson, 'Antiquarian Notices of Leprosy and Leper Hospitals in Scotland and England', *Edinburgh Medical and Surgical Journal*, 56 (1841); 57 (1842).

[27] *Edinburgh Medical Journal*, 1 (1855–6).

[28] Alexander Fiddes, 'Observations on Tubercular and Anaesthetic Leprosy, as They Occur in Jamaica', *Edinburgh Medical Journal*, 2 (1856–7), 1061.

unclean. And even these antitheses are less absolute than might at first seem. The Old Testament injunction to diagnose and expel the leprous did not rule out the possibility of recovery and return. And the modern missionary-led attempts to care for and protect the leper typically involved forms of segregation that amounted to an incommutable life sentence.

Although leprosy seems to have been linked with almost every imaginable aspect of human life, its most commonly recurring association has been with sex. Within literature, for example, the connection of leprosy and syphilis extends back at least as far as Henryson's *Testament of Cresseid* (1593) and could still be used by Somerset Maugham in his fictional treatment of Gauguin, *The Moon and Sixpence* (1919). When John Ford writes of 'The leprosy of lust' in *'Tis Pity She's a Whore* (1633) (I,i 74) the usage is commonplace. The association of leprosy and sex also occurs widely across different cultures and periods. According to Chinese legend leprosy was a divine punishment for necrophilia.[29] The idea that leprosy was a scourge for sexual licence recurs in parts of Africa where it was associated with incest.[30] In Marquesan society contact with menstruating women was believed to cause leprosy.[31] The German ethnographer Gunterh Tessmann described in *Die Pangwe* (1913) how in Cameroon, Equatorial Guinea and Gabon the active partner in male anal intercourse was thought to risk contracting leprosy.[32] Each of these random examples has its own cultural and historical specificity, but taken together they indicate broader patterns of response to the disease across cultures and through time.

In the modern colonial period leprosy was racialised as well as sexualised. This will be a recurring theme of subsequent chapters, but the theories of the American abolitionist Dr Benjamin Rush provide a useful starting point for my later discussions. In 1792 Rush presented a paper titled 'Observations intended to favour a supposition that the black Color (as it is called) of the Negroes is derived from the LEPROSY' to the American Philosophical Society. He argued that both the 'colour' and the 'figure' of Negroes were derived from a 'modification' of leprosy. A combination of tropical factors – 'unwholesome diet', 'greater heat', 'savage manners' and 'bilious fevers' – produced leprosy in Negroes. The visible symptoms of this were the Negro's physical features – the 'big lip', 'flat nose', 'woolly hair' and especially the black skin. Negroes were like lepers in their

---

[29] Nicholas Rankin, *Dead Man's Chest: Travels after Robert Louis Stevenson* (London: Phoenix Press, 2001), p. 275.
[30] Douglas, *Leviticus as Literature*, p. 185.
[31] Robert C. Suggs, *Marquesan Sexual Behaviour* (London: Constable, 1966), pp. 27–8.
[32] Rudi C. Bleys, *The Geography of Perversion: Male-to-Male Sexual Behaviour Outside the West and the Ethnographic Imagination 1750–1918* (London: Cassell, 1996), pp. 219–20.

'morbid insensitivity of the nerves' and in their unusually strong venereal desires. Rush also cited examples of white women living with Negroes acquiring a darker skin colour and Negroid features.[33] His paper strikes many of the keynotes that were to be heard in the increasingly racialised discourse of leprosy during the nineteenth century. It also demonstrates the continuity between traditional and emergent ways of figuring and explaining the disease, with a powerful libido linking the leper and the Negro.

Rush had pointed to 'unwholesome diet' as a cause of the 'leprous Negro' and, together with sex and race, food had a categorial association with the disease. Dutch settlers in Ceylon at the end of the eighteenth century decided that leprosy was caused by eating breadfruit and ordered all the trees to be cut down.[34] Dietary explanations of the disease flourished in the nineteenth century. W. Munro, some time medical officer in St Kitts, blamed vegetable diets and a want of salt.[35] Jonathan Hutchinson, former president of the Royal College of Physicians, on the other hand, put it down to eating fish, especially of the dried salted variety.[36] So convinced was Hutchinson of this theory that he partly attributed the disappearance of leprosy in Europe in the early modern period to the Reformation and its disavowal of Catholic dietary practices such as the compulsory use of fish on fast days.[37]

Sex, race and food are significant markers of boundaries. Many forms of sexual activity involve the mixing or penetration of bodies and hence the infringement of that most literal of boundaries between the self and what lies outside it. In the nineteenth century particularly, the construction and definition of racial boundaries was an intellectual industry. And food, it would seem, cannot help but invoke categories. That which is neither fish nor fowl is disturbing because it transgresses boundaries and threatens confusion. It is possible that in the examples above, breadfruit and dried fish were singled out because of their 'hybrid' nature, their apparently mixed form.

Leprosy, as I have already suggested, is a boundary disease par excellence. It can focus and dramatise the risk of trespass, serve as a punishment

---

[33] Ronald Takaki, *Iron Cages: Race and Culture in Nineteenth-Century America* (New York and Oxford: Oxford University Press, 1990), pp. 30–1.

[34] Charles Ker[r?] to Joseph Banks, 28 March 1793. Kew Banks Letters 2/94, Joseph Banks Archive of Letters, Royal Botanic Gardens Library, Kew, London. I am indebted to Dr Nigel Rigby of the National Maritime Museum, Greenwich, for this reference.

[35] W. Munro, *Leprosy* (Manchester: John Heywood, 1879), pp. 41, 93.

[36] Jonathan Hutchinson, *On Leprosy and Fish-Eating* (London: Constable, 1906), *passim*.

[37] Jonathan Hutchinson, 'Notes on Leprosy in Various Countries', *British Medical Journal*, 1 (1890), 651–6.

for such infringements, and help to re-establish the categories and boundaries that define our relation to the world by keeping the clean from the unclean, and thereby rescuing purity from danger. Concern with the maintenance and preservation of boundaries increased during the nineteenth century as European empires spread, and intensified at the end of the century with the growing understanding and acceptance of germ theory. As Laura Otis has argued, the imperial and the medical became closely imbricated. Beginning with mid-nineteenth-century cell theory – the idea that all living things were composed of individual cells – Otis emphasises the dependence of this on the existence of a membrane, a border that defined a cell by distinguishing it from its surroundings. This, in turn, intersected with 'inside/outside' thinking in the culture at large, a tendency greatly increased by the development of germ theory in the 1870s. The discovery that invisible germs spread by human contact could penetrate bodies and cause illness, according to Otis transformed human and social relations. And in the context of imperial expansion the anxieties produced by this changed understanding of the world intensified. As colonial powers extended their territorial control, while at the same time trying to keep their distance from the peoples, cultures and diseases of those territories, there was an acute need for further 'membranes'.[38] Imperial cell bodies might be in danger from colonised ones, even in metropolitan centres, and there was concern about the health and integrity of the national body at home and the imperial body overseas. As Otis puts it: 'The imperialist fantasy is to penetrate without being penetrated, to influence without being influenced. If one opens one's borders, however … the ensuing diffusion must proceed in both directions, and inevitably, one will take in more than oil, ivory and tea.'[39]

This very usefully opens up ways of seeing colonial and metropolitan worlds as cause and effect of each other, with a discourse of health and disease as central to the construction of boundaries in both nation and empire. Ann Laura Stoler and Frederick Cooper have spoken of the importance of a 'grammar of difference' in the construction of national and imperial identity in the nineteenth century, and have shown how this was established in terms of hierarchies of race, gender and class and articulated through relations of power.[40] Working within the very broad

---

[38] Laura Otis, *Membranes: Metaphors of Invasion in Nineteenth-Century Literature, Science, and Politics* (Baltimore and London: Johns Hopkins University Press, 1999), ch. 1.

[39] *Ibid.*, p. 168.

[40] Ann Laura Stoler and Frederick Cooper, 'Between Metropole and Colony: Rethinking a Research Agenda', in Frederick Cooper and Ann Laura Stoler (eds.), *Tensions of Empire: Colonial Cultures in a Bourgeois World* (Berkeley, Calif.: University of California Press, 1997), pp. 3–4.

terms of this formulation, this book will argue that the operation of a health/disease dichotomy was a crucial, but very unstable, marker of difference within and across these defining characteristics of race, gender and class. The complexity of this process must be kept in sight. Otis's elaboration of the 'membrane' metaphor is richly suggestive but not without problems. By emphasising the fear of 'invasion' and the need for 'defences' there is a danger of rendering the relation of colony and metropole more paranoid than it necessarily was. The postmodern and postcolonial accentuation of 'anxiety' can sometimes underplay the confidence upon which nineteenth-century imperialism was based and represent it as more vulnerable than, in truth, it normally felt.

Paul Gilroy is another whose work brings into focus the biopolitics upon which the modern imperial world was constructed. In *Between Camps: Race, Identity and Nationalism at the End of the Colour Line* (2000) (in the United States this book is titled *Against Race: Imagining Political Culture Beyond the Colour Line*) Gilroy argues that the 'antinomies of modernity' were first produced in the social order of the colony, which was sharply distinguished from that of the metropole in terms of culture, language, biology and race. He calls the resulting national and governmental formations 'camps', although, as I shall argue later, he might equally well call them colonies. 'Camp-thinking', articulated in terms of race, is for Gilroy the defining element of the distinctive nationalism produced by colonial expansion. Its 'biopolitical potency' derives from an appeal to national and ethnic purity, with questions of 'prophylaxis and hygiene', and the regulation of fertility and women's bodies at its centre.[41] He also follows Aimé Césaire and Frantz Fanon in seeing this model of inclusion and exclusion eventually brought home to Europe in the form of Nazi genocide.[42] Extending Gilroy's argument, I shall explore how disease, infection and contamination were closely associated aspects of this camp mentality. Gilroy's argument also has its problems, however. By ignoring the forms of exclusion and containment that were practised in nineteenth-century Europe he drives too strong a wedge between colonial margin and metropolitan centre, simplifying their relation in the process. In building on his arguments I shall suggest a more interactive model of relations between these two sites and across different colonised territories.

Giorgio Agamben is another whose writing on biopolitics and the boundary thinking this produces offers a productive context in which to understand better the place of disease in general, and leprosy in particular,

---

[41] Paul Gilroy, *Between Camps: Race, Identity, and Nationalism at the End of the Colour Line* (Harmondsworth: Allen Lane/Penguin, 2000), pp. 82–4.
[42] *Ibid.*, pp. 71, 81.

in modern colonial discourse. *Homo Sacer: Sovereign Power and Bare Life* (1998) also uses the idea of the camp as a biopolitical paradigm of the modern. Agamben argues that the biopolitics that characterise modernity require Western societies to set a threshold beyond which life loses intrinsic significance. This threshold defines 'bare life': that is, life that does not deserve to live and that can be eliminated without punishment.[43] It is an essential characteristic of modern politics that this threshold is constantly redefined as historical exigency demands the reassessment of what is inside and what is outside. Agamben uses Hannah Arendt's example of the refugee as a figure who, rather than embodying the rights of man, signals the breakdown of that idea and marks its limit. This figure of our time exemplifies 'bare life' and inhabits 'the pure space of exception' – the camp – that defines the boundary separating the human from its other.[44] In a later chapter I shall argue that the leper has frequently exemplified this state of bare life. Biologically alive but lacking the rights and expectations we normally attribute to human existence, this figure inhabited a no-man's-land, a limit zone between life and death, a camp or, as it became termed, a colony.

Here, too, there are problems. The cultural historians and theorists I am discussing write in the shadow of Foucault. Indeed *Homo Sacer* offers itself as a supplement to Foucault, arguing the need to complete his inquiry into the *grand renfermement* of hospitals and prisons that, for Agamben, should have culminated in those exemplary places of modern biopolitics, the concentration camp and the totalitarian state.[45] Even Edward Said's *Orientalism*, that founding text of postcolonial studies, is also very consciously a supplement to Foucault's analysis of the operation of power from the late eighteenth to the mid-twentieth century. Foucault's neglect of the colonial dimension of his archaeology of modernity, however, cannot simply be compensated by inference or supplement. The difficulties it presents run much deeper, as Ann Laura Stoler has shown.[46] This is a matter I shall return to later. The Foucauldian tradition can also too readily see *renfermement* wherever it looks, while forgetting the paradoxical ways in which Foucault understood power as having operated through this period and into our own. Tempting as it is to exploit the ease with which 'the leper' so readily becomes the ideal type of concepts such as Kristeva's abjection and Agamben's bare life, the reality for lepers in the

---

[43] Giorgio Agamben, *Homo Sacer: Sovereign Power and Bare Life* (Stanford, Calif.: Stanford University Press, 1998), pp. 131, 139.

[44] *Ibid.*, pp. 126–34.   [45] *Ibid.*, pp. 4, 119.

[46] Ann Laura Stoler, *Race and the Education of Desire: Foucault's History of Sexuality and the Colonial Order of Things* (Durham, N.C., and London: Duke University Press, 1995), *passim*.

modern period was often more complex. As we shall see, mid-nineteenth-century metropolitan medicine resisted the idea that lepers should be isolated and lose their human rights, and was supported in this by British governments of the time. Agamben argues that within the biopolitical horizon that characterises modernity, the physician and the scientist super-vise the camps of bare life,[47] but the integration of medicine with politics he is indicating was also resisted by liberal medicine for much of the nine-teenth century. And in the eyes of the missionary sent out to run a leper colony, Agamben's space of exception was the ante-room to a place of especial privilege with God. In other words, for much of the nineteenth century 'the leper' was less an emblem of bare life than a contested proto-type of an emergent biopolitics.

My aim is to historicise the processes that Foucauldian cultural history and theory conceptualise, and to suggest they were not always as total-itarian and clear-cut as Gilroy and Agamben, for example, assume. Reading back from the Nazi concentration camps into the nineteenth century can imply a more lethal biopolitics than is always strictly justified. This is not to deny many of the lines of continuity that Gilroy and Agamben trace, but to suggest a more conflicted genealogy and a more nuanced history. This argument will be picked up in later chapters.

These matters have a particular bearing on the kind of medico-cultural history I am attempting. Foucault's explorations of marginality have had a special appeal for interdisciplinary scholars, particularly for those practis-ing history at its boundaries whose infringements have often been resisted by academic historians.[48] There has been closely related border tension around the fringes of the history of medicine. This has been well discussed by Roger Cooter, who describes how on the one hand the historian of medicine has concentrated on the historical context of biomedical knowl-edge and practice, while, on the other, the literary-somatic turn in cultural studies has resulted in the appropriation of the body as a crucial element in the attempt at writing a conceptual history of modernity.[49] In a less polarised summary of this field he describes 'an intellectually and meth-odologically motley traffic of social, literary and cultural historians and critics pursuing, and ... reproblematising, the politics of the body and its representations'.[50] Despite his relative even-handedness, Cooter, a histor-ian of medicine himself, is critical of the 'historical emptiness' he discerns

[47] Agamben, *Homo Sacer*, 159.
[48] See Christopher Kent, 'Victorian Social History: Post-Thompson, Post-Foucault, Postmodern', *Victorian Studies*, 40: 1 (1996).
[49] Roger Cooter, 'The Traffic in Victorian Bodies: Medicine, Literature, and History', *Victorian Studies*, 45: 3 (2003), 514.
[50] *Ibid.*, p. 516.

in much literary-cultural 'body-work': 'One ends up with myriad revelations well described and often arresting, but no explanation either of
the genesis or the context in which particular discourses are sustained.
Aesthetics prevail.' And as he puts it more acerbically, by exceptionalising
and homogenising biomedicine, these 'literary champions of the discursive'
produce 'fictitious (if critically convenient) harmonious translations ...
between alleged social and scientific domains'.[51]

These strictures are not unfair. The somatic turn in Foucauldian-influenced
literary and cultural studies has resulted in some facile analogies between
the medical, the social and the ideological, the product of free-floating
metaphor rather than materially grounded history; whereas some recent
medical history of more conventional-seeming appearance has found
ways of avoiding the narrative of progress that the history of medicine
has often found difficult to escape, and employed versions of the indeter-
minacy favoured in theory, if not always in practice, by literary somati-
cians. One such is Michael Worboys' *Spreading Germs* (2000), which
demonstrates that the concept of 'germs' lacked any fixity of meaning
in the period leading up to the development of bacteriology, and that
even after this there was no 'single bacterial model for germs or their
actions in any branch of the profession'.[52] Worboys' scrupulous investigation of germ ideas and practices in the second half of the nineteenth
century should be an important check on metaphorically inclined cultural
critics who see infection, contagion and invasion wherever they look. Only
in the 1890s, Worboys argues, was the 'military analogy of invading germs
in conflict with the body's defences' becoming widely used.[53] Yet a history
such as Worboys' is confined to the medical profession and its local
cultures, and there is every reason for historians and others of a more
broadly cultural inclination to examine the ubiquity of disease and infection language in this period and beyond. The task should be to try and
bring these different worlds into more considered relation with each other.

The crossing of disciplinary fields, and the anti-disciplinary impulse at
the heart of my project, is fraught with difficulties. In the case of medicine
and literature some of the problems are structural. Anxiety about disease
has become a significant cultural matter and one especially congenial to
imaginative writers, while curing, allaying or dismissing these fears has
become one of the functions of medical science and the medical profession.
Imaginative writing has often been drawn to the power of disease-language

---

[51] *Ibid.*, pp. 520, 523.
[52] Michael Worboys, *Spreading Germs: Disease Theories and Medical Practice in Britain,
1865–1900* (Cambridge: Cambridge University Press, 2000), pp. 2–3.
[53] *Ibid.*, pp. 6–7.

as a means of expressing personal, social or national malaise, and since, say, Defoe's *A Journal of the Plague Year* (1722) this has been intensely so. Examples such as Mary Shelley, Thomas Mann, André Gide and others are too numerous to need extensive citation. Synonyms and related terms for ill-health and disease overwhelm those for health, as a glance at Roget's *Thesaurus* demonstrates. There appears to be something over-determined about the relation of literature to disease, and this is why a leprologist like Gussow, concerned to overcome the stigmatisation of leprosy, is suspicious of its distorting power and effects.

This over-determination, however, is not confined to literature and extends into most forms of social and political discourse, indeed into the language of public health and hygiene itself, as Alison Bashford has demonstrated.[54] In Foucauldian terms, disease is unstoppably discursive and irresistibly metaphoric. This, however, should not be an invitation for cultural historians to follow suit. Rather, the proliferating languages of disease should be returned to their sites and moment of production to be analysed and explored. The more figuratively extendable the disease, the more rigorously its elaboration needs to be scrutinised. This is particularly the case when writing about leprosy, a disease whose extraordinary signifying power has made it so amenable to cultural interpretation and application (whenever I have presented a paper on the history of leprosy someone has invariably drawn a parallel with AIDS). Such extreme susceptibility to cultural elaboration means that all metaphoric play with the disease should be viewed with suspicion rather than indulged. In this study I have tried to keep in mind the specificities of the disease at any one moment, and to analyse rather than augment its many different associations, parallels, analogues and applications.

The idea for this book grew from a chapter in my *Representing the South Pacific: Colonial Discourse from Cook to Gauguin* (1997) where I examined Jack London's account of his visit to the famous leper colony on the island of Molokai, in the Hawaiian group, and the several leprosy stories he subsequently wrote. My plan was to write something more like an essay, drawing on existing historical material, theorising this and including imaginative writing on the subject of leprosy. In the event, I could find no comprehensive history of leprosy in the nineteenth century so I had to construct one. As a result, the first two parts of this book are mainly a medical history of the disease from the late eighteenth to the early twentieth century.

---

[54] Alison Bashford, *Imperial Hygiene: A Critical History of Colonialism, Nationalism and Public Health* (Basingstoke and New York: Palgrave Macmillan, 2004), p. 7.

I am not, however, a historian of medicine, but a literary-cum-postcolonial critic of strongly historicist bent, and my approach across the whole book has been to situate the subject of leprosy within the entangled relations of metropole and colony during the period covered. Whereas historians of medicine have recently been relocating themselves at the colonial 'periphery', new imperial historians such as Ann Laura Stoler and Catherine Hall have questioned the very construct of 'centre' and 'periphery', arguing instead that metropole and colony were mutually constitutive. This, in turn, intersects with the deconstruction of its foundational terms of 'self' and 'other' that postcolonial studies has been undertaking, whereby self and other are both, though differently, understood as colonial subjects.

This book ranges across several different parts of the imperial world and no one colonial terrain receives particularly detailed treatment. The metropolis remains a central point of reference, which might seem at odds with my 'de-centring' purpose. Certainly greater concentration on a single colonial territory would have allowed more detailed attention to indigenous understandings of leprosy. Jane Buckingham's *Leprosy in Colonial South India* (2002) is an exemplary study of this kind. Her close examination of a single region allows her to trace the interaction between metropolitan and indigenous medical practices, between metropolitan and colonial medicine, and within colonial medicine itself (as in the power struggle between the Indian medical service and sanitary department).[55] But concentrating on a single colonial periphery risks eliding the broader imperial context in which the question of leprosy was debated. My intention in this book has been always to keep the imperial context in view while paying attention to the specificities of particular colonial terrains, and taking account of the interaction between different colonies, as well as that between colonies and the metropolitan centre.

My use of the terms 'leprosy' and 'leper', rather than the currently acceptable terms 'Hansen's disease' and 'patient' needs to be explained. The basic reason is historical veracity. This was how the disease and its victims were seen and referred to in the period covered by this book, and the terms have a resonance that captures both the fear and the compassion they provoked. 'Leper', in particular, has many possible inflections ranging through rejection, fear and abuse to pity and sympathy. To describe lepers as patients would dull this resonance and veil the fact that most lepers in this period were not treated as patients at all. 'Leprosy' is more neutral and has never really been replaced by 'Hansen's disease' anyway.

---

[55] Jane Buckingham, *Leprosy in Colonial South India: Medicine and Confinement* (Basingstoke: Palgrave, 2002), *passim*, especially pp. 148–50.

The main argument for dropping the term is to remove the stigma of the disease. Some present-day patients, however, prefer leprosy to Hansen's disease, arguing that the latter sanitises their condition and obscures the victimisation it has traditionally provoked. Such debates over usage are familiar from other contexts, particularly that of race, and will last as long as perceptions of these matters continue to change. In this book, the attempt to understand the disease historically has required that I should avoid describing it anachronistically.

Following this introduction, *Leprosy and Empire* divides into six chapters, each with several sections. Chapter 1 considers the re-emergence of European concern about leprosy in the late eighteenth and early nineteenth centuries. It commences with Johann Reinhold Forster, the scientist on Cook's second voyage to the Pacific (1772–5), caught in a protracted storm off the coast of New Zealand and musing on the different kinds of 'leprosy' he had observed on the islands of Tahiti and Tonga. Similar concerns are then found echoed in writing about the West Indies, with the association between leprosy and slavery much firmer in the Atlantic world. Consistent with my intention to trace the interconnections between empire and nation in respect of leprosy, and to demonstrate the involvement of literary culture in this process, I then discuss how leprosy figures in the writing of several of the Romantic poets, and in the life of Percy Shelley. This section, the first of several literary embedments, concludes with Mary Shelley's *The Last Man*, which, although not specifically about leprosy, presents a modern world without epidemiological borders in which Britain is vulnerable to the invasion of diseases from pathogenic tropical regions. With regard to disease, the fear of return was often to feature as prominently as the fear of encounter in colonial settings.

The focus of chapter 1 then becomes more narrowly medical, as early nineteenth-century physicians wrestle with the problem of how to distinguish 'true' leprosy from the very wide range of skin disorders with which it had so often been confused. Attention in this period was concentrated on the attempt to distinguish leprosy from elephantiasis, a persisting confusion that derived initially from the overlapping etymology of the terms. Accompanying this was the need for a clinical description of leprosy as a disease with a consistent set of symptoms. The first such account to be accepted as definitive came from Norway, Danielssen and Boeck's *On Leprosy* (1847), which established the terms within which leprosy was to be discussed for the rest of the century. Leprosy was classified as having two distinct forms, 'tubercular' and 'anaesthetic', and declared to be hereditary rather than contagious.

Norway was known to be the one country in Europe where leprosy had persisted. By the 1840s there was the beginning of concern about its reappearance in Britain, with several cases being reported in Scotland. Uncertainty as to why it had disappeared long ago now fed concern about its possible recrudescence. This, in turn, intersected with a growing conviction in many of Britain's tropical colonies that leprosy was spreading and threatening the health of native populations, settlers and colonial administrators. By the early 1860s this concern had prompted the British government to commission the Royal College of Physicians to conduct an empire-wide survey of the disease. Their 1867 Report endorsed the findings of Danielssen and Boeck, in particular that leprosy was hereditary rather than contagious. It also encouraged the idea that leprosy was a native disease unlikely to cross the boundaries of race or geography.

Chapter 2 covers the period following the 1867 Report to the end of the century. In respect of leprosy itself, this is the heart of my story. The College of Physicians' report on the disease was never widely accepted across the empire. For a while colonial insistence on the contagion of leprosy was dismissed in Britain as superstitious, but Hansen's isolation of the leprosy bacillus in 1874, and the spreading acceptance of the germ theory of medicine in the last decades of the century, together with the steady resistance of many colonial officials to the finding that leprosy was a hereditary disease, the collapse of a belief in European immunity, and anxiety at home about infection returning from the colonies, eventually resulted in the reconstruction of leprosy as contagious, a threat to Europeans, and a disease whose sufferers should be isolated.

By the 1880s the medical debate over leprosy had become a public matter, and concern was being expressed at the reinfection of the metropolis and the need to segregate sufferers at home as well as abroad. I look at several examples of leper scare stories in Britain, one involving a man working in the London meat market, the other a pupil at a Scottish public school. The death of Father Damien at the leper colony on the island of Molokai in 1889 became a particular focus of this public concern, and resulted more or less directly in a Leprosy Commission being sent to India to investigate the scale of the problem there and to reconsider the findings of the 1867 Report.

This report satisfied almost no one. Although it overturned the central finding of the 1867 Report that leprosy was a hereditary disease, it concluded that its degree of contagion was minimal. Segregation, therefore, was unnecessary and ineffectual. A very different conclusion was being reached at the same moment at the Cape, where an inquiry decided that the contagion level of leprosy was high and that isolation should be compulsory. This was more in tune with the times, and the first International Leprosy Conference held at Berlin in 1897 endorsed the contagionist position and declared that the strict isolation of leprosy sufferers was the key to preventing and eventually eliminating the disease.

Chapter 3 expands the discussion of leprosy as a focus of concern about the relations between metropole and colony to consider how it came to be conceptualised as a tropical disease. The category of tropical medicine was constructed and institutionalised at the end of the nineteenth century, just as the tropics were coming to be understood as a climatic zone uninhabitable by Europeans for any sustained period. This belief, derived from the fear of infection and the frequent breakdown in health experienced by those living in tropical regions, was inflected by a broader concern with degeneration at this time, and itself contributed to the *fin de siècle* degenerationist narrative. Although leprosy failed in most ways to conform to the emerging type of a tropical disease (not least because it was also found in cold climates), it was wrested into this category and made to fit. The disfiguring wrought by leprosy was an important element in the racialisation of the disease and its designation as 'tropical'. This also provided a significant point of connection between the concern with European degeneration in the tropics and urban degeneration in the cities of Europe.

A good deal of medical, sociological and literary writing about London in the late nineteenth century represented the metropolis as a pathological tropical environment. An existing discourse of urban degeneration was thereby intensified, and leprosy offered one vivid way of figuring this condition. This and allied descriptions of physical degeneration are examined in the writing of doctors and social investigators such as James Cantlie and William Booth, and in the work of novelists such as George Gissing and Oscar Wilde. A more developed discussion of *The Picture of Dorian Gray* in the light of these concerns draws together the different strands of this discussion.

Later nineteenth-century imaginative writers also dealt specifically with leprosy, reflecting wider public debate on the disease itself. The closing section of chapter 3 examines several literary texts of the period – Swinburne's poem 'The Leper', a story by Kipling and several by Arthur Conan Doyle – that dramatise different aspects of this specific concern. Kipling's 'The Mark of the Beast' is concerned with infection in the colonial world, while Conan Doyle's 'The Adventure of the Blanched Soldier' contemplates the possibility of leprosy being brought home. Swinburne's extraordinary poem has its own distinctive take on transgression, on the repulsion–attraction of the leprous body, and the psychosexual ambiguities of those drawn to the leper that were later to be constructed as leprophilia.

Chapter 3 argues that the new science of tropical medicine can be understood as an attempt to put a fence around Europe, and around the European in the tropics. It was, in Laura Otis's term, a membrane intended to distinguish and protect the metropole and the coloniser from the world they were colonising. The leper colony was a brutally literal form of this kind of thinking. Although isolation was a time-honoured way of responding to leprosy, the compulsory segregation of its victims in remote colonies, often on deserted islands, was the most striking characteristic of responses to the disease in the period between 1860 and 1940. Chapter 4 considers and compares several island leper colonies from different parts of the imperial world during these years. The first of these was the already mentioned colony on Molokai. This became the most famous of such colonies, partly because the comparatively rapid spread of leprosy in Hawaii between 1850 and 1900 was a significant influence in undermining the hereditary explanation for the disease, and more especially because of the life and death of Father Damien among 'the lepers of Molokai'. Damien, more than anyone else, brought leprosy to world attention, reminding it of the pariahs it had abandoned, and through his sacrifice alerting the world to the dangers of the disease. My second leper colony is Robben Island off the coast of Cape Town. Over almost two centuries this island has been quarantine for different kinds of groups or individuals perceived as threatening the social or physical health of the mainland. Initially a convict island for native populations, in the mid-nineteenth century it was used to isolate 'lepers, lunatics and the chronic sick'. By the closing decades of the century it had become almost exclusively a leper colony, and its type of detainee kept changing until the island eventually became world-famous as the site of Nelson Mandela's prolonged incarceration. Other island leper colonies to be considered include those established off the coast of Australia, and in several New Zealand harbours, around the turn of the century. This comparative study of island leper colonies across the imperial world is designed to draw out differences as well as similarities, and to examine how a familiar stigmatisation of the disease was inflected by local conditions and circumstance, especially the varying ethnic mix of different settler colonies.

Chapter 5 extends the discussion of the leper colony to other forms of physical exclusion and isolation characteristic of the high imperial era. It begins with a short history of the changing meanings of the word 'colony' and the proliferating applications of this term during the nineteenth century, almost all of which were concerned with spatial separation and management. The argument moves, via a consideration of Paul Gilroy's concept of 'camp-thinking', to the development of the concentration camp in the Anglo-Boer War, and the native reservation in the United States and Australia, as examples of the forced enclosure and containment of racially defined groups. The argument is then brought home to include analogous, usually class and/or gender-based, forms of quarantine or segregation in later nineteenth-century Britain. These include colonies for juvenile delinquents, lock hospitals for prostitutes thought to have venereal infections, tuberculosis sanatoria, and colonies for so-called mental defectives.

Common to these and other examples was a felt need to provide a cordon sanitaire to protect the fit from the unfit, the clean from the unclean. Chapter 5 therefore concludes by returning to the specific theme of leprosy, with a short history of the leper colony established in Essex in 1914. This helps bind the colonial and metropolitan examples of establishing colonies as forms of containment into a single argument. By elaborating and refining Gilroy's argument that practices developed and refined in the colonies were subsequently brought home and turned on pariah groups within Europe itself, and combining it with Agamben's preoccupation with the European antecedents of Hitler's camps and twentieth-century totalitarianism, I suggest a model in which metropole and colony can be seen as mutually constitutive, united by a concern with biopolitics that resulted in a markedly extended application of the idea of the colony to elements of the national population as well as to colonised peoples.

Chapter 6, which together with a Postscript concludes the book, looks back over almost a century during which the figure of the leper and the site of the leper colony exerted a fascinated pull on traveller-writers. In this way it is both a recapitulation and an updating. The boundaries established by the imperial world were an invitation to transgress as well as an injunction to keep away. Beginning with Charles Warren Stoddard, whose visits to Molokai in 1869 and again in 1884 resulted in the first book written about the colony, I examine the writing of several visitors to this island colony. Robert Louis Stevenson spent a week there in 1889, shortly after Damien's death. He wrote an account of his stay as well as a leprosy story, 'The Bottle Imp', both complex pieces of writing that dramatise an unusual range of conflicted response to the disease. Jack London makes up a trio of writers who visited Molokai and described and fictionalised their experience.

Finally I consider two post-Second World War writers who crossed the leper boundary. Graham Greene's visit to the leper colony of Yonda in the Belgian Congo in 1959 resulted in a novel, *A Burnt-Out Case* (1960), and *Congo Journal* (1961), the germ of his novel. *A Burnt-Out Case* describes a world in which leprosy has become curable, but the novel continues to feed off horror of the disease in a traditional manner that is by now anachronistic. It also identifies the spiritual malaise of its burnt-out European hero with the arrested physical deformation of the leper patients in a manner that has echoes of Swinburne. Greene's fascination with decay, salvation and the ambiguities of sainthood involves an uneasy blending of the medieval and the modern in his exploration of the leper and his carer. This brings Greene himself close to the type of the leprophil that he sees exemplified in Albert Schweitzer.

The last traveller-writer I discuss is Paul Theroux, whose autobiographical essay 'The Lepers of Moyo' (1994) looks back to the early 1960s when Theroux spent several months as a volunteer worker in a leper settlement in Malawi. The autobiographical narrator, Paul, breaches the last physical boundary between the clean and the unclean by having sexual intercourse with a young leper woman. But in a modern world of dapsone drug therapy the transgressive frisson of this action has dissipated, and Theroux's essay makes no attempt to pretend otherwise. By normalising this sexual encounter Theroux brings to an end a very long and old chapter in the history of writing about leprosy. The other main theme of 'The Lepers of Moyo' is the difficult relation of writing and leprosy, in discussing which I conclude my own account of this subject.

1   Describing, imagining and defining leprosy, 1770–1867

Leprosy in the Pacific and Atlantic worlds

In October 1773 Captain Cook's *Resolution* was caught in a violent and prolonged storm off the coast of New Zealand. The ship was returning to Cook's safe harbour at Queen Charlotte Sound after a sweep of the southern Pacific that had taken in Tahiti, the Society Islands and several islands in the Tongan group. Among those on board was Johann Reinhold Forster, the German-born scientist on Cook's second voyage (1772–5). On 26 October he recorded in his journal that 'The Sea is mountainous & the wind rages with the utmost fury.'[1] Water was coming through the door of his cabin, all the furniture was overturned and Forster could only remain in bed by holding on to the frame with both hands. Two days later the storm had not abated and Forster's discomfort had been compounded by his frustration at the ship's lack of progress: 'the longer we are out at Sea, the less time is left to us ... for our Observations on Plants & Animals'.[2] So he turned to 'the remarks of Prof. Michaelis on the Leprosy, and its various branches', and reflected on the different kinds of 'leprosy' he had observed on the recent voyage.[3]

In one of the longest single entries anywhere in his journals Forster described the three stages of leprosy he had observed. The slightest of these was 'a kind of scaly Exfoliation of the Skin of a white colour'; sometimes this extensive whiteness of the skin included ulcers that were red and surrounded by a 'spungy kind of flesh'.[4] The second stage involved 'brown or purple red ... elevated tumours' and more advanced ulceration.

---

[1] Michael E. Hoare (ed.), *The* Resolution *Journal of Johann Reinhold Forster, 1772–1775*, 4 vols. (London: Hakluyt Society, 1982), vol. III, p. 410.

[2] *Ibid.*, vol. III, p. 412.

[3] *Ibid.*, vol. III, p. 413. Michaelis was a leading figure of the early German Enlightenment, the guiding force behind a Danish expedition to Egypt and Arabia in the 1760s, and a life-long correspondent of Forster's.

[4] *Ibid.*, vol. III, p. 413.

24

Forster describes the 'third Degree of this Disease' in terms of two examples he had seen on Eua, in the Tongan group; a man with an extensively ulcerated back and shoulder, and a woman with an ulcerated face and 'the nose rotten away'.[5] Forster's entry then moves seamlessly into descriptions of what he takes to be elephantiasis, and concludes that these cases must have been introduced by the Spaniards at Tahiti: 'it is probable, that coming from Mauritius they had some Negro's [sic] on board, infected with that kind of *Elephantiasis* described by *Aretaeus & Paulus Aegineta*'.[6] Assuming that these cases have been 'communicated by cohabitation', he suspects they must therefore be a kind of venereal disease. Meanwhile, as Forster records next morning, 'The tempest [was] still raging.'[7]

Forster returned to the subject of leprosy in *Observations Made During a Voyage Round the World* (1778), written in more comfortable surroundings after his return to England. *Observations* systematises the scientific and ethnographic material Forster had gathered on the voyage into a coherent set of descriptions and reflections. On leprosy, for example, he is now careful to distinguish between the first stage of leprosy and other kinds of whitish 'scaly exfoliation' caused by sea salt or by excessive consumption of liquor prepared from the pepper-root.[8] He records that the natives have a single term, *e-pae*, to cover all skin disorders. On Cook's first voyage (1768–71) Joseph Banks had noted the susceptibility of Polynesians to 'cutaneous distempers',[9] and in the *Observations* Forster is trying to distinguish and classify the various kinds of skin disease he had seen. Forster was particularly sensitive to the possibility that many of the skin diseases he observed had been introduced by recent European ships. Venereal disease was an especial focus of this concern, with British, French and Spanish voyagers blaming each other for its introduction to the Pacific. The *Observations*, therefore, refines the suggestion in the journal that 'Negro's' had somehow introduced leprosy into Tahiti. Forster reports that following the visit of a Spanish ship a disease had broken out that caused ulcers and hair loss, and resulted in death. The Tahitians had called it *e-pae-no-peppe* (Peppe's disease or sore), and believed it was sexually communicated. At first Forster had thought this to be a venereal disease, but on reflection had concluded that as the Spanish ship had come from Lima and Callao, where there were a great many negro slaves with various kinds of 'leprosis and elephantiasis', a member of the crew might

[5] *Ibid.*, vol. III, p. 414.   [6] *Ibid.*, vol. III, p. 415.   [7] *Ibid.*, vol. III, p. 415.

[8] Johann Reinhold Forster, *Observations Made during a Voyage Round the World*, ed. Nicholas Thomas, Harriet Guest and Michael Dettelbach (Honolulu: University of Hawaii Press, 1996), p. 295.

[9] *The* Endeavour *Journal of Joseph Banks, 1768–1771*, ed. J. C. Beaglehole, 2 vols. (Sydney: Angus and Robertson/Public Library of New South Wales, 1962), vol. I, p. 373.

have been infected with 'elephantiasis' which they communicated to the Tahitians: 'for it is well known, that some species of leprosy may be communicated by cohabitation, that many lepers are very immoderate in venery, even a few moments before they expire, and that especially the elephantiasis described by Aretaeus and Paulus Aeginita, had some symptoms that are perfectly corresponding with those pointed out by the natives'.[10]

Forster adds that he cannot be positive about this chain of infection because diseases are often unfairly blamed on visitors when in truth they are indigenous. Uneasy at the charge that Cook's voyages were leaving venereal and other diseases in their wake, Forster concludes that this disease was prevalent in the Pacific long before the arrival of Europeans, so that when he describes a youth seen on Huahine (but not mentioned in the journal) 'covered with ulcers . . . His eyes . . . almost extinct', this young man is said to be 'the sad victim of brutal appetite and libidinous desire', in other words the agent of his own misfortune.[11]

Even today, diseases involving the skin and its underlying tissue are impossible to diagnose accurately with the eye. Late eighteenth-century medicine had few means of distinguishing between syphilis, yaws, lesions caused by fungi, scabies and so on. Leprosy, whose Latin name *elephantiasis graecorum* added further confusion, was commonly used as a generic term for a wide range of skin disorders. Forster's son, George, wrote of Tahiti: 'there are several sorts of leprous complaints existing among the inhabitants, such as the elephantiasis, which resembles the yaws'.[12] Today it is possible, with some confidence, to conclude that on Tahiti and Tonga yaws was often mistaken for syphilis. Yaws, an indigenous disease, gave near-total immunity to syphilis. Gonorrhoea, therefore, was the most common venereal disease introduced by European ships (syphilis and gonorrhoea had not yet been established as distinct diseases). Leprosy was not an indigenous disease and was not introduced until the mid-nineteenth century.[13]

In his efforts to distinguish between different kinds and degrees of leprosy, and to assign the disease an origin, J. R. Forster was all at sea.

---

[10] Forster, *Observations*, p. 297.   [11] *Ibid.*, pp. 298–9.

[12] George Forster, *A Voyage Round the World*, ed. Nicholas Thomas and Oliver Berghof, 2 vols. (Honolulu: University of Hawaii Press, 2000), vol. I, pp. 201–2.

[13] For more detailed discussion of the confusion about disease in the Pacific, see Howard M. Smith, 'The Introduction of Venereal Disease into Tahiti: A Re-examination', *Journal of Pacific History*, 10 (1975), 38–45; Sir James Watt, 'Medical Aspects and Consequences of Cook's Voyages', in Robin Fisher and Hugh Johnston (eds.), *Captain James Cook and his Times* (Vancouver and London: Douglas and McIntyre and Croom Helm, 1979); John Miles, *Infectious Diseases: Colonising the Pacific* (Dunedin: University of Otago Press, 1997).

The attempt to do so, however, is full of interest. On the one hand there is the scrupulous observation and description of various skin disorders, with the intention of distinguishing between them. On the other is the use of leprosy as a generic term for all such symptoms, and the indiscriminate racialisation and sexualisation of this disease. Forster is simultaneously as obsessive as the author of the Book of Leviticus and as careless as subsequent commentators on leprosy and empire.

His immediate successor in this latter respect was Sir William Jones, the famed Orientalist, whose *Collected Works* were published in 1799 and widely discussed. In his essay 'On the cure of the elephantiasis and other disorders of the blood', Jones describes leprosy as the holistic disease par excellence: 'it is in truth a distemper corrupting the whole mass of blood, and therefore considered by Paul of Aegina as an universal ulcer'. An Indian physician has assured Jones 'that it is frequently a consequence of the *venereal infection*', and Jones has no doubt that the negro is responsible for its alarming spread across the globe. He refutes the belief that leprosy is confined to the Nile; it has 'been imported from *Africa* into the *West-India* Islands by the black slaves, who carried with them their resentment and their revenge'.[14]

By the end of the eighteenth century the West Indies had become an especial focus of concern about leprosy. The first of several slave medical manuals to express this was James Grainger's *An Essay on the More Common West Indian Diseases, and the Remedies which that Country Itself Produces. To Which are added some hints on the management, etc. of Negroes* (1764). Grainger is best known for his very long poem *The Sugar Cane* (1764), the notes to which formed the basis of his medical manual.[15] Grainger's *Essay*, like subsequent slave medical manuals such as those by David Collins (1803) and James Thomson (1820), was intended to maximise the profitability of the plantation through the maintenance of slave health.[16] For Grainger, of those 'distempers ... [which] peculiarly affect the Negroes ... the leprosy is the most dreadful'. It has no remedy and 'continues to spread its ravages daily, to the disgrace of art, and the detriment of the planter'. Although primarily a Negro disease, 'the White

---

[14] *Works of Sir William Jones*, ed. Lord Teignmouth, 13 vols. (London: John Stockale and John Walker, 1807), vol. IV, pp. 368–9.

[15] Alan Bewell (ed.), *Medicine and the West Indian Slave Trade* (London: Pickering and Chatto, 1999), p. 277. On Grainger's *The Sugar Cane*, see Tobias Doring, *Caribbean-English Passages: Intertextuality in a Postcolonial Tradition* (London: Routledge, 2002), pp. 53–64; Markman Ellis, ' "The Cane-land Isles": Commerce and Empire in Late Eighteenth-Century Georgic and Pastoral Poetry', in Rod Edmond and Vanessa Smith (eds.), *Islands in History and Representation* (London: Routledge, 2003), pp. 43–62.

[16] Bewell, *Medicine and the West Indian Slave Trade*, p. 277.

people in the West-Indies are not exempted from this dreadful calamity'.[17] Grainger's discussion of leprosy expresses unease at ignorance of its origin and transmission, as well as its incurability. It is unclear whether or not it is infectious; children and spouses of infected adults do not necessarily contract it. Nevertheless it is prudent 'to remove the distempered from the sound'. The disease 'oftenest breaks out without any visible cause', but it also 'frequently arises from being overheated, and getting too suddenly cool'. The 'art' that it 'disgraces' is the art of medicine and healing, which is unable to explain or cure the disease. Grainger describes a leprous 'Negroe man' he once saw: 'He was a hideous spectacle. His appetite was good.'[18] The stark juxtaposition of these two sentences, one signalling decay, the other health, represents leprosy as a puzzling contradiction.

Grainger's essay also expresses confusion over what is and is not leprosy. His first four entries under distempers most likely to affect slaves are leprosy, elephantiasis, the joint-evil and yaws. I have already noted the recurring confusion of leprosy, elephantiasis and yaws. The joint-evil was another leprous condition that attacked the toes, in which, as Grainger describes it, 'the joints ... successively drop off'. It was commonly known by its African name *coco bays*, and also as king's evil, both also synonyms for leprosy.[19] Matthew (Monk) Lewis, for example, visiting his Jamaican estates in 1816, described the sad condition of one of his slaves, 'a poor creature named Bessie ... afflicted with the *cocoa-bay*': 'It shows itself in large blotches and swellings ... which ... by degrees, moulder away the joints of the toes and fingers, til they rot and drop off; sometimes as much as half a foot will go at once. As the disease is communicable by contact, the person so afflicted is necessarily shunned by society.'[20]

Informants to the 'Parliamentary Inquiry into the Treatment of Slaves in the West Indies' in 1789 listed those diseases to which negro slaves were subject but from which white inhabitants were immune: 'The Coco-bays, The Leprosy of the Greeks, The Leprosy of the Arabians, The Elephantiasis.' Within a few lines, however, the Report describes 'Coco-bea' as another name for Arabian leprosy. The 'Seeds of such Diseases' are described as having been brought by the slaves from Africa 'and entailed on their Posterity'. That said, however, 'There is no Doubt but the Negroes in Jamaica, whether Free or Slave, would live healthier, and for a much longer Term than they do in general, if it were not for their vicious and irregular Practices.'[21]

---

[17] *Ibid.*, pp. 279–80.   [18] *Ibid.*, p. 282.   [19] *Ibid.*, p. 283, and n. 320.

[20] Matthew Lewis, *Journal of a West India Proprietor*, ed. Judith Terry, (Oxford: World's Classics, 1999), pp. 90–1.

[21] Bewell, *Medicine and the West Indian Slave Trade*, p. 189.

Amid all this confusion of names, aetiology and mode of transmission are certain features that will recur in discussions of leprosy throughout the nineteenth century. On the one hand, it is a native and hereditary disease with pronounced and distinctive symptoms; on the other, Europeans are not immune from the disease, it is infectious, indeed communicable by touch, and its symptoms are impossible to distinguish from many other conditions. Further, although leprosy is easily contracted by slaves, it is also the fault of those natives who catch it.

Leprosy and Romantic writing

This contradictory, shape-shifting and most resonant of diseases was being deployed by imaginative writers at the time, particularly the Romantic poets. In Blake's 'America a Prophecy' (1793) Albion's Angel sends the plagues of the Book of Revelation against the rebel Americans, only to have these turn back on their perpetrator:

> ... the plagues recoil'd! then rolld they back with fury
> On Albions Angels; then the Pestilence began in streaks of red
> Across the limbs of Albions Guardian, the spotted plague smote Bristols
> And the Leprosy Londons Spirit, sickening all their bands:
>
> (14: 20; 15: 1–3)

As the plagues spread across Britain, the 'leprous head' of Urizen emerges from the heavens (16: 3): 'Leprous his limbs, all over white, and hoary was his visage' (16: 11). As Urizen weeps and howls 'before the stern Americans' (16: 12), the thrones of France, Spain and Italy shudder in terror at the sight of Albion and its 'ancient Guardians / Fainting upon the elements, smitten with their own plagues' (16: 17–18).[22] Leprosy and plague figure disease in the body politic. David Erdman has shown that in choosing Bristol and London, Blake is reflecting precise contemporary detail, namely the riots against the war in those two merchant cities that were most involved in the American trade.[23]

This view of Albion itself as leprous is distinctive. Later Romantic writers – Southey, Shelley and De Quincey, for example – locate and challenge despotism in terms of a confrontation with 'the East', as represented by the diseases of that ill-defined but capacious zone.[24] Blake,

---

[22] *The Complete Poetry and Prose of William Blake*, ed. David V. Erdman, commentary by Harold Bloom (New York: Anchor Books, 1982), pp. 56–7.

[23] David V. Erdman, *Blake: Prophet Against Empire*, third edn (Princeton, N.J.: Princeton University Press, 1977), pp. 59–60.

[24] Alan Bewell, *Romanticism and Colonial Disease* (Baltimore and London: Johns Hopkins University Press, 1999), p. 222.

however, applies these diseases directly to the *anciens régimes* of Europe. In doing so he is drawing on the traditional idea of leprosy as retributive justice, a judgement on the sins of rulers. In 'America' leprosy bites back, infecting a 'mildewed' and repressive state that had thought to punish its rebel colony with disease. Elsewhere Blake seems to associate leprosy with the punishing aspect of Jehovah, apparently in contrast to Jesus who healed lepers.[25] The ancient idea of leprosy as a retributive disease therefore seems to have been reviving around the turn of the nineteenth century. We have already seen it in William Jones's essay where it figures as an expression of slave resentment and revenge. 'America', with its careful identification of Bristol as the first target of the 'spotted plague', would seem to be making a similar association, although in this case with a pronounced anti-slavery bias. Indeed the idea of leprosy as revenge was ubiquitous. Matthew Lewis records that Bessie believed her cocoa-bay to be the result of a curse by an Obeah man.[26]

Coleridge's 'Lecture on the Slave Trade', delivered in Bristol in 1795, and the reworked version published in *The Watchman* the following year, associates slavery with disease in general and leprosy in particular. The 'Luxury ... [and] imaginary wants' that depend on the slave trade are 'pestilent inventions'.[27] Africans complicit in this trade have been 'innoculate[d]' with European vices.[28] The ravages of disease infect without discrimination everyone involved in the slave trade. British seamen are to be found begging on the streets of Jamaica, 'dying daily in an ulcerated state'.[29] On the ships 'the hot & pestilent vapours' arising from the bodies of slaves confined in such 'a crowded and cramped state' rot the very timbers.[30] Having summarised the common arguments used to justify the slave trade, Coleridge concludes: 'Such have been the cosmetics with which our parliamentary orators have endeavoured to conceal the deformities of a commerce, which is blotched all over with one leprosy of evil.'[31]

'The Rime of the Ancient Mariner' expresses a paranoid view of infection as retribution for the injuries of slavery, with leprosy once again the focus. The association between the skeleton ship with its crew of Death ('a fleshless Man') and Life-in-Death ('Her skin was as white as leprosy'), and the plankless hulks of slaving ships was pointed out by William

---

[25] See 'The Four Zoas', Night the Eighth, 405–6. I am indebted to Dr Andrew Lincoln for this reference and suggestion.
[26] Lewis, *Journal of a West India Proprietor*, p. 91.
[27] Samuel Taylor Coleridge, *Lectures 1795 On Politics and Religion*, ed. Lewis Patton and Peter Mann (London: Routledge and Kegan Paul, 1971), p. 236.
[28] *Ibid.*, p. 241.   [29] *Ibid.*, p. 239.   [30] *Ibid.*, p. 241.
[31] Samuel Taylor Coleridge, 'On the Slave Trade', *The Watchman*, 25 March 1796, ed. Lewis Patton (London: Routledge and Kegan Paul, 1970), p. 136.

Empson. He quoted Coleridge's description in *The Watchman* of the bodies of slaves rotting the planks of the vessel, adding: 'Everybody in Bristol knew that you could smell a Slaver five (or ten) miles to windward, and that planks only lasted for five (or ten) voyages.'[32] The figure of Life-in-Death that dices with her 'mate' Death for the mariner and the ship's crew is of particular interest here. Empson describes her as 'among other things ... the bad girl sailors meet in port'.[33]

> Her lips were red, her looks were free,
> Her locks were yellow as gold;
> Her skin was as white as leprosy.

Empson, though, passes over the way in which slavery, leprosy and sexuality are brought together in this figure into a densely packed image of temptation and retribution; the similes 'yellow as gold' and 'white as leprosy' condense and assimilate the evils of empire to the poem's catalogue of horrors. As Alan Bewell points out, disease in 'The Rime of the Ancient Mariner' is concentrated in a slave ship whose reach 'extends to the limits of the known world'.[34] Bewell also suggests that the poem is a narrative of colonial return. Like Wordworth's *Salisbury Plain* (1793–4), it features an outcast and wandering 'tropical invalid', a new kind of social pariah whose experiences abroad render him a disturbing and potentially infecting presence at home.[35] It therefore becomes another example of Blake's 'rolling back' of disease, of metropolitan centres being 'smitten with their own plagues'.

Southey's *The Curse of Kehama*, begun in 1801, resumed in 1808 and published in 1810 is another contemporary narrative poem in which plague and leprosy figure. Indeed it has echoes of several Coleridge poems. In *The Curse of Kehama* the mighty Rajah Kehama, 'King of the World', places a curse on Ladurlad who has killed the Rajah's son to protect his daughter Kailyal. The curse denies Ladurlad food and water while protecting him from death, condemning him to live in pain. However, his immunity from death also enables him to save his daughter from the many dangers that repeatedly threaten her. One such danger comes from the vengeful enchantress Lorrinte, whose specialty is disease:

> Her look hath crippling in it, and her curse
> All plagues which on mortality can light;
> Death is his doom if she behold ... or worse ...

[32] William Empson and David Pirie (eds.), *Coleridge's Verse: A Selection* (London: Faber, 1972), pp. 28–30.
[33] *Ibid.*, p. 29.   [34] Bewell, *Romanticism and Colonial Disease*, p. 104.
[35] *Ibid.*, pp. 101, 108–9.

> Diseases loathsome and incurable,
> And inward sufferings that no tongue can tell.[36]

(XI, 4, 60–4).

Lorrinte's corrosive gaze consumes her victim's 'vital parts / Eating his very core of life away' (XI, 4, 69–70), but Ladurlad manages to protect his daughter from the power of this enchantress. However, when Kailyal rejects an offer of marriage from Kehama, the Rajah takes revenge by infecting the young woman with leprosy, that 'O'er all her frame with quick contagion spread' (XIX, 1, 10). Kailyal the Virgin is innocence personified and threatened, and she welcomes this latest curse as a defence against further assault: 'this scurf and scale / Of dire deformity, whose loathsomeness / Surer than panoply of strongest mail / Arms me against all such foes' (XIX, 2, 25–8).

The contrast of Kailyal and Lorrinte the enchantress resembles that in Coleridge's 'Christabel' (composed between 1798 and 1801) between the eponymous heroine and Geraldine, a confrontation of virginal innocence with malignant infection. When the Lamia-like Geraldine undresses before lying down with Christabel, 'her bosom and half her side' is described as, 'A sight to dream of, not to tell!'[37] The manuscript text of 1800 is more explicit, describing the uncovered part of her body as 'lean and old and foul of hue'. Geraldine herself describes her deformity as 'This mark of my shame, this seal of my sorrow.' In Southey's poem virtue is rewarded, and when, eventually, Kailyal and her father travel beyond the range of Kehama's power her 'leprous stain' disappears. Leprosy, comfortingly, comes to emblematise the truth that beauty is but skin deep. Kailyal has taken comfort in the purity of her soul, which is 'Exempt from age and wasting maladies / And undeform'd, while pure and free from sin.' Her leprosy might be 'a loathsome sight to human eyes / But not to eyes divine' (XIX, 3, 57–60), and as a consequence her beauty is restored. Coleridge's unfinished poem, on the other hand, stops with Geraldine having succeeded in alienating Christabel from her father; malignity and disease have done their worst.

Percy Shelley knew *The Curse of Kehama*, and having sent it to Elizabeth Hitchener was pleased that she had enjoyed it: 'I am happy that you like Kehama. Is not the Chapter where Kailyal despises the leprosy grand?'[38]

---

[36] Maurice H. Fitzgerald (ed.), *Poems of Robert Southey* (London: Oxford University Press, 1909), p. 154.

[37] Ernest Hartley Coleridge (ed.), *Coleridge: Poetical Works* (London: Oxford University Press, 1969), p. 224 and note.

[38] Frederick L. Jones (ed.), *The Letters of Percy Bysshe Shelley*, 2 vols. (Oxford: Clarendon Press, 1964), vol. I, pp. 97–8, 126.

There is nothing surprising about Shelley's interest in this particular episode. Nora Crook and Derek Guiton have shown that Shelley's often discussed and apparently inexplicable fear at this time that he had contracted elephantiasis was actually an alarm about *Elephantiasis graecorum*, or leprosy, rather than filiaris, or 'Barbados leg'.[39] Their detailed examination of this curious incident concludes that Shelley was frightened he had contracted syphilis that was degenerating into leprosy. Shelley owned and was familiar with William Jones's essays from which source, or from others available at the time, he would have learned that the terminal stage of syphilis was believed to combine with and mutate into leprosy.[40]

The most up-to-date medical text on the subject, Thomas Bateman's *A Practical Synopsis of Cutaneous Diseases* (1813) claimed that leprosy 'was almost unknown in this country'. Almost immediately two instances of leprosy were reported in London. One of these involved a boy of European parentage recently arrived from the Bahamas; the other, a daughter of an English officer and a Hindu woman. The first was treated by William Lawrence, almost certainly the doctor Shelley had consulted over his suspected elephantiasis; the second was attended by H. H. Southey, the poet's brother, and also someone known to Shelley.[41] Together these two doctors wrote a paper on the cases in *The Transactions of the London Medico-Chirurgical Society*.[42] Crook and Guiton demonstrate that Shelley's seemingly paranoid delusion about having contracted leprosy becomes more understandable in the imperial and medical context of the day. They also suggest that the pathological imagery of Shelley's famous sonnet 'Ozymandius' (1817–18) – in which the 'passions ... yet survive, stamped on these lifeless things', and 'Two vast and trunkless legs of stone' remain – can be read as drawing together disease with the ruins of empire.[43]

By Shelley's time it was obvious that diseases as well as people were colonising the globe. There was, as Alan Bewell puts it, 'deepening concern about the epidemiological consequences of colonialism'. At first this concern was with the impact of disease on Europeans in colonial settings, but it ramified as increasing numbers of invalid colonists returned to metropolitan centres, and especially when the worldwide spread of cholera in the 1820s threatened the bio-geographical boundary between a healthy Europe and a pathogenic colonial world.[44]

---

[39] Nora Crook and Derek Guiton, *Shelley's Venomed Melody* (Cambridge: Cambridge University Press, 1985), ch. 6.

[40] *Ibid.*, pp. 90–1.   [41] *Ibid.*, pp. 86, 94.

[42] 'Two Cases of the True Elephantiasis or Lepra Arabum', *Transactions of the London Medico-Chirurgical Society*, 6 (1815), 210–17.

[43] Crook and Guiton, *Shelley's Venomed Melody*, p. 99.

[44] Bewell, *Romanticism and Colonial Disease*, p. 307.

The text of the period that more than any other highlights this concern is Mary Shelley's *The Last Man* (1826). Mary Shelley's novel differs from older plague narratives such as Defoe's *A Journal of the Plague Year* (1720) in treating disease as a global phenomenon rather than as internal to a national culture.[45] In this way it brings together the view of non-European countries as pathogenic and threatening, with the idea of disease recoiling and 'rolling back' that we saw in Blake. In the rapidly colonising and embryonically globalised world of the early nineteenth century, there was a growing fear of tropical and other diseases travelling back along the trade and communication routes and infecting the metropolitan centres of Europe. *The Last Man* gives powerful expression to this. Written against the background of the spread of cholera across the world from Britain's Indian possessions during the 1820s, the slow progress of the disease towards Britain reinforced a growing awareness of vulnerability to the epidemiological forces that were reshaping the globe. In Shelley's novel, as the plague reaches London the narrator reflects on the self-deluding comfort the English have always taken from a mere strip of water:

[W]e fancied that the little channel between our island and the rest of the earth was to preserve us alive among the dead. It were no mighty leap methinks from Calais to Dover. The eye easily discerns the sister land; they were united once; and the little path that runs between looks in a map but as a trodden footway through high grass. Yet this small interval was to save us: the sea was to rise a wall of adamant – without, disease and misery – within, a shelter from evil, a nook of the garden of paradise – a particle of celestial soil, which no evil could invade.[46]

This passage dismantles the rhetoric of John of Gaunt's 'sceptred Isle' speech in *Richard II*, with its serenely confident picture of England's natural bio-geographical immunity:

> This Fortresse built by Nature for her selfe,
> Against infection, and the hand of warre.

(II, 1)

In *The Last Man* the Channel is no longer the cordon sanitaire of a 'demy paradise'. As the small group of survivors trapped on the disease-ridden island of Britain gather in Dover with the hope of escaping back across the Channel, the town is engulfed by a tidal wave. From the cliff-top they watch the approaching wave with apprehension: 'Would not our little island be deluged by its approach?'[47] Different versions of this question continue to be asked.

---

[45] *Ibid.*, pp. 299–300.

[46] Mary Shelley, *The Last Man* (Lincoln, Nebr., and London: University of Nebraska Press, 1993), pp. 179–80.

[47] *Ibid.*, p. 270.

There is one scene in particular that dramatises the intimate connection between the spread of empire and the death of England. The plague in *The Last Man* is a new disease whose nature and mode of transmission are never discovered. That is with one exception. The novel's narrator, Verney, contracts the disease when he stumbles across an infected, dying negro in a London house. Hearing a groan, and entering a darkened room from which emanates 'a pernicious scent', Verney feels his leg clasped:

I lowered my lamp, and saw a negro half clad, writhing under the agony of disease, while he held me with a convulsive grasp. With mixed horror and impatience I strove to disengage myself, and fell on the sufferer; he wound his naked festering arms round me, his face was close to mine, and his breath, death-laden, entered my vitals.[48]

The only clear-cut example of infection in the novel involves the only non-European character even glimpsed in the text. The breath of the negro has brought disease back to the centre of empire, reversing the narrative of infection spread by colonial expansion and turning fortress England into a doomed fever camp.

The non-specific nature of the plague in *The Last Man* generalises the anxiety about infection coming from warm zones, variously referred to as the tropics or the East, that was becoming apparent at the turn of the nineteenth century. At different moments during the nineteenth century different diseases would become the focus of such fears. Cholera, which would have been recognised as the unnamed point of reference in Mary Shelley's novel, was the most important and recurring of these and became the defining disease of concern about guarding the shores of Britain from the arrival of infection. Although cholera as traditionally named and understood was familiar to English medical practitioners both at home and in India, *The Lancet* insisted that the cholera of Mary Shelley's day was a new type to which it was misleading to apply the same name.[49] It differed from previous forms of the disease in its persistence, its degree of contagion, and especially in the fact that it travelled. The *Quarterly Review* described how it 'has mastered every variety of climate, surmounted every natural barrier, conquered every people ... the cholera, like the small-pox or plague, takes root in the soil which it has at once possessed'.[50] Cholera was becoming the classic type of a tropical disease, in which the geographical distinction between Europe and the tropics, or West and East, was articulated in terms of the geography of the body. Western diseases like tuberculosis invaded the upper part of the body while those of the East

[48] *Ibid.*, p. 245.   [49] Bewell, *Romanticism and Colonial Disease*, pp. 242–3.
[50] *Ibid.*, p. 243.

such as cholera attacked the lower. As Alan Bewell puts it: 'To move from West to East is to move from the lungs to the bowels, from the soul to the body, from diseases of respiration to those of excretion, from breath to dirt.'[51] Successive waves of cholera invasion in 1831–2, 1848–9, 1853–4 and 1866 had the effect, on one hand, of collapsing such distinctions and, on the other, making it all the more imperative they should be reinforced.

Any particular disease thought to be contagious was liable to be assimilated to a more general concern with preserving the nation's health from the threat of infection. Each, however, had its own specific resonance. Leprosy, as we have seen, was especially associated with retribution. This was not only because it had traditionally been understood as a punishment or curse. Unlike cholera, or other diseases emanating from tropical zones, leprosy was a European disease that was thought to have been eliminated, and now threatened to return. This gave it an atavistic character well suited to the idea of 'rolling back' and of retribution. It reminded Europe of a past that was assumed to have been outlived, of a present that brought home the cost of its colonial expansion, and the intertwining of these two. James Martin, in arguing that tropical countries were sick but curable, pointed out that Britain itself had once been an insalubrious place.[52] This recalls Marlow's famous remark at the beginning of Conrad's *Heart of Darkness* that London, too, 'has been one of the dark places of the earth'. The underside of Martin's confidence was that Britain might also regress, threatened by the very things it had once expelled. Leprosy also resisted the attempt to divide the world in terms of the upper and lower body. It could not readily be restricted to any single zone of either the body or the world, and its indiscriminate and inconsistent character was unsettling, threatening as it did to obliterate the differences upon which nineteenth-century colonialism was being constructed.

Benjamin Moseley, in *A Treatise on Tropical Diseases* (1787), had remarked that 'diseases undergo changes and revolutions. Some continue for a succession of years, and vanish when they have exhausted the temporary, but secret, cause which produced them. Others have appeared and disappeared suddenly; and others have their periodical returns.'[53] Southey, a recurring point of reference for the disease fears of this period, asks in *Sir Thomas More* (1831) whether there is any reason why the mysterious sweating sickness that was epidemic in the first half of the sixteenth century before mysteriously disappearing should not reappear in the nineteenth.[54] Uncertainty as to whether diseases were new or old, tropical or domestic, and about how they were spread and caught, was a defining feature of early nineteenth-century metropolitan and colonial

---

[51] *Ibid.*, p. 250.   [52] *Ibid.*, p. 39.   [53] *Ibid.*, p. 308.   [54] *Ibid.*, p. 309.

worlds. My earlier example of the scene from *The Last Man* when Verney wrestles with the plague-stricken negro illustrates this. Although the one moment in the novel when the transmission of infection is actually described, Verney is also the only person in the novel to contract and survive the disease. In this, the scene anticipates a leprosy story by Jack London, 'The Sheriff of Kona' (1912), to be discussed again in chapter 6, in which the narrator struggles with a native leper while trying to free a European friend from enforced isolation in a leper colony. In the course of the struggle the leper's face is suddenly revealed by a lantern:

> It was not a face – only wasted or wasting features – a living ravage, noseless, lipless, with one ear swollen and distorted, hanging down to the shoulder ... In a clinch he hugged me close to him until that ear flapped in my face. Then I guess I went insane ... I began striking him with my revolver ... just as I was getting clear he fastened upon me with his teeth. The whole side of my hand was in that lipless mouth.[55]

Even though the narrator's hand is left looking 'as if it had been mangled by a dog', seven years later (the period it was commonly believed the disease took to incubate) he has not been infected by leprosy. Whereas the cause of the incarcerated friend's infection is unknown and mysterious, the narrator seems certain to become infected but escapes this. Apart from the obvious point that narrators usually survive, both scenes illustrate the uncertainty and caprice of infection. Far from being comforting, this blurred the distinction between health and disease that was integral to the grammar of difference that colonial and domestic discourses were seeking to establish while simultaneously being compelled to defend.

Classifying leprosy

The intense metaphorical power of leprosy at this time was reinforced and legitimated by its unstable and confusing medical usage. Thomas Bateman's *A Practical Synopsis of Cutaneous Diseases* (1813) sought to clear up the muddle. Bateman employed a classification of eight categories of skin diseases: pimples, scales, rashes, bullae, pustules, vesicles, tubercles and spots. Scaly diseases have four genera, one of which is lepra. Bateman then distinguishes three different kinds of lepra. The first is *vulgaris,* 'one of the most common affections of the skin, at least in the metropolis, and occurs at all periods, and under every circumstance of life. It is certainly not communicable by contagion.'[56] Bateman notes a hereditary predisposition

---

[55] Jack London, *Tales of the Pacific* (Harmondsworth: Penguin, 1989), p. 133.
[56] Thomas Bateman, *A Practical Synopsis of Cutaneous Diseases, According to the Arrangement of Dr. Willan* (London: Longman, Hurst, Rees, Orme, and Brown, 1813), p. 28.

in some individuals. The second kind, *alphoides* is less severe and extensive, and is most common in children.[57] The third, *nigricans*, is darker in colour and associated with outdoor work and poor diet.[58]

Bateman then distinguishes these different kinds of leprosy from the tubercular disease elephantiasis, with which it has persistently been conflated. This confusion has arisen from a mistake in translation from Greek to Latin whereby leprosy has been misapplied to elephantiasis.[59] Elephantiasis, wrongly known as leprosy, is virtually unknown in Britain, Bateman never having seen an instance of it.[60] Aretaeus and succeeding Greek writers probably named it such because it results in diseased skin resembling the hide of an elephant: 'For it is disgusting to the sight, and in all respects terrible, like the beast of a similar name.'[61] It is also known as satyriasis, because the facial disfiguration it causes suggests the features of a satyr, and possibly also because of the 'excessive libidinous disposition said to be connected with it'.[62] Yet another term, leontiasis, again connects this disease with the animal world. Greek writers attribute this term to the wrinkling of the forehead, Arabian writers to the reddening of the eyes and the similarity of the whole visage to that of a lion.[63] Common to all three names is a sense of the disease as breaking down the division between the human and animal worlds.

Bateman distances himself from this animalisation of the disease. The ancients' view of elephantiasis as 'an universal cancer of the body', and their emphasis on its hideous character, contagion and fatality, is expressed in such 'strong metaphorical language' that Bateman questions the fidelity of their description. He is suspicious of the 'poetical appropriation' of these names, and ridicules Aretaeus for prefixing to his description of the disease an account of the elephant in order to make the analogy explicit. Bateman suggests that terror of the disease led the writer ' to adopt the popular opinion respecting the malady, without the correction of personal observation', and that modern accounts (he cites Hilary's *Diseases of Barbadoes*, 1766) have copied this tradition.[64] The isolation of lepers, Bateman continues, has been enforced in compliance with this ancient opinion, whereas 'there is great reason to believe that Elephantiasis is *not contagious*'.[65] Another received opinion Bateman questions is that of *libido inexplebilis*, the heightened libido of the leper asserted by Aretaeus and others. Against this he cites the observations of Dr Adams in Madeira on the wasting of the generative organs among those with the disease.

---

[57] *Ibid.*, pp. 30–1.   [58] *Ibid.*, p. 36.   [59] *Ibid.*, pp. 25–6.   [60] *Ibid.*, p. 292.
[61] *Ibid.*, p. 293.   [62] *Ibid.*, p. 294.   [63] *Ibid.*, pp. 294–5.   [64] *Ibid.*, pp. 295–6.
[65] *Ibid.*, p. 297.

There is yet more confusion for Bateman to clear. The misleading identification of leprosy with elephantiasis, he continues, has recently been compounded by the use of 'elephantiasis' to describe a tumid condition of the leg accompanied by a thickening and roughening of the skin. This application is suggested by the resemblance of a leg so affected to that of an elephant; it is the condition also commonly known as 'Barbadoes leg' (filiariasis).[66] Even as Bateman struggles to tidy up the disorder, his classification threatens to unravel:

Elephantiasis and Lepra have been ... confounded. The word Lepra (which should be confined to a scaly disease) has been erroneously applied to the proper Elephantiasis (a *tubercular* disease). Elephantiasis ... has been transferred ... to the local affection of the leg ... But it has also been misapplied to the white disease of the skin, called by the Greeks, Romans, and Arabians, Leuce, Vitiligo and Baras (or Beras) respectively; and thence by an easy step, it has been again transferred, by some unlearned persons, even to the scaly Lepra; while the term Lepra has been often indiscriminantly applied to all these affections.[67]

Bateman has already conceded that some Greeks and Arabians thought that Leuce or Baras had affinities with elephantiasis and sometimes terminated in it.[68] And all this apparently without him knowing of the further confusion between yaws, syphilis and leprosy that Pacific voyagers had contributed.

In such circumstances, Bateman concludes, the prevalence of leprosy in Europe in the Middle Ages is impossible to determine: 'every species of cachectic disease, accompanied with ulceration, gangrene, or any superficial derangement, was deemed *leprous*'.[69] Many observers still 'confound every foul cutaneous disease under the term Leprosy', and the closest modern approximation to accuracy is the distinction between *lepra graecorum* (scales) and *lepra arabum* (elephantiasis).[70]

Bateman's determination to distinguish between leprosy and elephantiasis appears to have had immediate success. Lawrence and Southey, in their joint report of two cases of the disease that Bateman had never seen, and which would seem to have caused Shelley such alarm, consistently use 'elephantiasis' and not 'leprosy'. These two cases are worth looking at in more detail because their history and documentation is characteristic of most instances of 'leprosy' that were to be reported in Britain from time to time throughout the nineteenth century. Lawrence's case concerned an adolescent male, Charles Uncle, aged fourteen. Charles had been born in Augusta, in the United States, of an English father and an American mother. His childhood was spent in the Bahamas, where he frequently worked outdoors and ate food

---

[66] *Ibid.*, pp. 304–5.   [67] *Ibid.*, p. 307.   [68] *Ibid.*, p. 302.   [69] *Ibid.*, p. 301.
[70] *Ibid.*, pp. 25–6.

'of a coarse kind, the same that was given to the negroes'.[71] During his passage to England, when he worked on the ship, he developed 'prodigious swelling' of his head and face, followed by the appearance of tubercles on his ears and face and stiffening of the limbs. When he first saw Lawrence at St Bartholomew's Hospital in April 1814 the tubercles were covering the whole of his face and had spread to the upper and lower limbs. Other symptoms included a flattened and expanded nose, loss of eyebrows, tuber-culated palate, hoarseness of voice, swelling of toes and feet, and a shrivelling of the genital organs, especially the testes.[72] Charles was admitted to St Bartholomew's where he does not seem to have been isolated as he caught measles from a patient in the same ward. He was treated externally with poultices and internally with mercury and arsenic; the latter treatment was soon abandoned because it disturbed his general health. By February 1815 the elephantiasis appeared to be declining and he was discharged, although the remains of ulceration were visible, his features permanently deformed and his genital organs still diminished. However, letters in May and June from Devonshire, where he had gone to convalesce, reported the return of facial ulceration and the appearance of pulmonary symptoms. Lawrence was also told of the recent death of Charles's brother from consumption.[73]

Lawrence made no attempt to explain how his patient might have con-tracted the disease, but his account selects certain features of Charles's history that were to become common in reporting leprosy cases. This is an offshore disease that almost certainly originated in a tropical island setting. It is also a native disease that has somehow been contracted by a European; Lawrence reports that elephantiasis was otherwise unknown among the white inhabitants of the Bahamas.[74] The implication is that Charles has had a semi-native upbringing, working outdoors and eating 'negro' food. The detail about working his passage reinforces this. Lawrence shares Bateman's interest in *libido inexplebilis*, emphasising the diminution of the boy's genitalia and the persistence of this symptom.

Southey's account essentially only differs to the extent that his patient is female. Miss R., aged twenty-two, is a native of Bombay, the daughter of an English officer and 'a Hindoo woman'. At the age of ten red blotches had appeared on various parts of her body. These were temporarily removed by 'mercurial medicines' but kept returning, and for the last five years tubercles had appeared and spread. When Southey saw her in January 1814 her body was badly ulcerated and her face 'horribly disfig-ured', with the eyebrows gone, the eyelids tuberculated but the eyelashes

---

[71] William Lawrence and H. H. Southey, 'Two Cases of the True Elephantiasis or Lepra Arabum', *Medico-Chirurgical Transactions*, 6 (1815), 211.
[72] *Ibid.*, pp. 211–14.   [73] *Ibid.*, pp. 215–17.   [74] *Ibid.*, p. 211.

remaining (Lawrence had also noted this last feature in Charles). The woman's nose was flattened, her ears had thickened and her voice was hoarse. Although her menstrual discharge was regular it 'was found ... to coagulate upon exposure to air'. And, Southey continued: 'With regard to the libido inexplebilis, or the absence of sexual passion; it may be proper to state, that an offer of marriage was made to this unfortunate female within the last two years, which she was inclined to accept.' Southey also notes that her breasts have disappeared.[75]

Whereas Charles has been forced by economic circumstances to cross the colour line, Miss R. is actually of 'mixed blood'. This seems to free Southey of the need to find any environmental explanation for the disease; in this case there are no details of upbringing, work or diet. The focus on sexual organs and their functioning is even sharper in this history; the *libido inexplebilis* question has been gendered, although Southey's contribution to this topical debate is not entirely clear. While the inclination to marriage might imply sexual passion, the disappearance of the woman's breasts could suggest otherwise. However we interpret these details, the question of the relation of leprosy to sexuality is clearly pressing.

Bateman's insistence on the difference between leprosy and elephantiasis is still holding in James Robinson's 'On the Elephantiasis, as it appears in Hindostan' (1819).[76] Robinson, however, nuances Bateman's classification by arguing that there are two distinct varieties of elephantiasis or *lepra arabum*. The first of these, which he terms *elephantiasis anaisthetus*, begins with the appearance of lightly coloured and insensitive patches of skin. Within a few years this is followed by symptoms of internal disease such as torpid bowels, slow pulse and a torpid and inactive mind. As the disease progresses, the fingers and toes become numb, skin cracks, arms and legs swell, joints ulcerate, muscles are destroyed and joints begin to fall off. In this condition the leper 'will ... crawl about with little but his trunk remaining, until old age comes on, and at last he is carried off by diarrhoea or dysentry, which the enfeebled constitution has no stamina to resist'.[77] The second variety Robinson terms *elephantiasis tuberculata*, the variety described by Bateman and 'now occasionally seen in this country'.[78]

---

[75] *Ibid.*, pp. 218–19.
[76] First published in *Medico-Chirurgical Transactions*, 10 (1819), this was reprinted in James Johnson and James Ranald Martin, *The Influence of Tropical Climates on European Constitutions* (London: S. Highley, 1841). This compendium had been started by Johnson in 1813; Martin became its co-editor at the time of the sixth edition in 1841, and its sole editor after Johnson's death in 1845.
[77] Johnson and Martin, *The Influence of Tropical Climates on European Constitutions*, pp. 373–4.
[78] *Ibid.*, p. 375.

Although this form of the disease sometimes supervenes in cases of *elephantiasis anaisthetus*, it is 'by no means connected with, caused by, or necessarily subsequent to this disease'.[79] Robinson is here contributing to the emerging distinction between two main forms of leprosy, anaesthetic and tubercular.

Whitelaw Ainslie's 'Observations on the Lepra Arabum, or Elephantiasis of the Greeks, as it appears in India' (1826) denies this distinction.[80] Ainslie has never seen a case in which both tubercles and a lack of feeling in the extremities has not been present. He follows Bateman and others in the emerging early nineteenth-century consensus that the disease is unlikely to be contagious. Ainslie has seen three Europeans die of elephantiasis under his care but their wives and servants have not been infected.[81] Instead he believes it to be hereditary, and claims support for this view from Hindu doctors. But he also allows that it can occur independently of any constitutional predisposition, 'under a particular combination of causes, in most regions of the Torrid Zone'. Although he has met instances of the disease among Europeans, he has never seen a case in an Englishman.[82]

Ainslie also engages in the debate about the alleged 'salacity of lepers'. Acknowledging that current medical opinion is divided on this question, he cites two recent cases in Britain (one at Brighton, so this is not Charles Uncle) in which there was wasting of the testicles.[83] The leper 'immoderate in venery' remained a pressing issue at least until Aretaeus and the classical tradition were no longer regarded as authoritative. Bateman had challenged their authority by asserting the primacy of empirical observation over myth and metaphor, but the influence of this tradition persisted. Ainslie's description of the progress of the disease also blurs the line dividing the human sufferer from an animal. As the eyes become inflamed, rheumy, and rounder from the pressure of the surrounding face, they come to 'resemble those of some wild animal'; a 'most offensive ichor ... distils from the nose'; 'the already ugly become loathsome'.[84] Different kinds of discourse jostle uneasily against each other in Ainslie's essay; on the following page, for example, Ainslie makes the modern sanitarian point that poor living conditions and want of cleanliness are 'constant attendants of this dreadful affliction'.[85]

---

[79] *Ibid.*, p. 374.

[80] First published in *Transactions of the Royal Asiatic Society*, 1 (1826), this was reprinted in Johnson and Martin, *The Influence of Tropical Climates on European Constitutions*, where it was grouped with Robinson's article under the heading 'Elephantiasis'.

[81] Johnson and Martin, *The Influence of Tropical Climates on European Constitutions*, p. 376.

[82] *Ibid.*, p. 379.   [83] *Ibid.*, p. 376.   [84] *Ibid.*, p. 378.   [85] *Ibid.*, p. 380.

In 1841–2 James Simpson published a series of three articles on the history and nature of leprosy in the *Edinburgh Medical and Surgical Journal*. Simpson argued that leprosy had persisted in Scotland after it had disappeared from England, and in the northern islands of Scotland even after its disappearance from the Scottish mainland.[86] This Scottish dimension to the history of leprosy in Britain was to figure in discussions of the disease in the 1850s. The main purpose of Simpson's articles, however, was to establish that the leprosy of the ancient and medieval periods was identical to that of today. In spite of the terminological confusion that Bateman had analysed, and which Simpson himself discusses, the elephantiasis of the Greeks, the Arabic juzam, the lepra of the Latin translators, the simple leprosy of the Middle Ages and the tubercular leprosy of modern European medicine once more become one and the same disease. Simpson's historical researches have revealed more scrupulous concern with the correct diagnosis of leprosy in the later Middle Ages than Bateman allowed, and he is therefore less inclined to accept that leprosy had been merely a generic term for a wide range of skin diseases. Simpson explains the minutely detailed description of symptoms he has discovered as a result of the extremely severe consequences of being diagnosed as a leper.[87] This repeats the obsessive concern of the Leviticus writer with accurate diagnosis, but it certainly does not preclude a wide range of different kinds of skin disease from having been described as leprosy.

Simpson's argument that leprosy had remained a constant entity in spite of the confusion of its naming had the effect of blurring the distinction between leprosy and elephantiasis that Bateman had insisted upon. Simpson refers variously to 'European leprosy', 'tubercular elephantiasis', and 'tubercular leprosy (lepra tuberculosa)', commonly summarising these, together with their Greek, Arabic and Latin antecedents, as leprosy. Elephantiasis is hardly used, and then mainly in passing reference to the condition otherwise known as Barbados or Cochin leg. So although Simpson accepts Bateman's etymological history, the original Greek distinction between leprosy and elephantiasis is once again being lost. From now on, leprosy would be the dominant term, with elephantiasis normally applied to Barbados leg.

Perhaps because of his concern to establish the unity and constancy of leprosy, Simpson takes no account of Robinson's argument that leprosy had tuberculated and anaesthetic forms. Another contributor to the

---

[86] James Simpson, 'Antiquarian Notices of Leprosy and Leper Hospitals in Scotland and England', 1, *Edinburgh Medical and Surgical Journal*, 56 (1841), 327–8.

[87] James Simpson, 'Antiquarian Notices of Leprosy and Leper Hospitals in Scotland and England', 2, *Edinburgh Medical and Surgical Journal*, 57 (1842), 130.

Edinburgh Medical and Surgical Journal at this time, however, clearly distinguished between 'tubercular elephantiasis' and 'leprosy of the joints'.[88] Otherwise, Simpson concurs with the growing consensus that the theory of the contagious origin of leprosy is merely a superstition that modern science has overturned, although he acknowledges that some pathologists believe it was imported into the West Indies and other parts of the New World by 'subjects brought from Africa'. He cites Hillary's *Diseases of Barbadoes* (1766) and Schilling's *Commentationes de Lepra* (1778) as supporting this view, clear anticipations of Jones's use of the same theory.[89] According to Simpson, leprosy is a hereditary disease which, like other such disease, is selective and may lie dormant for several generations. Where it still lingers in Europe, it is 'transmitted through an old hereditary taint in particular families, rather than generated by existing external circumstances acting on the bodies of those who now become its victims'.[90] In other words, there are no longer endemic or environmental factors at work in Europe, although Simpson does concede the difficulty of isolating 'external exciting causes' in a disease that is found in so many different latitudes and climates.[91]

Simpson, therefore, consolidates Bateman's view of leprosy as non-contagious and provides historical depth to his predecessor's essentially clinical account of the disease. Although he endorses Bateman's account of the confusion over its naming, Simpson ignores the insistence that leprosy should be confined to a scaly disease and effectively defeats the rear-guard attempt to reinstate elephantiasis as the correct term. Simpson is virtually free of the influence of classical medical commentators but the fascination with *libido inexplebilis* remains. On this subject his observations do not accord with the wasting of the generative organs described by Adams, in fact 'quite the reverse', a remark that he leaves unexplained.[92]

Leprosy in Norway

It is likely that Simpson's researches into the persistence of leprosy in Scotland well after its disappearance from the more southern latitudes of Britain, and his concern about its possible return, were prompted by rediscovery of the disease in Norway during the first half of the nineteenth century. Not only had leprosy lingered in that country, but at the time

---

[88] James Kinnis, 'Observations on Tubercular Elephantiasis as it Appears in Madeira and Ceylon, and on Leprosy of the Joints as it Appears in Ceylon', *Edinburgh Medical and Surgical Journal*, 58 (1843), 142.

[89] James Simpson, 'Antiquarian Notices of Leprosy and Leper Hospitals in Scotland and England', 3, *Edinburgh Medical and Surgical Journal*, 57 (1842), 411n.

[90] *Ibid.*, 406.   [91] *Ibid.*, 407–9.   [92] Simpson, 'Antiquarian Notices of Leprosy', 2, 124.

Simpson was writing it appeared to be spreading. Simpson regarded Norwegian leprosy (*spedalskhed*) as identical with 'true tubercular leprosy' or 'Arabian leprosy',[93] and his concern about its presence across the North Sea was shared by other Scottish doctors during the 1840s and 50s.

Leprosy had been rediscovered among the Norwegian peasantry during the early years of the nineteenth century at a time when emergent nationalism had kindled a new interest in this hitherto ignored section of the population.[94] Eventually the Norwegian government commissioned an investigation, and a report was published by its Home Department in 1847. Accompanying the written report of more than 400 pages was an Atlas of 24 coloured plates illustrating different facets of the disease. The Report and the Atlas were translated into French the following year, in which form the work became widely known in Britain. Authored by D. C. Danielssen and C. W. Boeck, it became the definitive European medical account of leprosy until the discovery of the leprosy bacillus in the 1870s began to disturb one of its two main findings.

Danielssen and Boeck reached two basic conclusions. They established the distinct types of 'tubercular' and 'anaesthetic' leprosy, providing detailed accounts of both, and organising the plates in the Atlas in such a way as to reinforce this classification, with tubercular examples grouped separately from the anaesthetic ones.[95] And they dismissed the idea that leprosy was contagious, arguing that it was predominantly hereditary but sometimes spontaneously prompted by environmental factors. Although, as we have seen, these new ideas about leprosy were already in circulation, Danielssen and Boeck provided detailed conclusions based upon carefully gathered evidence from an environment conducive to a controlled experiment. Their investigations were focused on remote and self-contained communities, ethnically homogeneous, within a sparsely populated European country that had no colonial territories. Unlike the West Indies, for example, where an imported slave population lived alongside a white settler elite, there was little coming, going or mixing in the small worlds that Danielssen and Boeck examined. Norway was to remain a crucial point of reference in leprosy debates throughout the nineteenth century, its differentiating feature always being the absence of a colonial dimension.

---

[93] Simpson, 'Antiquarian Notices of Leprosy', 1, 330.

[94] Zachary Gussow, *Leprosy, Racism, and Public Health: Social Policy in Chronic Disease Control* (Boulder, Colo.: Westview Press, 1989), pp. 67–9.

[95] D. C. Danielssen og C. W. Boeck, *Om Spedalskhed: Atlas*, udgivet efter Foranstaltning afden Kongelige Norske Regjerings Departement for det Indre (Bergen, 1847).

Danielssen's and Boeck's findings, however, were not quite as clear-cut as this summary suggests. Despite the categorical account of two distinct forms of leprosy, Danielssen and Boeck acknowledged a mixed form of the disease in which tubercular and anaesthetic symptoms were simultaneously present. This received much less attention in the Report, but the Atlas included several illustrations of mixed cases. The question as to whether there really were two distinct forms of the disease had been a matter of discussion before the Norwegian investigation, and would go on being debated. And although Danielssen and Boeck regarded the idea that leprosy was contagious as old-fashioned and superstitious, a view that was to remain dominant in Europe until at least the 1870s, there was an interesting anticipation of Hansen's eventual discovery of the leprosy bacillus in their description of the composition of leprous tubercules. Danielssen and Boeck discovered in both the surface and interior of raised tubercules, when placed under magnification, 'millions of acarides, which we believe to be identical with acarus scabiei. These crusts are almost wholly composed of the dead bodies of these animalcules.'[96] In retrospect, these 'animalcules' can be seen as proto-bacilli.

In time the example of Norway as proof of the hereditary explanation of leprosy was to become increasingly contradictory. As the surveillance, registration and voluntary isolation of lepers followed the 1847 Report, this home of anti-contagionism also came to be seen as the place where isolation policies were having some effect in containing and beginning to reduce the disease. There were answers to this, as we shall see, but nevertheless both within the Report itself, and in the public health policies it prompted, anti-contagionism contained the seeds of its own eventual undermining.

Danielssen and Boeck's findings were made available to British doctors through a series of eight articles by Erasmus Wilson that appeared in *The Lancet* in 1856 and were essentially a summary of the Norwegian report. On the question of causation, Wilson declared with absolute confidence: 'The doctrine of infection and contagion ... has long been abandoned.'[97] Leprosy, Wilson argued, was the result of a not fully understood interaction of heredity with geography, or seed and soil to borrow the concept

---

[96] *Ibid.*, commentary on plates 4 and 21. The translation is by W. E. Nourse, FRCS whose copy of *Om Spedalskhed* is held by the Wellcome Institute Library, London. Nourse's handwritten translation is bound into the Atlas. His notes to the translation reveal that Nourse visited the leper hospital in Bergen in 1850 and observed one of the patients whose face was illustrated in the Atlas.

[97] Erasmus Wilson, 'On the Nature and Treatment of Leprosy, Ancient and Modern', 4, *The Lancet*, 1 (1856), 226.

that Michael Worboys has elaborated to explain the dominant understanding of infection in the second half of the nineteenth century.[98]

The cause of elephantiasis is an animal poison generated in, or received into the
blood ... The nature and origin of the poison are wholly unknown, certain conditions of the human body, and of the elements around it, must have co-operated at
its first production, and those conditions ... may still be in action more strongly in
some countries than in others, for the maintenance of the poison, and for the
perpetuation of the disease. This constitutes the spontaneous or endemic origin
of elephantiasis.[99]

We have already seen in Simpson the idea that certain environments are
more likely to trigger the inherited disease than others. Wilson provides
examples from among his own cases to suggest that hot climates were
far more likely to do this than temperate ones. Four of the five cases
he summarises are of Europeans born in tropical climates: Mauritius,
Jamaica and India. A fifth, however, is of a young woman who had
never been out of Britain.[100] Cases such as this troubled the idea that
Europe had been cleansed of the environmental factors, whatever these
might be, that interacted with a hereditary taint to bring about the disease.
At the end of his summary of the causes of leprosy Wilson added that
although most of Europe was free of the disease, 'there is no reason why at
some later day it may not regain all its old power, and become a second
time one of the epidemic pestilences which ... affect mankind'.[101]

This fear of return is emphasised in the later articles of Wilson's series
where he goes well beyond his previous careful summaries of Danielssen
and Boeck: 'Leprosy exists amongst us still, but only as a faint trace of a
worn-out disease, or as an ember of the burnt-out fire. God forbid that the
spark should be rekindled!'[102] This idea of a vestigial taint, already seen in
Simpson, then mutates into an embryonic form of leprosy, a shadow or
sign of the disease, still commonly found in Britain. This is *morphoea alba
lardacea* and *morphoea alba atrophica*. According to Wilson, in countries
where leprosy exists the first form of *morphoea* often develops into tubercular leprosy, the second into anaesthetic leprosy. In Britain it remains
arrested at this preliminary stage, but Wilson implies there is no guarantee
this will always be so.[103] And not only is '*morphoea* ... a relict of that
bygone scourge of this country, the great leprosy', but so too is another

[98] Michael Worboys, *Spreading Germs: Disease Theories and Medical Practice in Britain,
1865–1900* (Cambridge: Cambridge University Press, 2000), *passim*.
[99] Wilson, 'On the Nature and Treatment of Leprosy', 4, 226.
[100] Wilson, 'On the Nature and Treatment of Leprosy', 3, 146–50.
[101] Wilson, 'On the Nature and Treatment of Leprosy', 4, 227.
[102] Wilson, 'On the Nature and Treatment of Leprosy', 7, 450.
[103] Wilson, 'On the Nature and Treatment of Leprosy', 7, 450–1.

very common condition, *alopecia areata*. Wilson believes *alopecia* to be a *morphoea* of the scalp and hair-bearing skin with the same relation to leprosy as the other *morphoea* he has already described.[104] In other words, the *'materies morbi'* of leprosy has persisted despite the apparent disappearance of the disease itself. As leprosy became a growing concern in the imperial world, this prompted fears that it might also be reactivated within Europe itself. The fear of its possible importation was hardly yet an issue, and was only to become pressing much later in the century. Around mid-century the fear was that leprosy might never have been fully eliminated and was merely hibernating.

Otherwise, however, Wilson stays close to paraphrasing Danielssen and Boeck, merely adding cases of his own by way of example. He regards the division of leprosy into tubercular and anaesthetic forms as axiomatic. His first article describes the tubercular form, his second the anaesthetic, and, following Danielssen and Boeck, he declares the tubercular form to be the more common. Of the five cases he describes, only one is anaesthetic: that of a young woman from Wiltshire, referred to above, who had never left Britain. Wilson describes her, a year before she died: 'her skin [was] so much contracted as to appear too small for her body.'[105] But the sharp distinction between these two forms of the disease easily blurs. Still following the Norwegian report, Wilson concedes that not only do the two forms often blend, but that parents with one form may have children in whom the other form develops. The taxonomy of leprosy was to remain problematic. Although Danielssen and Boeck established the terms in which the disease was to be discussed for the next three decades, there were always those who, like Ainslie, would dispute that leprosy could be classifed according to the Norwegian schema. This was to figure in further medical discussion of the disease in Scotland at this time.

In 1855 Dr Broadbent exhibited a Scottish leprosy patient to the Medico-Chirurgical Society of Edinburgh. He was a nineteen-year-old male from the island of Lewis, born and bred on the island where his father managed the salmon fisheries. Broadbent reported that 'no hereditary taint can be made out', and that 'his diet has been good, although he has lived much upon fish'. His patient had undergone three months' treatment at Edinburgh Royal Infirmary but there had been no improvement in his condition and after the patient became despondent he was allowed to return home.[106] In the discussion following Broadbent's presentation the alarming spread of leprosy in Norway and Canada, emphatically

---

[104] Wilson, 'On the Nature and Treatment of Leprosy', 8, 506.
[105] Wilson, 'On the Nature and Treatment of Leprosy', 3, 150.
[106] *Edinburgh Medical Journal*, 1 (1855–6), 424–6.

non-tropical countries with comparable climates to Scotland, was noted, and it was agreed that 'the question as to its probable reappearance on our shores was a startling one, and should not be lost sight of'.[107] At the same meeting Dr Simpson referred to another recent case in Scotland concerning a young woman of English parentage who had been born in Jamaica and also spent time in a convent in the Himalayas. The possibility of the return of leprosy had become a matter of concern. The 'great mystery' surrounding its previous disappearance from Scotland added to the 'great doubts [that] rested on the cause of its present reappearance'.[108]

In the following year the Edinburgh Medico-Chirurgical Society heard a paper from Alexander Fiddes on leprosy in Jamaica, prompting further discussion of the mystery of the disappearance of leprosy and the possibility of its return. Fiddes referred to Erasmus Wilson's view that conditions such as *alopecia areata* were 'lingering remains' of the disease; it was therefore, he suggested, 'not unreasonable to suppose that ... as the scourge declined spontaneously in the sixteenth and seventeenth centuries, so it may resume its activity at a future time, should the external causes which favour its development ever regain their ancient ascendancy'.[109]

Fiddes also emphasised the racial character of the disease, reporting that in Jamaica Jews were the most susceptible, those born in Europe the least, with the 'dark races' and Jamaican-born Europeans coming somewhere between. Fiddes added that the Jewish race had been 'liable to leprosy' since biblical times, 'and it is remarkable they should be still peculiarly subject to it'. He speculated that not only did different races have their 'peculiar mental and physical endowments, but possess likewise a special liability to certain diseases, or a comparative exemption from others'.[110]

Fiddes accepted the conclusions of Danielssen and Boeck on the question of causation and the distinction between tubercular and anaesthetic forms. He insisted there was no evidence of contagion, and that the seclusion of lepers was unjust and deprived them of care.[111] Also following Danielssen and Boeck, or Wilson's account of their report, he argued that leprosy was more intense in the second generation than the first, and even more so when the second and fourth generations was conjoined rather than the first and third. Leprosy, he insisted, was hereditary to a greater degree than perhaps any other disease. This added to the worrying sense of its hidden or lingering nature that had surrounded the discussion of Broadbent's paper. Fiddes compared leprosy to those cases of 'family likeness, or ... abnormal or morbid conditions of the body, where the person resembles a remote ancestor, and not the parent from which he has

---

[107] *Ibid.*, 77.   [108] *Ibid.*, 76–7.   [109] *Edinburgh Medical Journal*, 2 (1856–7), 1061.
[110] *Ibid.*, 1063–4.   [111] *Ibid.*, 1066.

immediately sprung'.[112] This, in turn, echoed a much wider nineteenth-century concern with the biological return of the repressed. Thomas Hardy's poem 'Heredity' captures this perfectly:

I am the family face;
Flesh perishes, I live on,
Projecting trait and trace
Through time to times anon,
And leaping from place to place
Over oblivion.

Fiddes's paper prompted further discussion of the classification of the disease. W. T. Gairdner, who is to figure later, questioned whether the tubercular and anaesthetic forms were even the same disease. Fiddes allowed they were more distinct than Danielssen and Boeck had suggested: 'the two species are so far independent, that the one does not usurp the place of the other – each form pursues its own career ... in cases where they appear in combination ... the development of one species keeps the other in abeyance, and prevents its advance further than a slight appearance only'.[113] Clear-cut classification of leprosy remained problematic. Previously the question had been of how distinct these two forms actually were. Now it was being asked if they even shared a common clinical identity.

A final point to emerge from the discussion of Fiddes's paper was the contrast between the attention paid to leprosy by the Norwegian government and the neglect of the problem in India. The 'recrudescence' of the disease in India was noted with alarm, and for all that Fiddes had insisted that leprosy was not contagious, and that segregation of its victims was unjustified, the *Edinburgh Medical Journal* envisaged the need in India for 'forcible concentration ... into districts specially appointed by the State, so that the healthy population may not run the risk of contamination'.[114] Here, as later, anti-contagionism did not necessarily preclude segregation. The contrast between Norway and tropical countries was to be a recurring one. The policies of the Norwegian government were frequently held up as a model of how to contain and treat the disease, and were sometimes misrepresented as more strongly segregationist than in fact they were. India, in particular, was constructed as Norway's antithesis: hot, teeming, disorderly and full of contagion. Climate, race and colonial status made for a very different attitude to the disease. Norway became a Mecca for leprologists, and the presence of leprosy in a relatively homogeneous and isolated northern culture was seen as less alarming than its hold in the tropical zones of European empires. This also held true in the United

---

[112] *Ibid.*, 1065.   [113] *Ibid.*, 1043.   [114] *Ibid.*, 280.

States, where the settlement of Norwegians with leprosy in the Upper Mississippi Valley was regarded with far greater equanimity than were cases of the disease among Black Americans in Louisiana or among Chinese immigrants to California.[115]

The 1867 Royal College of Physicians' Report

It was against this backdrop that in 1862 the Colonial Secretary, the Duke of Newcastle, asked the Royal College of Physicians for advice on how to control leprosy in Britain's West Indian colonies. His request was prompted by a letter from the Governor of the Windward Islands, Barbados about the spread of the disease in those islands.[116] The College of Physicians was asked whether the degree of communicability of the disease justified the compulsory segregation of lepers. Newcastle observed that:

[I]n respect to the treatment of lepers, there arise questions other than medical, and yet depending much on medical and physiological data – namely, respecting laws and regulations for the restraint or seclusion of lepers founded on the popular notion of the disease being contagious, and partly ... on the notion that, being transmissible from parent to child, and in these times rarely otherwise generated, the propagation of it should be ... prevented by separation of the sexes.[117]

The terms in which Newcastle put the central question – was leprosy contagious or was it transmissible from parent to child? – was in tune with metropolitan medical thinking. The idea that leprosy was a contagious disease is virtually dismissed as an outmoded theory. In fact Newcastle's letter was an embryonic version of the official line on the disease that the Colonial Office and the College of Physicians were to hold almost to the end of the century.

Newcastle also wanted to know if leprosy was common in other colonies apart from the West Indies.[118] In response, the College of Physicians set up a Leprosy Committee that drew up a list of seventeen questions for the Colonial Office to send around the Empire. As the replies came back they were forwarded to the Leprosy Committee for processing and analysis. At first this Committee comprised six doctors, but after the first year only three of these were regularly attending meetings, and the drafting of both

---

[115] Gussow, *Leprosy, Racism, and Public Health*, pp. 53–4, 125, 132.

[116] Governor Walker to the Duke of Newcastle, 19 February 1862, in *Report on Leprosy by the Royal College of Physicians, Prepared for Her Majesty's Secretary of State for the Colonies* (London: Eyre and Spottiswoode, 1867), p. 2.

[117] Frederic Rogers, Colonial Office to Henry Pitman, Royal College of Physicians, 14 April 1863, *ibid.*, p. vi.

[118] Frederic Rogers, Colonial Office, to Henry Pitman, Royal College of Physicians, 1 July 1862, *ibid.*, p. iv.

the interim reports and the final one was effectively the work of one man, Gavin Milroy, the College's acknowledged expert on leprosy and Honorary Secretary to the Committee.[119]

Milroy, a physician and epidemiologist born and trained in Edinburgh, had made his name as a critic of the quarantine system.[120] As medical officer with the government's Mail Packet Service in the 1840s he had experienced the use of quarantine as a precaution against plague on vessels. He believed this to be an unnecessary restriction on trade and liberty and, further, that the contagionist theories on which quarantine was based could not sufficiently account for the spread of diseases such as plague and cholera. As Mark Harrison points out, Milroy's views were at one with the prevailing ethos of free trade. Milroy became a superintendent medical inspector of the General Board of Health during the cholera epidemics of the late 1840s and early 1850s, and the Colonial Office sent him to Jamaica to report on sanitary conditions after an outbreak of cholera. It was here that Milroy first encountered leprosy, a disease he wrote, 'respecting which I have never ceased to feel much concern'.[121] He then became one of the commissioners who investigated the health of the British Army in the Crimea, after which he continued to write reports and advise governments on matters of quarantine and controlling the spread of disease. By the 1860s, when he was sifting leprosy reports from around the Empire, he was also Secretary of the Epidemiological Society of London.

Although the findings of the leprosy inquiry were not published until 1867, several interim reports anticipated its conclusions. By mid-1863, with a number of responses already in, the Leprosy Committee was being pressed by the Colonial Office for a decision on 'the question of the contagiousness, or otherwise, of Leprosy'.[122] The Committee replied that on the basis of fifty replies received so far there was little evidence of its contagiousness, and none that 'would justify any measures for the compulsory segregation of Lepers'.[123] Newcastle immediately proposed advising all colonial governors 'that any Laws affecting the personal liberty of

---

[119] *Leprosy Committee Minute Book*, 4119/361, Wellcome Library, Royal College of Physicians, London.

[120] For biographical material on Milroy see Mark Harrison's entry in H. C. G. Matthew and Brian Harrison (eds.), *Oxford Dictionary of National Biography, From Earliest Times to the Year 2000* (Oxford: Oxford University Press, 2004), vol. xxxviii, pp. 330–1.

[121] Gavin Milroy, *Report on Leprosy and Yaws in the West Indies*, 1873, p. 27. This report is bound into Milroy's copy of the *Report on Leprosy by the Royal College of Physicians 1867*, among Milroy's papers at the Wellcome Library, Royal College of Physicians, London.

[122] C. Fortescue, Colonial Office, to Henry Pitman, Royal College of Physicians, 21 May 1863, *Leprosy Committee Minute Book*, 4119/361.

[123] Pitman to Fortescue, 10 June 1863, *Leprosy Committee Minute Book*.

Lepers ought to be repealed', and requested the support of the College of Physicians for this instruction.[124] This was forthcoming,[125] and by the end of the year Newcastle was again pressing the Committee, this time to make their final report without waiting for any more replies.[126]

The Committee responded by agreeing to prepare an Abstract of Replies from those received so far. Printed by the Colonial Office, this constituted in effect an interim report.[127] Another such interim report was issued in 1865 as outstanding replies from known sites of leprosy such as Bengal and Ceylon continued to delay its final conclusions.[128] In effect, however, these conclusions had already been decided. The final Report, published in 1867, declared that leprosy was non-contagious, and that any reported cases to the contrary rested on 'imperfect observation'.[129] Leprosy, it concluded, was 'essentially a constitutional disorder', and was best tackled by improving the health, diet and living conditions of native populations. Such improvements, the Report argued, had formerly brought about its decline in Europe and a similar decline could be 'confidently anticipated' in Britain's colonies.[130] The disease was most frequent among 'dark populations', and those few Europeans who were afflicted had usually been born and had grown up in a tropical colony.[131]

Although these conclusions reflected the views that Milroy held before the inquiry, and although it is clear that by 1865, if not earlier, the Committee was a one-man band, the Report was more than a summary of Milroy's firmly held beliefs. In the first place, much of the evidence gathered from around the empire did support its conclusions, although, as later commentators were to remark, evidence pointing the other way was discounted. And there was constant pressure from the Colonial Office. Newcastle had encouraged Milroy to jump the gun, and although Milroy was undoubtedly in sympathy with Newcastle, he had resisted the demand for a premature final report. His response, which was to provide interim reports instead, had the short-term effect of restraining Colonial Office impatience to have the disease conclusively declared as hereditary.

---

[124] Fortescue to Pitman, 9 July 1863, Correspondence re. Leprosy 1862–1887, 4119/302, Wellcome Library, Royal College of Physicians, London.

[125] Pitman to Fortescue, 17 July 1863, *Leprosy Committee Minute Book*.

[126] Frederic Rogers to Henry Pitman, 30 December 1863, as reported to Leprosy Committee, 8 January 1864, *Leprosy Committee Minute Book*.

[127] *Leprosy Committee Minute Book*, 19 January 1864. Gavin Milroy to Henry Pitman, 5 March 1864, Correspondence re. Leprosy 1862–1887, 4119/303.

[128] *Leprosy Committee Minute Book*, 16 December 1864; 3 July 1865.

[129] *Report on Leprosy by the Royal College of Physicians 1867*, p. lxix.

[130] *Ibid.*, p. lxxiv.   [131] *Ibid.*, p. lxvi.

On the face of it this impatience was strange. Leprosy was traditionally thought to be highly contagious; indeed was still commonly believed to be communicable by touch. Why, at a time of growing concern about its spread in Britain's overseas empire, should the Colonial Office and the College of Physicians have been so keen to declare the disease non-contagious and to free its sufferers who were being held in isolation? A number of different answers suggest themselves: medical, ideological and imperial.

The first is purely medical. As Michael Worboys has shown, by the 1850s and 60s anti-contagionists had the upper hand in their long-running debate with contagionists over public health policy. The failure of quarantine measures to halt the spread of cholera in 1848–9 had resulted in a number of diseases being refashioned as non-contagious and therefore best prevented by environmental and sanitary reform.[132] By the 1860s it was increasingly believed that pathological change originated internally, and was the result of physiological weakness derived from inherited tendencies, poor nutrition or other obscure internal forces.[133] The role of external causes in the aetiology of disease was thought to be indirect,[134] and the idea that infection came externally from some kind of 'organic-germ' was widely seen as old-fashioned, even Aristotelian;[135] hence, I take it, Newcastle's dismissal of the contagious nature of leprosy as a 'popular notion'. This, then, was the immediate medical context in which leprosy was declared a hereditary disease. As Milroy was to put it several years later: 'Leprosy is a constitutional cachexy . . . not of any one part or texture of the body, but of its whole framework and system.'[136] A similar debate over consumption in the later 1860s also resulted in the conclusion that it was constitutional and non-contagious.[137]

Second, the rights of colonial subjects in British colonies were a matter of real concern. Since emancipation, anti-slavery had become a movement for the civil rights of freed slaves. This was intensely topical in the mid-1860s because of the Governor Eyre case, with arguments for Eyre's prosecution deriving from the idea of the equality of British subjects across the Empire. Of course the failure to prosecute Eyre made clear that any such formal equality was often belied by the informal practices of colonial rule.[138] Nevertheless, Newcastle's concern was real enough and contributed to his impatience to advise all colonial governors 'that any Laws affecting the personal liberty of Lepers ought to be repealed'.

---

[132] Worboys, *Spreading Germs*, pp. 39–42.   [133] *Ibid.*, p. 33.   [134] *Ibid.*, p. 76.
[135] *Ibid.*, p. 38.   [136] Milroy, *Report on Leprosy and Yaws in the West Indies*, p. 37.
[137] Worboys, *Spreading Germs*, p. 199.
[138] Catherine Hall, *Civilising Subjects: Metropole and Colony in the English Imagination 1830–1867* (Oxford: Polity, 2002), pp. 127, 263.

In this, as in most things, the Colonial Office and the College of Physicians in the person of Milroy were at one. One communication that prompted concern in the Colonial Office was from New Brunswick, an acknowledged leprosy black-spot. As the Governor wrote, expressing his unease: 'I assume that the contagious character of the disease is so clearly proved as to render the seclusion of those affected with it within the walls of a lazaretto indispensable ... nothing short of an imperative public necessity would justify the horrible mental torture which such a confinement ... must inflict.'[139] Milroy, who had no doubt that the contagious character of leprosy was a myth, reprinted this letter in one of a series of articles he wrote for *The Medical Times and Gazette* between 1874 and 1880.[140] Milroy's objection to compulsory detainment was consistent and insistent. After witnessing the conditions in which lepers in British Guiana were kept, he wrote:

I could not but feel that the case of the leper at the present time is much like that of the poor lunatic at the close of the last century; a hopeless outcast, regarded as a burden and possibly a danger to society, to be immured and kept apart ... The sight, too, of so many human beings living in complete idleness, though most of them were far from being incapable of some useful occupation, left a most painful impression on me.[141]

In a subsequent letter to the Colonial Office dismissing alleged evidence of contagion in British Guiana, Milroy wrote that compulsory seclusion was 'unjust towards the sufferers ... [and] serves to sanction & perpetuate a delusion which has had, & still leads, to much evil'.[142] In 1877, advising the Colonial Office on the treatment of lepers in Surinam, he wrote: 'They are treated as dangerous outcasts, being expelled and rigorously excluded (for the rest of their lives) from society, deprived not only of personal liberty but also of sundry civil rights.'[143]

This language of 'personal liberty' and 'civil rights' had its limits, however. Responding to another Colonial Office request for advice, this time on leprosy in Mauritius, Milroy advised: 'On grounds of public health alone, there is no necessity for excluding the leprous sick from admission into any institution designed for the reception of the suffering or disabled poor.'[144]

---

[139] Lieutenant-Governor Gordon to the Duke of Newcastle, 13 April 1863, in *Report on Leprosy by the Royal College of Physicians 1867*, p. 204.
[140] Gavin Milroy, 'Is Leprosy Contagious?' 2, *Medical Times and Gazette*, 2 (1875), 65.
[141] Milroy, *Report on Leprosy and Yaws in the West Indies*, p. 4.
[142] Gavin Milroy to R. H. Meade, 9 October 1874, Dr Gavin Milroy's MS: 464, Wellcome Library, Royal College of Physicians, London.
[143] Gavin Milroy to Robert G. W. Herbert, 22 October 1877, *ibid.*
[144] Gavin Milroy to John Branston, 2 November 1878, *ibid.*

Even more striking than the class bias within Milroy's liberalism revealed by this advice, was his advocacy of compulsory gender segregation. During a tour of leper asylums in the West Indies in 1871–2, to be discussed in Chapter 2, Milroy repeatedly insisted on the need to decontrol relations between lepers and others, while enforcing strict gender segregation between leprous males and females. In British Guiana, for example, he opposed a plan to move all lepers to Kaow Island, wanting instead a mainland site where male leprosy sufferers would be free to come and go, and to use Kaow Island for the female lepers.[145] In the event, gender segregation was introduced in the existing site at Mahaica. In Jamaica Milroy recommended a new site within easy reach of Spanish Town or Kingston so that it should not be isolated, but also wanted strict segregation within the asylum: 'The huts or buildings for the males should be separated from those for the families and children by the houses of the Resident Manager being interposed between the two sets.'[146] In Trinidad, where Milroy wrote a new set of regulations for the leper asylum, he was successful in getting a ward exclusively for female lepers built in the asylum grounds but outside the enclosure, 'so as to separate them more effectually from the male patients'.[147]

For all Milroy's strong anti-contagionism there appears to be some idea of differential gender-based infection at work here. Even though leprosy was thought to be more common in men than women, the latter were frequently regarded as conduits or contaminants. Of course this alternative form of segregation also followed logically enough from Milroy's hereditarian position on the disease. If leprosy was non-contagious there was no need to keep lepers away from non-lepers. But if, as Milroy was convinced, it was the result of inherited constitutional defects, then it was imperative to stop leprosy sufferers from reproducing. The likelihood of this occurring between a sufferer and a non-sufferer was, he must have assumed, remote. Some form of segregation also squared with Milroy's belief that public health was an important secondary factor in the aetiology and transmission of the disease. The regimen Milroy introduced at Trinidad, and advocated elsewhere, was based on the sanitary benefits of healthy living, exercise and hard work. As he wrote to the Colonial Office in 1878: 'the indigent leper in tropical climates should be in Industrial Houses where occupations, indoor & outdoor, shall be required of all the inmates who are not

---

[145] Governor Scott to Earl of Kimberley, 1 November 1871, *ibid*.

[146] Gavin Milroy to R. H. Meade, 16 November 1872, *ibid*.

[147] Name illegible, Trinidad, to Gavin Milroy, 6 September 1873; Meade to Milroy, 13 April 1874, *ibid*.

bedridden'.[148] Once again the limits to Milroy's dislike of coercion are apparent.

A third explanation for the conclusions of the 1867 Report is imperial or, one might say, postcolonial. The evidence upon which its findings were based came from precisely those groups that had the strongest interest in believing that Europeans were virtually immune to the disease. Consciously or not, the Report offered reassurance to colonial administrators and settlers. Among the questions asked about leprosy in the Physicians' interrogatories was: 'Is it more frequent among certain races? Among the white, the coloured, or the black population? And in what relative proportions?'[149] This elicited some elaborate replies. That from Crete, for example, identified three different forms of the disease – Arab, Greek and Jewish.[150] In its conclusions the Report had noted the widely varying accounts of Jewish susceptibility to the disease.[151] However, this and other such attempts at racialising the disease repeatedly broke down. Having carefully distinguished the three forms to be found on Crete, the respondent added: 'These forms are, however, often blended and combined in one patient, so that it is difficult to disassociate them.'[152]

Another example of the threat to racial difference that leprosy could embody was provided by Erasmus Wilson in an essay 'Observations on the True Leprosy or Elephantiasis, with Cases', included in the lengthy appendices to the 1867 Report. One of these cases concerned a young medical officer in the Indian Army, born in India but of English parents, whose anaesthetic leprosy had caused a significant darkening of his skin. Wilson reported that as a result of leprosy, occurring after syphilis, this young man 'has become swarthy, and at present is darker than a native of India, the swarthiness not being limited to the exposed parts of the body – the face and the hands, but pervading the whole skin'.[153]

The threatened collapse of racial distinctions typically resulted in greater insistence upon them. The 1867 Report officially encouraged the idea that leprosy was a native disease, transmitted indigenously, and unlikely to jump the barriers of race or geography. In doing so it helped to reinforce the distinctions between coloniser and indigene that

---

[148] Gavin Milroy to John Branston, 2 November 1878; also Milroy, *Report on Leprosy and Yaws in the West Indies*, pp. 22–4.
[149] *Report on Leprosy by the Royal College of Physicians 1867*, p. iv.
[150] *Ibid.*, p. xii.   [151] *Ibid.*, p. lxvi.   [152] *Ibid.*, p. xii.
[153] *Ibid.*, p. 240. Wilson's diagnosis of this case as one of anaesthetic leprosy had been confirmed by Boeck who was visiting the capital at the time.

became more urgent as colonial powers extended their territories while attempting to keep their distance from the peoples and diseases of those territories. Leprosy was becoming part of that evolving 'grammar of difference' that, as Ann Laura Stoler and Frederick Cooper have argued, became central to the construction of national and imperial identity in the nineteenth century.[154] The primary differences were established within the hierarchies of race, gender and class, but within each of these categories the operation of a health/sickness dichotomy became a significant, though highly unstable, marker of difference. By the 1860s leprosy was becoming one particular focus of this general way of thinking.

For all the carefully gathered evidence about leprosy from around the Empire upon which the 1867 Report was based, its method of inquiry and its conclusions were firmly based upon Boeck and Danielssen's report of twenty years earlier. The Physicians' Report was quite explicit about this, announcing at the beginning: 'In foot notes appended to most of the conclusions, the leading results of the observations of MM. Danielssen and Boeck on the several questions discussed are given, from the Norwegian Official Report on Leprosy in 1847.'[155] On the crucial matter of contagion, for example, the Report's emphatic conclusion that leprosy was non-contagious was reinforced by a long quotation from Danielssen and Boeck on how long-term marriage or cohabitation had never in their experience resulted in the partner of a leper becoming infected.[156] In a long review of the Report, the *Edinburgh Medical Journal* concluded that its main significance lay in confirming the general accuracy of the research of Danielssen and Boeck, 'to whom the profession is so much indebted for the light they have thrown on the nature and medical history of leprosy', and whose 'masterly work' the journal commends.[157] Even here, however, the *Edinburgh Medical Journal* points up material in the Report that sits uneasily with its main conclusions. Erasmus Wilson's essay in the Appendix to the Report had suggested the possibility of contagion through inoculation, lactation and syphilis, and the *Edinburgh Medical Journal* pointed to this when discussing how it was

---

[154] See Ann Laura Stoler and Frederick Cooper, 'Between Metropole and Colony: Rethinking a Research Agenda', in Frederick Cooper and Ann Laura Stoler (eds.), *Tensions of Empire: Colonial Cultures in a Bourgeois World* (Berkeley, Calif.: University of California Press, 1997), pp. 3–4.

[155] *Report on Leprosy by the Royal College of Physicians 1867*, p. vii.

[156] *Ibid.*, p. lxix.

[157] Review of *Report on Leprosy by the Royal College of Physicians 1867*, *Edinburgh Medical Journal*, 14 (1868–9), 547–8.

that leprosy sometimes occurred when there was no apparent hereditary tendency.[158]

Another uncertainty raised but not dispelled by the 1867 Report was leprosy at home. Britain itself was not included in the Empire-wide survey, but the Report did include a short section on indigenous cases. These included Broadbent's case from the island of Lewis, discussed earlier, and a more recent one in London involving 'a poor Irishwoman long resident in London … who had never been abroad'.[159] The Report also referred to a case in Brighton, recently described by W. E. Nourse. This concerned a fifty-two-year-old charwoman with five healthy children, who had never been out of England. Her symptoms had first appeared when she was around forty, and included tubercles, ulceration and hoarseness of voice. Nourse elsewhere explained the case as the result of 'hard work, beyond the person's strength, poor living, and the marine atmosphere (a condition seldom absent in the history of the leper)'. This, he concluded, had caused 'a changed and deteriorated condition of the mass of the blood. This being the *fons et origio mali* in leprosy.'[160] Such cases were to appear and disappear in the history of leprosy in the second half of the century. Although Wilson's essay in the 1867 Report included four of the five case histories from his 1856 *Lancet* articles, the fifth, the indigenous one of the young woman, has disappeared from his portfolio. Much later in the century, when the absence of indigenous examples of the disease was frequently asserted, examples such as Nourse's case had also fallen out of sight.

To conclude: Danielssen and Boeck provided the foundation for the 1867 Report by the Royal College of Physicians. Prompted by concern in the West Indies, the College of Physicians' empire-wide survey of leprosy concluded that although the disease was endemic in many colonies it posed almost no risk to European settlers and officials. This was because of its hereditarian and non-contagious nature. These findings were in accord with the anti-contagionist views of the Report's author, Gavin Milroy, and more generally with current medical thinking about the cause of disease. Nevertheless, for all the certainty with which its findings were presented the Report left unanswered questions, such as how to explain the disease in cases where the hereditary factor seemed to be missing. It also contained evidence of examples of apparent infection that were at odds with its

---

[158] Erasmus Wilson, 'Observations on the True Leprosy or Elephantiasis, with Cases', in *Report on Leprosy by the Royal College of Physicians 1867*, p. 231. Review of *Report on Leprosy, Edinburgh Medical Journal*, 14 (1868–9), 543.

[159] *Report on Leprosy by the Royal College of Physicians 1867*, p. lxxiii.

[160] W. E. C. Nourse, 'Case of True Leprosy, or Elephantiasis Graecorum', *Medical Times and Gazette*, 2 September 1865, 251–2. For more on Nourse, see n. 96.

conclusions. And the isolated instances of leprosy in Britain were difficult to reconcile with the Report's confidence that leprosy was primarily a tropical and native disease. Norway, after all, was a conspicuous exception, even if it was doing something about the problem. If the example of Norway offered some reassurance that in Europe leprosy could be managed and perhaps brought under control, it was also a permanent reminder of its enduring presence in Europe.

2   Scientists discuss the causes of leprosy, and the disease becomes a public issue in Britain and its empire, 1867–1898

Milroy in the West Indies

The Royal College of Physicians' *Report on Leprosy 1867* was based on information gathered across the empire as interpreted by advanced metropolitan thinking on leprosy in particular and disease in general. Its findings, however, made little difference to how the disease was regarded in most colonial territories. In the West Indies particularly its conclusions were ignored or resisted, and in the decade following the report Milroy was frequently called upon to endorse and restate its findings.

The most common challenge to the report came in the form of claims to have found a cure for the disease. Having declared that leprosy was non-infectious, the College of Physicians was bound to regard such claims with deep scepticism. In the years following the Report local remedies such as gurjun and cashew nut oil were often suggested to the Colonial Office from various colonial territories. These would be passed on to Milroy, who was consistently dismissive of such claims. As he wrote to the Colonial Office in 1878: 'It is vain to look for any permanent benefit from empirical medicaments in a bad form of Cachexia, or chronic malady connected with constitutional depravation. Unhappily, the public is, every now and then, being misled by the announcements of specific remedies which are speedily found to be utterly fallacious, if not also positively mischievous.'[1] One such claim, a decade earlier, had taken Milroy to the West Indies. Although this journey consolidated his position with the Colonial Office as the last word on leprosy and its treatment, Milroy also discovered that the 1867 Report, insofar as it was known at all, commanded little respect in the West Indies.

A doctor in Venezuela, L. D. Beauperthuy, claimed to have discovered a successful treatment for leprosy. This aroused interest in London and the

---

[1] Gavin Milroy to John Branston, 2 November 1878, Dr. Gavin Milroy's MSS: 464, Wellcome Library, Royal College of Physicians, London.

West Indies, and in 1868 Dr. R. H. Bakewell, Medical Superintendent of the Leper Asylum in Trinidad, was sent to investigate. He reported enthusiastically on Beauperthuy's methods but the College of Physicians was unconvinced: 'the alleged cures are said to have been effected by secret remedies, in the employment of which there is notoriously much room for deception'.[2] Bakewell was asked to revisit and follow up the cases he had examined. By now the French authorities in Guadeloupe were also interested and had sent a doctor of their own to investigate the alleged cure. Beauperthuy was jealous of his secret and the Colonial Office reluctantly agreed a six-month trial during which secrecy would be maintained, and promised to provide 'ample compensation for the disclosure of his discovery if he insists on a condition so unusual and regarded in so unfavourable a light by the Medical Profession at large', if the cure proved to work.[3] Bakewell's second report was more qualified, and the College of Physicians, still unconvinced, advised that 'some competent and disinterested person' should now be sent to investigate. This proved to be Milroy, who left for the West Indies in July 1871. Bakewell, by now in England giving evidence to a parliamentary inquiry into vaccination, was extremely put out.[4]

Milroy's first port of call was British Guiana where Beauperthuy was now under temporary engagement to the colonial government. He spent more than three weeks observing Beauperthuy's methods before moving on to Barbados. Curiously, Beauperthuy died suddenly the day after Milroy left, and interest in his remedy seems more or less to have died with him.[5] Milroy himself had little to say about Beauperthuy's method, predisposed as he was to disregard it. Bakewell, however, had reported that it consisted of the external application of cashew nut oil to the diseased part, supplemented by the internal administration of mercury.[6]

---

[2] Henry Pitman to Sir Frederic Rogers, 28 January 1869, Correspondence re. Dr. Bakewell's Report 1868–70, 4119/294, Wellcome Library.

[3] J. Scott Bushe, Colonial Secretary of Trinidad, to Dr Bakewell, 7 May 1869, Correspondence re. Dr. Bakewell's enquiry into Dr. Beauperthuy's method of treating leprosy, 4119/337, Wellcome Library.

[4] R. H. Bakewell to Royal College of Physicians, 4 May 1871, Correspondence re. Leprosy 1870 with reference to Dr. Beauperthuy's method of treating leprosy, 4119/334, Wellcome Library.

[5] Milroy, *Report on Leprosy and Yaws in the West Indies*, pp. 6, 11. This report is bound into Milroy's copy of the *Report on Leprosy by the Royal College of Physicians 1867*, among Milroy's papers at the Wellcome Library.

[6] R. H. Bakewell to the Earl of Granville, 25 May 1870, Correspondence relating to the discovery of an alleged cure of leprosy, *House of Commons Sessional Papers 1871*, vol. LVI, p. 691. Jane Buckingham, *Leprosy in Colonial South India: Medicine and Confinement* (Basingstoke: Palgrave, 2002), pp. 135–40, gives a detailed account of the negotiation

Milroy continued on his tour, but with an altered agenda. As he travelled from British Guiana to Barbados, Antigua, Trinidad, Dominica and Jamaica, Milroy was alarmed to discover that the 1867 Report was virtually unknown. It 'had been seen by very few; most of the medical men even had not read it ... It seemed as if not above two or three copies had ever reached each colony; in more than one, the Government offices were without a copy.'[7] Milroy's task now became one of spreading the word according to the College of Physicians to a superstitious and incredulous colonial world. Throughout his tour he drummed home the message that leprosy was hereditary and not contagious, and therefore that strict isolation was unwarranted and the neglect of patients inhumane. He wanted lepers to be treated alongside other chronically ill patients, and for the 'leprosy' label to be dropped from the title of institutions:

As long as the terms 'leper', 'leprosy', are continually being repeated, it will be very difficult to disabuse the public mind of the dread and aversion which the words have hitherto suggested. These feelings have led to the perpetuation of opinions which, on strict investigation, have been shown to be the offspring of mere traditional belief rather than of unprejudiced observation.[8]

Another theme of Milroy's Report, and one that grew from more than his distaste for incarceration, was the need for lepers to be put to work: 'it is the want of will, much more than the want of ability, that generally lies at the root of the inaction and indolence of leprous patients ... Even when great mutilation of the extremities exists, it is surprising how much the poor sufferers can do if they are but willing to make the effort.'[9] This aim, however, was frustrated by the 'superstitious' horror of the disease that Milroy so deplored. In Trinidad Asylum, for example, where Milroy was impressed to discover that work-therapy had been introduced, the public refused to purchase or use articles made by lepers for fear of infection.[10] Another frustration for Milroy in the West Indies was the widespread belief that leprosy was spread by smallpox vaccination. Bakewell, who was also Vaccinator-General for Trinidad, was in England giving evidence to this effect as Milroy toured the West Indies. A circular on the matter had been sent by the Colonial Office to 'Governors of the principal Colonies in which Leprosy prevails' in September 1871, just as Milroy was beginning his island-hopping.[11] It sought information about the

---

between the Colonial Office and the Royal College of Physicians over how best to respond to Beauperthuy's claims, and includes material on how the alleged cure was given trials in Madras and other presidencies in India.

[7] Milroy, *Report on Leprosy and Yaws in the West Indies*, p. 65.   [8] *Ibid.*, p. 30.

[9] *Ibid.*, p. 14.   [10] *Ibid.*, p. 23.

[11] R. H. Meade to Gavin Milroy, 5 August 1872, Dr Gavin Milroy's MSS: 464.

possibility of infection through vaccination and wet nursing, subjects that were to recur time and again in Milroy's discussions with the various colonial administrations in the Caribbean islands. These were important issues because they bore directly on the question of person-to-person contagion, and encouraged comparisons between leprosy and syphilis that Milroy was always determined to resist. It was commonly accepted that syphilis could be communicated by vaccination if the lymph included blood. But for Milroy leprosy was not a poison, was not contagious, and was therefore quite unlike syphilis.

In his report Milroy conceded that leprosy could occur even when there was no hereditary trace; it is 'liable to be acquired or become developed, independently of congenital trait or predisposition', he wrote, as the result of 'a weakened vital action in the system generally'.[12] Diet was therefore of primary importance in preventing, retarding or mitigating the disease: 'In leprosy, as in scrofula, it is by renovating the system, not by seeking to counteract or to eliminate a morbific element, that we can reasonably hope to effect the greatest amount of good.'[13] Bad diet, he added, was mainly a problem amongst 'the negro & imported Hindoo & Chinese labourers' where the leprosy problem was worst. This meant that the 'food question . . . concerns the planter and the economist quite as much as it does the sanitarian';[14] hygiene and profitability went hand in hand. In the series of articles Milroy subsequently wrote on leprosy and contagion for the *Medical Times and Gazette*, however, he made much less of the spontaneous origin of leprosy. These were nine articles appearing between 1874 and 1880 under the collective title 'Is Leprosy Contagious?' Here Milroy was much more concerned to defend the hereditarian position against a new kind of challenge from the contagionists, and it must have seemed that the spontaneous origin theory would leave open a door through which they might push.

Although the title page of Milroy's Report described it as being 'In continuation of the Paper presented to both Houses of Parliament in 1871' (an earlier one on Beauperthuy's alleged cure), it was essentially a reiteration and sequel to the 1867 Report. As if to underline this, the interrogatories and conclusions of the 1867 Report were appended to Milroy's West Indian one. This was certainly how the Colonial Office received and endorsed it. Their letter to colonial governors that followed the official circulation of Milroy's Report instructed them to implement Milroy's recommendations for the arrangement of asylums. It concluded:

---

[12] Milroy, *Report on Leprosy and Yaws in the West Indies*, pp. 37–8.   [13] *Ibid.*, p. 44.
[14] *Ibid.*, pp. 48–9.

The fact that Leprosy is transmitted from parent to child is indisputable, and as Leprosy by descent is often through a natural error mistaken for Leprosy by contagion (the members of one family being naturally in contact), it is important that this fact should be borne in mind. It is a fact which points also to the expediency of placing Asylums for Females at a distance from Asylums for Males when circumstances permit, and when the numbers are such as to justify separate establishments.[15]

These recommendations, however, were frequently resisted or ignored and Milroy continued to complain about the inability of the West Indian colonies 'to modify the old views which had been for so many years universally accepted as true'.[16] The failure of the 1867 Report to win acceptance in many parts of the empire also troubled the Colonial Office during the 1870s, although for slightly different reasons. The Colonial Secretary, Kimberley, had hesitated before accepting Milroy's recommendations for the treatment of lepers in British Guiana: 'I have come to the conclusion (though with much doubt) no longer to insist on the resumption of the system of isolation.'[17] During the next few years the Colonial Office repeatedly sought reassurance from the College of Physicians on the question of contagion. The answer was always the same: 'The College thinks it very desirable that, on all occasions, the hereditary character of the disease should be kept steadily in view.'[18] Alleged instances of the transmission of leprosy by vaccination or breast-feeding, for example, were always rejected on the grounds of inadequate evidence, with Milroy reminding the Colonial Office of the necessity for 'minute and accurate details from the local observers, including dates and localities of the occurrences'.[19] The absence, or sheer impossibility, of such detailed and conclusive evidence left the authority of the 1867 Report officially intact.

Meanwhile, discussion of leprosy in Britain in the early 1870s was beginning to turn away from unequivocal adherence to the hereditary explanation. Robert Liveing's 1873 Goulstonian Lectures, revised and published the following year as *Elephantiasis Graecorum, or True Leprosy*, accepted without question the hereditary origin of leprosy, while at the same time showing this theory starting to come under pressure. Although Liveing regarded the idea that leprosy was contagious as the product

[15] Earl of Kimberley to Colonial Governments, 4 September 1873, letter bound into Milroy's copy of *Report on Leprosy and Yaws in the West Indies*.
[16] Gavin Milroy to Robert G. W. Herbert, 27 February 1875, Dr Gavin Milroy's MSS: 464.
[17] Earl of Kimberley to Governor Scott, British Guiana, 18 December 1871, *ibid.*
[18] Dr. Pitman to R. H. Meade, 16 September 1873, Correspondence re. Leprosy 1862–1887, 4119/321, Wellcome Library.
[19] Leprosy Committee of Royal College of Physicians to Lord Carnarvon, 20 December 1875, Correspondence relating to the Leprosy Committee of Royal College of Physicians 1873–6, 2248/51, Wellcome Library.

of medieval superstition and ignorance, he also subscribed to the belief that it had spread from Africa and established itself in tropical America as a result of the slave trade.[20] This required a modified theory of heredity, for which he turned to Virchow's distinction between 'true hereditariness', as with syphilis, and 'hereditary predisposition'.[21] Liveing also argued, as others had, that Indian marriage customs, particularly intermarriage within lower-caste families, intensified the hereditary tendency of the disease.[22] In fact he elaborated this instance of leprosy as a disease of closed social groups into a totalising theory:

[L]eprosy exists … in exact inverse proportion to the amount of commercial exchange, intermixture of races, and other elements of civilisation; and it persists among communities shut in by the sea, or by the social barriers of prejudice and caste, which have not been able to eliminate the specific element of the disease by natural selection.[23]

This endogamous theory of leprosy was the antithesis of the exogamous theories that were to flourish in the 1880s and 90s. Whereas these were to see leprosy as a product of the transgression of borders, Liveing regarded it as a consequence of being contained within them. It was very definitely a pre-germ theory and sat oddly with the fear of the disease spreading that he sometimes voiced.

On the other hand, Liveing's lectures also demonstrated that the apparent spread of leprosy in many parts of the colonised world was making unqualified acceptance of the 1867 Report difficult. He noted it was beginning to appear that inoculation was one of the means by which the disease spread.[24] This, of course, had been suggested by Erasmus Wilson in his appended essay to the 1867 Report and given further publicity by the vaccination hearings. Crucially, the example of Hawaii was beginning to trouble the hereditarian explanation. Liveing cited both C. N. Macnamara's *Leprosy* (1865), and a recent series of lectures by Erasmus Wilson to the College of Surgeons on the spread of leprosy in the Hawaiian islands, and suggested that the disease might be contagious in tropical countries though not in Europe. He also mentioned unconfirmed reports of leprosy spreading beyond the Chinese population in Australia.[25] Living's rather strained conclusion was that although leprosy was 'not contagious in the ordinary sense of the word, it is propagated by the imbibition of the excretions of those affected, much in the same way (not in the same degree) as typhoid fever or cholera are

---

[20] Robert Liveing, *Elephantiasis Graecorum, or True Leprosy* (London: Longmans, Green, and Co., 1873), p. 48.
[21] *Ibid.*, p. 87. [22] *Ibid.*, p. 68. [23] *Ibid.*, p. 86. [24] *Ibid.*, p. 90.
[25] *Ibid.*, pp. 91–2. (Wilson's lectures were reported in *The Lancet*, 1 (1873), 240, 358–9.)

propagated ... [However] as leprosy is developed but slowly, there is far greater difficulty in tracing it home to its true source'.[26] Finding himself virtually in the contagionist camp, Liveing turned to Milroy himself in a long footnote to the passage just quoted:

Since writing the above I have come upon the following remark in Dr. G. Milroy's report on 'Leprosy in the West Indies', 1873, which to a limited extent bears out my own view, though he evidently thinks the disease less liable to spread than I do. 'In conclusion I would say in respect of ... the communicability of the disease by contact with the afflicted – that having carefully considered the whole evidence ... and wishing to avoid even the appearance of dogmatism upon a matter which does not admit of absolute certainty, leprosy appears to me to be neither more nor less contagious than scrofula (Phthisis?). What Dr Williams, whose authority no one will question, has stated in regard of pulmonary consumption, one form of tuberculosis disease, is, in my opinion, equally applicable to the other cachexy.'[27]

What Dr Williams had said was to be elaborated the following year in a highly influential work by Henry Vandyke Carter, and this passage from Milroy's report was to be seized upon by other contagionists.

Hansen and *Mycobacterium leprae*

There was also a new kind of challenge to the hereditarian explanation during the 1870s, one that was less easily ascribed to backward colonial doctors and administrators and superstitious colonial subjects. In 1873 the Norwegian scientist Armaeur Hansen isolated what would prove to be the leprosy bacillus, a discovery that soon made the advanced thinking of the previous decade itself seem out of date. Hansen's work first entered British debate on leprosy through two books by Henry Vandyke Carter, *Report on Leprosy and Leper-Asylums in Norway; with reference to India* and *On Leprosy and Elephantiasis*, both published in 1874.

Carter had worked in the Indian Medical Service since 1858. His evidence to the College of Physicians' inquiry had figured prominently in the 1867 Report and added to his reputation as an experienced and respected leprologist. Liveing's argument about the interaction of heredity and caste in perpetuating leprosy in India had come from another of Carter's publications, his *Report on Leprosy in the Bombay Presidency* (1872). In 1872 he had been sent on paid furlough by the government of India to study leprosy in Europe and the Middle East. Visiting Norway, Carter had investigated their asylum system for lepers, and consulted with Boeck

---

[26] *Ibid.*, pp. 93–4.
[27] *Ibid.*, p. 94. The passage Liveing cites is in Milroy, *Report on Leprosy and Yaws in the West Indies*, p. 41.

and Hansen. Most significantly, he had observed Hansen's laboratory investigation of the micro-organisms in leprous tissue that the Norwegian leprologist was coming to believe were the cause of leprosy. Following his visit to Norway Carter produced two books. The first and much shorter was *Report on Leprosy and Leper-Asylums in Norway; with reference to India*, which concentrated on the practical measures adopted by the Norwegian government to contain the spread of leprosy. Carter approved of its asylum policy and argued that a similar practice should be followed in India.[28] On contagion he was more cautious. He claimed still to be emphasising the importance of heredity,[29] and the Appendix included a report by Boeck who had continued to disparage the contagion hypothesis. Elsewhere, however, Carter introduced the case for contagion, asking, for example, whether leprosy had spread 'in a new and healthy country where it had been directly introduced by known lepers, in a manner quicker and wider than was possible in the ordinary process of generation?'[30] Although conceding that Boeck's American researches suggested not, and that evidence from Australia was still wanting, Carter is clearly referring to the example of Hawaii, though without actually naming the islands. And, tucked away in a footnote, he mentions Hansen's latest investigations that pointed to 'the parasitic origin of the disease'.[31]

Carter's report on leprosy in Norway seemed to face both ways on the question of contagion. Milroy noted a little uneasily that although Carter had failed to make clear his position on contagion, the 'general evidence' of his findings corroborated the 1867 Report.[32] Nevertheless, when the Colonial Office informed Milroy it was to circulate Carter's report to 'the Colonies in which Leprosy prevails' (this, by now, was a quasi-official category) he requested that his current article in the *Medical Times and Gazette* should also be included as an official printed addition. This was to defend the 1867 Report from some of Carter's imputations, and also to ensure that his newly equivocal position on contagion was outweighed by Milroy's insistence that the hereditary character of the disease remained undisturbed.[33]

Carter's *On Leprosy and Elephantiasis* was a large, detailed, illustrated monograph that must have been years in the making.[34] The very layout of

---

[28] Henry Vandyke Carter, *Report on Leprosy and Leper-Asylums in Norway; with reference to India* (London: Eyre and Spottiswoode, 1874), pp. 23, 29–30.

[29] *Ibid.*, p. 12.   [30] *Ibid.*, pp. 26–7.   [31] *Ibid.*, p. 27n.

[32] Gavin Milroy, 'Is Leprosy Contagious?', *Medical Times and Gazette*, 1 (1874), 727.

[33] R.H. Meade to Gavin Milroy, 29 August 1874; Milroy to Meade, 8 September 1874, Dr Gavin Milroy's MSS: 464, Wellcome Library.

[34] Carter, the son of an artist, was a skilled illustrator who had previously drawn all the illustrations for the seventeenth edition of *Grays Anatomy* (1856).

this work demonstrated the recent conversion to contagion that Carter had undergone. Thus, while the text maintained that 'heredity is the common cause of the complaint', a series of long footnotes add that his recent acquaintance with investigations in Bergen has led him to believe that the contagion case is 'tolerably definite'. Hansen's description of 'rounded masses or collections, which closely resemble the so-called Bacteria – or Microccus – colonies, now so well known in Medicine', together with the 'rapid spread of the disease in recent time' (Hawaii is now specifically mentioned), suggest that contagion should replace heredity as the primary cause of leprosy.[35] In one of these footnotes Carter turned to the passage from Milroy that Liveing had quoted, in which the arch-hereditarian seemed to concede an element of extraneous origin and communicability in the spread of leprosy. Carter provided the full quotation from Dr Williams that Milroy had cited and added his own telling gloss:

Although I concur in the opinion that we have no evidence that pulmonary consumption is infectious like small-pox, scarlatina, or typhus, or that it depends on a specific poison, yet I think that both reason and experience indicate that a noxious influence may pass from a patient in advanced consumption to a healthy person in close communication, and may produce the same disease, just as foul pus or putrid muscle will produce tubercles in an inoculated animal.

To which Carter adds: 'If such passage [sic] and the comment preceding have ... a precise meaning, this seems to be practically in favour of the extraneous origin, and the possible communicability of scrofula; and no other admission could be desired with respect to leprosy, by the earnest advocate of the later views touching that disease.'[36]

Carter, like Liveing before him, is enlisting support from an unlikely and unwilling quarter. The copy of *On Leprosy and Elephantiasis* held by the Wellcome Institute Library in London had been Milroy's own (an inscription records that the India Office sent it to him in April 1875), and has been annotated in Milroy's hand to highlight those passages in the body of the text that support the hereditarian position. Phrases such as 'leprous germ' that contradict this position have been underlined.[37] Milroy's resistance to Carter's conclusions, and to being represented as lending them support, were developed later that year in the fourth of his 'Is Leprosy Contagious?' articles in the *Medical Times and Gazette*.

Carter's end-point, reached in long footnotes that run across several pages, was that prima facie the contagion argument was true, and that

---

[35] H. Vandyke Carter, *On Leprosy and Elephantiasis* (London: Eyre and Spottiswoode, 1874), pp. 169, 178–9.
[36] *Ibid.*, p. 176. [37] *Ibid.*, p. 175.

'in practice, one ought to act as if contagion were possible'.[38] These notes must have been added very soon before the book went to press and they form a sub-text that contradicts the argument of the main text. The visit to Norway had resulted in a fundamental revision in Carter's thinking on the vexed problem of the aetiology of leprosy that was to be pivotal in the subsequent British turn against the 1867 Report. Both Carter's 1874 volumes, however, also demonstrate the difficulty in abandoning a long-held position and challenging the orthodoxy laid down by Danielssen and Boeck and underwritten by the College of Physicians. Carter, a long-term hereditarian, had travelled to Norway, the fount of that belief, to meet and work with its leading proponents. In doing so he had also discovered Hansen's work and recognised its potential significance. In *Report on Leprosy and Leper-Asylums in Norway* the hereditary explanation is still dominant, and Carter makes clear that the voluntary asylum policy in Norway is not based on the idea that the disease was contagious.[39] In *On Leprosy and Elephantiasis* the hereditary theory has been undercut, although it continues to inform the main body of the text. Both, therefore, fascinatingly reveal the tensions around the time that Hansen's discovery threw into question the position that modern science had for several decades regarded as incontrovertible.

After the publication of *On Leprosy and Elephantiasis* it was no longer possible to see Carter as an anti-contagionist, and Milroy went on to the attack. In his fourth 'Is Leprosy Contagious?' article he argued that Carter's revised position was based on hearsay and imprecise and deficient evidence, much of it derived from a misinterpretation of the rapid spread of leprosy in Hawaii. Neither in this article, nor the following one which returned to Carter's apostasy, did Milroy even refer to Carter's interest in the clusters of identical micro-organisms that Hansen had recently been discovering in leprous tissue.[40]

Hansen's own account of his research first appeared in Britain in an article published in the *British and Foreign Medico-Chirurgical Review* in 1875. This began with a discussion of the difficulty of challenging the hereditary explanation with one based on contagion: 'As ... heredity in leprosy is said to manifest itself until the fourth generation, and perhaps longer, nay even that it can operate without leprous ancestors, it is ... impossible absolutely to exclude this hypothetical heredity.'[41] And further, as leprosy patients often suffer from the disease for years without knowing

---

[38] *Ibid.*, p. 179.   [39] Carter, *Report on Leprosy and Leper-Asylums in Norway*, pp. 23, 25.
[40] Milroy, 'Is Leprosy Contagious?', *Medical Times and Gazette* 2 (1875), 66–7; 3 (1875), 593.
[41] Armaeur Hansen, 'On the Etiology of Leprosy', *British and Foreign Medico-Chirurgical Review*, 55 (1875), 469.

it, discovering the particular occasion of contagion in an already leprous setting is extremely difficult.[42] The bulk of the article is a detailed examination of the disease in Norway based on the family history and other demographic features of individual cases. This leaves Hansen unable to prove either heredity or contagion as their cause, but able to point to a number of factors 'which find a natural explanation by supposing contagion, but which ... remain unexplained under the supposition of heredity'.[43] On the final page of his article Hansen gives up trying to prove a negative and turns to his intimation of a direct proof:

I will briefly mention what seems to indicate that such proof is, perhaps, attainable. There are to be found in every leprous tubercle extirpated from a living individual ... small staff-like bodies, much resembling bacteria, lying within the cells; not in all but in many of them. Though unable to discover any difference between these bodies and true bacteria, I will not venture to declare them to be actually identical. Further, while it seems evident that these low forms of organic life engender some of the most acute infectious diseases, the attributing of the origin of such a chronic disease as leprosy to the apparently same matter must ... be attended with still greater doubts.[44]

This tentative announcement of a possible discovery, held back until the closing paragraph of the article, could hardly be more different from the conclusive tone of Milroy's statements of the alternative position.

For all the hesitancy of its claims, the article caught the attention of the Colonial Office which wrote to the College of Physicians asking if it had in any way 'led the College to modify their views on this matter' of contagion. A reconvened Leprosy Committee could find 'no such minute and accurate details of well observed facts as to afford reason for modifying the opinion it has before expressed'.[45] In fact Milroy had already replied to Hansen's essay in the third of his *Medical Times and Gazette* articles, dismissing the idea that leprosy derived from a germ as 'merely ingenious speculation': 'I can see no greater reason for presuming the existence of a distinct or special virus or morbific parasitic germ ... for the development of leprosy than of scrofula, rickets, cretinism, or cancer.' Milroy had contrasted all these conditions with that of syphilis which 'always originates primarily from a palpable poisonous matter, cognisable by the senses'.[46] In fact, whereas Hansen had actually discovered the leprosy bacillus, that for syphilis would not be identified for another thirty years.

[42] *Ibid.*, 470. [43] *Ibid.*, 487. [44] *Ibid.*, 489.

[45] Report of the Leprosy Committee, 20 December 1875, Correspondence relating to the Leprosy Committee of the Royal College of Physicians 1873–6, 2248/51, Wellcome Library.

[46] Milroy, 'Is Leprosy Contagious?', *Medical Times and Gazette*, 1 (1875), 658.

Meanwhile, challenges to the College of Physicians' line continued to come in from around the empire. The most persistent of these were from British Guiana, where Milroy had been disturbed by the spread of the disease among 'its working population', and by his discovery that 'the doctrine as to the contagiousness of Leprosy was very prevalent among the educated classes at the Colony'.[47] Neither his circulation of the 1867 Report, nor the publication of his *Report on Leprosy in the West Indies* was to change this. In 1874 the Colonial Office sent Milroy a report from British Guiana regarding alleged cases of contagion at Kaow Island, and proposing that there should be a medical inquiry into these claims.[48] In reply Milroy pointed out the lack of evidence for the claims – as usual, he wanted to know details such as age, parentage, family history, and case history – and voiced his frustration at the backwardness of medical and other opinion in the colony: 'As long as the uninformed public believes that a leper is to be shunned, from the dread of his communicating his malady by mere proximity or casual intercourse, he will be tabooed and treated as an outcast. This has been and is the case in the W. Indies.'[49]

The British Guiana inquiry went ahead, nevertheless, and reported to the Colonial Office the following year. It concluded that:

[L]eprosy in many cases is propagated by immediate contact; the term 'contact' not being accepted in the ordinary sense of the word, but as meaning a protracted intercourse of the healthy and the unhealthy, by which contact is produced by the inhalation by the healthy of the exhalations of the unclean, as well as the immediate juxtaposition of the parties by which diseased fluids may be inoculated from one to the other.[50]

Authored by three local doctors, the report had taken account of recent lectures by Erasmus Wilson to the Royal College of Surgeons, the experimental work of Hansen and Carter, and the recent history of the disease in Hawaii. In fact, the wording of the conclusion echoed Wilson's first lecture: 'in its endemic haunts a special poison may be exhaled from the leper, which might convey infection to others, and ... the disease might

---

[47] Gavin Milroy to Henry Pitman, 19 October 1871, Correspondence re. Leprosy 1862–1887, 4119/313, Wellcome Library.

[48] R. H. Meade to Gavin Milroy, 29 September 1874, Dr Gavin Milroy's MSS: 464, Wellcome Library.

[49] Milroy to Meade, 9 October 1874, *ibid.*

[50] Governor Longden to Earl of Carnavon, 28 August 1875. This letter accompanied the *Report as to the Contagion or Transmission of Leprosy, British Guiana*, 1875. Both letter and report are bound into Milroy's copy of the 1867 *Report on Leprosy by the Royal College of Physicians*, together with Milroy's own *Report on Leprosy and Yaws in the West Indies* and other related papers, held in the Wellcome Library.

possibly be given to a child from a nurse through the lung exhalations, or through the breast milk'.[51]

In another of his *Medical Times and Gazette* articles, Milroy remarked of this Report that 'some writers hastily grasp at unverified data which seem to favour their theoretical views'.[52] This was unfair. The British Guiana Report was very conscious of the weight of medical opinion against it. It acknowledged that the hereditary explanation was difficult to establish because families did not like admitting to being 'tainted' by the disease. It also accepted Milroy's argument in his *Report on Leprosy in the West Indies* that 'the disease seems to develope [sic] itself often spontaneously without any appreciable cause'.[53] Its conclusion on the weighting to be given the three likely causes of the disease was almost apologetic: 'leprosy, although in a great many cases due to hereditary taint, in the majority of cases arising spontaneously without any appreciable cause, is propagated in not a few instances by contagion'.[54] There is, however, a note of muted defiance in its anticipation of Milroy's response: 'Those who hold the opinion that the disease is not contagious are too often prone to disregard the cases brought forward by those who entertain a different opinion as based on imperfect observation or inattention to hereditary taint, mode of living, locality, etc.'[55] The letter from Governor Longden accompanying the Report was similarly apologetic. It reminded the Colonial Office that as Governor of Trinidad in 1872 he had followed their instructions based on the assumption that the disease was not contagious, and had allowed free ingress and egress of patients from Trinidad Asylum. Nevertheless, he now argued, dread of the disease was not unreasonable for those living in 'tropical colonies' where the question of contagion involved 'momentous consequences'.[56]

During the 1870s Milroy became permanent defence counsel for the 1867 Report. Although Erasmus Wilson's lectures had drawn openly on Milroy's West Indian Report,[57] his suggestion that leprosy might be contagious in tropical climates utterly discredited him in Milroy's view. When the epithet 'distinguished' was attached to Wilson's name in a report from the leper asylum in Trinidad, Milroy pencilled it out in his own copy.[58] And the fact that the British Guiana Report not only referred to Wilson's

[51] Reported in *The Lancet*, 1 (1873), 240.
[52] Gavin Milroy, 'Is Leprosy Contagious?', *Medical Times and Gazette*, 2 (1876), 85.
[53] *Report as to the Contagion or Transmission of Leprosy, British Guiana*, 1875, p. 7; see n. 50 above.
[54] *Ibid.*, p. 10.   [55] *Ibid.*, p. 7.   [56] Longden to Carnarvon, 28 August 1875, see. n. 50 above.
[57] *The Lancet*, 1 (1873), 358.
[58] Report from the Leper Asylum, Port of Spain, Trinidad 1872, Dr Gavin Milroy's MSS: 464.

lectures but also to Hansen's research, Carter's apparent endorsement of this, and the rapid spread of leprosy in Hawaii 'amongst a population previously untainted with the malady' put it beyond the pale.

The Colonial Office did circulate the British Guiana Report around the colonies, together with the College of Physicians' rebuttal of its findings. This had become the pattern. Alternative points of view on the question of contagion – Bakewell's, Carter's, and now the report from British Guiana – were circulated but always accompanied by a corrective from the College of Physicians. Responses to the Report were predictably varied. The Chief Medical Officer for the State of Victoria reported that his experience was 'entirely against its being contagious', the disease there being confined to Chinese immigrants. Unlike Milroy, he also attacked the conclusions being drawn from Hansen's laboratory work, arguing that those who cited it were 'apparently ignorant that bacteria and micro-cocci abound in nearly every tissue in which disease of any kind exists'.[59] The response from Jamaica, however, without denying the hereditary character of the disease, also claimed that its propagation by intermarriage and cohabitation was 'clearly established', by inoculation distinctly possible, and added: 'persons free from any leprous taint may ultimately become victims of the disease, if when suffering from the effects of much privation and exposure to the debilitating and prejudicial influences of an unhealthy tropical climate, they are subjected to frequent intercourse in ill ventilated rooms with Lepers, the additional insanitary condition of insufficient and unwholesome food being also present'. Therefore, both isolation of the disease and strict segregation of the sexes were 'of the first importance'.[60] This inclusive formulation rather elegantly accepted Milroy's position, while at the same time going well beyond it. It also demonstrated the difficulty for colonial officials of reconciling the still authoritative 1867 Report with their own local experience and observation.

The College of Physicians shored up its position on contagion by drawing attention once again to Milroy's report on leprosy in the West Indies, while Milroy continued to advise the Colonial Office on every reported instance of the contagious nature of leprosy that came their way. From 1876 he was receiving a fee for every such piece of advice.[61] Reports from British Guiana continued to trouble the College line on contagion and isolation. In 1879 Milroy responded sharply to claims by the Medical

[59] W. McCrea, to Sir George Bowen, 21 December 1876, *ibid.* This letter was then relayed to Carnarvon who copied it to Milroy, the usual pattern.
[60] Superintending Medical Officer to the Colonial Secretary, 29 December 1876, *ibid.*
[61] Henry Pitman to Robert G. W. Herbert, 16 February 1876, Correspondence Relating to the Contagious Nature of Leprosy 1876–9, 4119/323, Wellcome Library. Herbert to Milroy, 27 March 1877, Dr Gavin Milroy's MSS: 464.

Officer of the asylum at Mahaica, John Hillis, that leprosy was contagious, could be propagated by vaccination and wet-nursing, and that strict segregation was required to control the spread of the disease. Milroy had already explained the increase of leprosy in the colony as a result of the influx of indentured labourers, 'Coolies or Chinese',[62] and he now informed the Colonial Office there was no 'logical connection' between Hillis's data and his conclusions. He suggested that Hillis should be 'directed by the Government Authorities into a more promising channel than the attempt to revive an exploded doctrine', recommending 'serious Practical Hygiene' in which he said the colony was badly deficient.[63]

Milroy was always a root-and-branch hygienist, believing in public health, sanitation, good diet, cleanliness, discipline and work as the counter to a wide range of diseases he was convinced derived from inherited constitutional defects. He described his own method as 'attaching ... the utmost importance to exact information concerning the geographical prevalence of the malady in respect of the discovery of its etiological relations'; and he contrasted this 'patient, inductive research' with bacteriological investigations which he dismissed as 'the hasty offspring of a superficial and biased consideration of the subject'.[64] Whenever alleged examples of contagious transmission were presented to him he would always request information about family and environmental factors. Whether available or not, the effect was always to throw serious doubt on the possibility of contagion; negative data would be taken as a sign of insufficient research.

Milroy's antipathy to laboratory investigation of the disease meant that he refused to distinguish between traditional attitudes to the disease as dangerously infectious and the contemporary research of Hansen and subsequent micro-biologists. There was no Latourian accommodation between hygienists and Pasteurians in Milroy's world, no readiness to admit the co-existence of different points of view or of different systems of medical knowledge.[65] Contagionists in the 1870s were trying to include Milroy's hygienism in their arguments but Milroy would have none of it. Scientifically, therefore, he was sidelining himself. On the other hand he continued to determine colonial policy towards leprosy.

For Milroy, the 1867 Report had inaugurated a progressive and liberal approach to leprosy based on a repudiation of the traditional superstitious

---

[62] Milroy to Herbert, 5 April 1877, *ibid.*
[63] Milroy to John Branston, 10 October 1879, *ibid.*
[64] Gavin Milroy, 'Is Leprosy Contagious?', *Medical Times and Gazette*, 2 (1880), 264–6.
[65] Bruno Latour, *The Pasteurization of France* (Cambridge, Mass. and London: Harvard University Press, 1988), pp. 55ff. describes how in France the hygienists assimilated rather than opposed contagionism.

belief that it was communicated by touch and that its sufferers should therefore be strictly isolated. Setting his face against the stigmatisation that made the life of leprosy sufferers in many parts of the empire a living hell, he also refused to consider the possibility that Hansen's discovery might be crucial in discovering the obscure aetiology of the disease. For Milroy, all suggestions of contagion were based on superstition and ignorance. So fundamental was his opposition to contagion and germ theory that he never made the point that Hansen and others had failed to establish a causal relation between the bacillus and the disease. To concede this possibility would also have been to acknowledge the inherent plausibility of germ theory. Milroy was clearly and justifiably horrified at the attitudes to leprosy he met on his tour of the West Indies, although he was somewhat insensitive to the alarm of colonial subjects, doctors and officials at rising levels of the disease. By the mid-1870s, however, the form of hereditary explanation he subscribed to was becoming as outmoded and superstitious as the misapprehensions he deplored in British Guiana and elsewhere. He admitted no distinction between superstition and prejudice on one hand, and emergent micro-biology on the other, and ran together all the different kinds of disagreement with the 1867 Report. Medical contagionists, there-fore, were no better than superstitious natives.

The inflexibility of Milroy's position also meant that he was committed to minimising the incidence of the disease because hereditary transmission could not explain a rapid spread of leprosy such as that being experienced in Hawaii. Milroy's response to the Hawaiian example was to argue that leprosy must have existed on the islands prior to its supposed introduction in the 1840s; in other words, it was an indigenous rather than an intro-duced disease that was only now being recorded. Evidence to the contrary was, as usual, said to lack precision and to be deficient in detail.[66] When Milroy, under pressure from the Colonial Office over the report from British Guiana, was collecting material in support of his position he suggested the College of Physicians should 'leave out the communi-cation ... about Honolulu', presumably because it seemed to lend weight to the contagionist position.[67]

Thus, for fifteen years or so following the 1867 Report the Colonial Office, advised by Milroy in the name of the College of Physicians, main-tained that leprosy was hereditary and non-infective. Although the colo-nies were repeatedly advised of this, and were asked to adapt their treatment of leprosy suffers accordingly, they had little or no belief in the

---

[66] Gavin Milroy, 'Is Leprosy Contagious?', *Medical Times and Gazette*, 2 (1875), 66–7.

[67] Gavin Milroy to Henry Pitman, 16 February 1876, Correspondence re. Leprosy 1872–1887, 4119/322, Wellcome Library.

official explanation of the disease and made only minimal efforts to implement the policies they were instructed to follow. Whereas in Britain news
of Hansen's bacillus eventually prompted a reaction against the 1867
Report, there was no equivalent backlash in the colonies because they
had never accepted the hereditary explanation in the first place. Insofar as
micro-biology was known to them at all, it merely confirmed what they
already believed.

Heredity or contagion? Overlapping positions

By the end of the 1870s criticism of the anti-contagionist position was
spreading in medical circles at home, often led by former colonial medical
officers. W. Munro's *Leprosy* (1879) was far more direct in its criticisms of
the 1867 Report and the hereditary argument than Liveing had been.
Munro was a former Medical Officer in St Kitts, in the West Indies, and
his book had first appeared as a series of articles in the *Edinburgh Medical
Journal* between 1876 and 1879. He produced the familiar argument that
leprosy had been spread from Africa to America and the West Indies by
negroes, but elaborated this into a more general theory about race and
empire: wherever 'indigenous tribes have come into constant contact with
the blacks or Portuguese they have become infected'.[68] Hawaii was presented as compelling proof that leprosy always spreads from an infected to
an uninfected people. Munro contradicted Milroy's claim that leprosy was
indigenous in Hawaii, arguing instead that it had spread through the
islands without any possibility of hereditary taint, and must therefore
have been conveyed by contagion.[69]

Munro was sceptical of contemporary reports of leprosy in Britain, such
as those by Broadbent and Wilson. These cases, in fact, presented problems for contagionists; if there really were instances of leprosy in contemporary Britain, why had the disease not spread? Munro conceded one
authentic contemporary case, that of Johanna Crawley who had allegedly
died of leprosy in 1874, but he argued that although this was indigenous it
was not autochthonous. Crawley was a sail-maker living and working
close to the London docks, 'in a district crowded with people *in constant
communication* with the East and West Indies, and in which there are many
coloured people'.[70] Unlike Liveing's endogamous explanation, Munro
saw the disease as spreading through the promiscuous mingling of different races, something that was occurring at the heart of empire as well as its

[68] W. Munro, *Leprosy* (Manchester: John Heywood, 1879), pp. 28–9, 31.
[69] *Ibid.*, pp. 36–8.   [70] *Ibid.*, p. 47.

outposts. This view of leprosy was to be increasingly emphasised in the next two decades.

Munro set out the case against Milroy and the 1867 Report, seizing on Milroy's apparent concession to the contagionist point of view that Liveing and Carter had already highlighted. Rather than enlisting Milroy on his side of the argument as Liveing and Carter had attempted, Munro openly attacked Milroy's 'vacillating indecision' and compared him unfavourably with experts such as Wilson and Carter who had openly changed their position.[71] Munro summed up the case against the hereditary theory: 'leprosy is ... only very rarely transmitted from generation to generation, has never been proved to be transmitted without contact ... and goes back from child to parent when in contact'.[72] As a result he came down strongly in favour of segregation: 'in the later ... ulcerative stages, it is the undoubted duty of every government, with the well-being of the population at heart, to insist on such a measure just as strictly as they would against smallpox'.[73] Curiously, he made no mention of Hansen's discovery of the leprosy bacillus, even though he was familiar with Carter's recent work. This was probably because Munro had his own dietary explanation for the aetiology of the disease, believing the want of salt and a heavily vegetable diet to be its primary cause. In Australia, for example, he argued that white settlers had been protected from catching leprosy from Chinese immigrants because of the unusually large amounts of mutton in their diet.[74] The Chinese, of course, were associated with the growing and marketing of fruit and vegetables. This also indicates how it is possible retrospectively to exaggerate the significance of Hansen's discovery at the time. Although Munro was pleased to have Carter on his side, the crucial element in Carter's change of mind was ignored. The causal connection between the bacillus and the disease remained unproven, and the growing fears of infection were detachable from the germ theory of disease.

It was also possible to have an informed and sympathetic understanding of Hansen's work while retaining some belief in the hereditarian explanation, as John D. Hillis's *Leprosy in British Guiana: An Account of West Indian Leprosy* (1881) illustrates. On one hand, Hillis assumes 'that hereditary influence in this disease is now generally acknowledged', and that 'a predisposition to the disease may be transmitted'.[75] On the other, he was conversant with Hansen's, Carter's and Neisser's work on the leprosy bacillus and saw it as going 'to prove that leprosy is essentially a

---

[71] *Ibid.*, pp. 48n, 77n.   [72] *Ibid.*, p. 79.   [73] *Ibid.*, p. 94.   [74] *Ibid.*, p. 41.
[75] John D. Hillis, *Leprosy in British Guiana: An Account of West Indian Leprosy* (London: J. and A. Churchill, 1881), pp. 47n, 106.

contagious disease'. He dismissed other explanations such as diet, geography and spontaneous occurrence but, unlike Munro, believed that leprosy could be transmitted by vaccination with tainted lymph.[76] Like many others in the West Indies he believed that leprosy had been introduced to British Guiana by African slaves, and reintroduced in the nineteenth century by indentured labourers from China and India.[77] On this latter point, of course, he was in agreement with Milroy, although the two interpreted the implications of this rather differently. Hillis offered a more developed and considered criticism of the 1867 Report than Munro. Of its anti-contagionist conclusion, he claimed there was 'hardly sufficient evidence ... to warrant so decided an opinion', and he pointed to evidence of contagion from within the report itself.[78] Contrasting Hansen's recent investigations with the report's heavy dependence on Danielssen and Boeck, he argued that anti-contagionism had proved short-lived, that centuries of experience indicated that isolation helped control the disease, and that if segregation were abandoned leprosy would spread.[79] On the basis of his own experience he regarded desegregation policies with 'horror'.[80]

For all this, however, Hillis remained in some senses an hereditarian, and he felt it necessary to separate the value of Hansen's bacteriological research from the Norwegian's rejection of heredity: 'His denial of the influence of heredity in leprosy in no way detracts from the value of the practical information he brings forward.'[81] This illustrates the range of overlapping positions in the debate around the causes of leprosy in the 1870s and early 80s. Between the hereditarian camp represented by Danielssen and Boeck, Milroy and the 1867 Report, and the contagion camp of Hansen, were a variety of intermediate positions. Planck, for example, admitted the possibility of contagion while denying it played a significant part in propagating the disease.[82] Hillis, although a contagionist, retained a belief in the hereditary factor as a predisposing condition. Carter moved from the conclusions of the Physicians' Report towards Hansen's position with some difficulty. More eccentric dietary explanations such as too many vegetables or too much fish continued to play a part within the debates and were compatible with a belief in either heredity or contagion. The onus was still on contagionists to disprove the hereditarian explanation. The very existence of *Mycobacterium leprae* was disputed, its role in causing the disease had not been conclusively established, and segregation was still widely regarded as irrelevant or an unjustified infringement of individual liberties.

---

[76] *Ibid.*, pp. 146, 208.   [77] *Ibid.*, pp. 158, 161.   [78] *Ibid.*, pp. 176ff.
[79] *Ibid.*, pp. 183, 185ff.   [80] *Ibid.*, p. 207.   [81] *Ibid.*, p. 188.   [82] Munro, *Leprosy*, p. 80.

When T. R. Lewis and D. D. Cunningham were commissioned by the government of India in the mid-1870s to investigate leprosy in the northern region of Kumaun they approached their task on the basis of complete faith in the conclusions of the 1867 Report. Their report, somewhat mis-leadingly titled *Leprosy in India* (1877), found 'little or no evidence' to support the 'recent revival of contagion theory'.[83] Indeed they found evidence to correct a misleading suggestion of contagion from the area that had been reported to the College of Physicians in 1867,[84] thus strengthening as well as reaffirming the 1867 Report. Throughout the region they discovered distribution of the disease by family, and therefore, they concluded, by hereditary predisposition. Indeed they believed that the figures they gathered probably understated the actual proportion of lep-rous kindred.[85] Although accepting that asylums could provide necessary shelter for those in dire need and thereby reduce beggary, they opposed compulsory confinement on the grounds of its inefficiency, impracticabil-ity and 'tyranny'.[86] Although their Report reaffirmed the position of the College of Physicians against recent criticism, there was nothing beleag-uered in its tone. The correctness of the heredity position was confidently assumed throughout.

The fear of return

Medical debate about leprosy continued into the 1880s and 90s. The question of whether it was hereditary or contagious remained, but the discovery of *Mycobacterium leprae* had opened up further problems with contagionists unable to explain how the disease was transmitted and contracted, and why the leprosy bacillus resisted cultivation *in vitro* and transmission by inoculation. Nevertheless, Hansen's discovery of the bacillus at the same time as the germ theory of disease was being elabo-rated reinvigorated the traditional idea that leprosy was contagious and carried debate about the disease into a wider public sphere. In the final decades of the century leprosy became far more than a medical question. Concern about the disease moved beyond specialist medical discussion to the periodical and newspaper press, and into popular and imaginative writing as well. Leprosy was believed to be spreading across the imperial world and threatening to return to metropolitan centres from which it had long ago disappeared. Reports of its rising incidence came in not only from

---

[83] T. R. Lewis and D. D. Cunningham, *Leprosy in India: A Report* (Calcutta: Office of the Superintendent of Government Printing, 1877), pp. 56–8.
[84] *Ibid.*, p. 58n.   [85] *Ibid.*, p. 60.   [86] *Ibid.*, p. 68.

Hawaii, the Caribbean and India, but also from so-called white settler colonies such as New South Wales and the Cape.

Disease travelled easily in the global imperial world of the late nineteenth century. Cases of leprosy contracted abroad, most commonly in India, were being diagnosed in London, demonstrated to medical audiences, and reported in metropolitan newspapers. Reported cases from the Cape and from the Australian colonies undermined the idea of the white settler colony as a healthy offspring of the metropolitan parent. It was increasingly feared that the flow of people and goods between colony and metropole was helping to spread disease. Leprosy had always been the boundary disease par excellence and at this moment in Western imperial history it became a particular focus for concern about the geographical and cultural relation of Europe to its others. Anxiety about the movement of leprosy between different countries and climatic zones was paralleled by concern about its transmission between people. Was leprosy essentially a tropical disease? Were some kinds of bodies, native ones in particular, more susceptible to the disease than others? If leprosy was contagious, how did it pass from one body to another? Was the leprosy bacillus internal or external to the human body (perhaps it existed in food or in water)?[87] Was the disease located in the world or in the body?

Even within the body itself the boundaries were unclear. The *British Medical Journal* discussed the problem of the uneven spread of leprosy within the body. Why was it that leprosy bacilli could grow 'with the greatest luxuriance at one point, and at a part immediately adjoining no bacilli are found at all?'[88] Leprosy was capricious. It seemed to resist explanation in terms of geographical and somatic boundaries, or else to practise some inexplicable boundary behaviour of its own devising. In this way the new micro-bacterial world of the late nineteenth century was rediscovering in its own terms the age-old view of the disease as transgressing the boundary between life and death. Eduard Arning, a German leprologist who was employed by the Hawaiian government in the mid-1880s to investigate the spread of the disease in their islands, claimed 'that the bacillus seems to multiply in the bodies of dead lepers months after they have been buried'.[89] Modern science could thus be seen to augment the traditional idea of the leprous body as a prototypical corpse, and leprosy as a disease that operated across the divide between life and death. The *British Medical Journal* cited Arning's research as a powerful argument for segregation: 'it ought to be accepted as a matter of common prudence that

---

[87] 'The Spread of Leprosy', *British Medical Journal*, 2 (1887), 1056.
[88] *British Medical Journal*, 2 (1884), 111.   [89] *Ibid.*, 2 (1887), 1056.

healthy persons should avoid as far as possible contact with lepers living or dead'.[90]

Arguments in favour of segregation were now increasingly common, prompted by the growing conviction that leprosy was contagious, and by the many boundary uncertainties this caused. Another work of Carter's, published by the Bombay government in 1884, drew attention to the 'enlightened proceedings of the Government of Norway' and recommended both the isolation of lepers and segregation of the sexes. On the pathology of leprosy, the *British Medical Journal* reported Carter as having written that 'he has long regarded this malady as one of the great chronic infective diseases of the human race: a view which he considers to be confirmed by Hansen's discovery of the bacillus leprae'.[91] Several years later *The Lancet* reported that Carter was urging the Bombay government to take heed of the correlation between the increasing number of leper patients living in government asylums and the declining incidence of the disease that the recent quinquennial on leprosy in Norway had highlighted (Hansen had sent a summary of this report to Carter). He also reported that Hansen 'has probably succeeded in inoculating rabbits with *perfectly fresh* leprous material, but these experiments require confirmation'.[92] This was incorrect but similar reports were to circulate over the next decade or so as leprologists sought to cultivate *mycobacterium leprae* and reintroduce it into living tissue.

The imperial dimension and implications of leprosy were by now central to most discussions of the disease. A report in 1887 by M. Besnier of the French Academy of Medicine drew attention to the rapid spread of the disease that had accompanied the extension of French colonial possessions, with soldier, sailors, traders and missionaries falling victim in large numbers. This was the occasion for a leading article in the *British Medical Journal*. Claiming that leprosy had formerly been eliminated from Britain and Europe because of the segregation of its victims, it argued that the hereditary explanation, officially endorsed by the 1867 Report, was now being disproved by investigators such as Besnier.[93] The *British Medical Journal* returned to the subject the following week in a long leading article under the title 'Is Leprosy Contagious?' This is worth pausing on because it provides a useful context for understanding the leprosy narratives that were soon to become a matter of public debate and which are to be discussed below.

The article begins with an account of the disease that could have been written in almost any previous century:

[90] *Ibid.*   [91] *Ibid.*, 2 (1884), 429–30.   [92] *The Lancet*, 2 (1887), 429–30.
[93] *British Medical Journal*, 2 (1887), 1055.

Leprosy is, perhaps, the most terrible disease that afflicts the human race. It is hideously disfiguring, destructive to the tissues and organs in an unusual degree, and is hopelessly incurable, the fate of its victims being, indeed, the most deplorable that the strongest imagination can conceive, and many years often passing before death rids the unhappy sufferer from a life of misery to which there is scarcely any alleviation.

It turns to the 1867 Report and describes how its conclusions have drawn into the open several cases in which contagion was either probable or certain. It looks in particular at a case of Dr Hawtrey Benson's in Dublin in 1872. This had been, and would continue to be, cited as the most clear-cut example of leprosy having been brought back from the empire and infecting a European. An Irishman who had lived in the West Indies for twenty-two years had come home to Dublin where he had died of tubercular leprosy. For the last year and a half of the man's life his brother had shared his bed and his clothing. This brother had only been out of Ireland once, a visit to England forty-six years earlier. There was no other leprosy in the family, nor indeed in Ireland, but the brother had somehow contracted the disease and had later been exhibited to the Dublin Medical Society. This apparently telling example was supplemented by others from around the imperial world, with Hawaii providing the most recent and extensive evidence for the contagionist argument: 'The rapid spread of leprosy in the Sandwich Islands cannot be explained in any other way than by contagion.'

The article concluded by drawing attention to the growing public interest in the disease: 'The whole question is one of such world-wide importance that its discussion can hardly be limited to professional journals, and we are not surprised that reviews and newspapers have recently taken it up.' As this happens, belief in the contagious nature of the disease will spread, and with it the demand for 'strict segregation': 'The instinct of self-preservation is too strong in all communities to allow vital matters of this kind to be settled on the purely abstract principles applicable to personal freedom.'[94] In other words, the liberal ideology that underpinned the 1867 Report and the whole of Milroy's work must now be set aside in the public interest.

One prominent example of the wider public discussion noted by the *British Medical Journal* was a pair of articles by Agnes Lambert published in *The Nineteenth Century* in 1884. The first of these highlighted the protracted horror and the historical persistence of the disease:

[I]t distorts and scars, and hacks, and maims, and destroys its victim inch by inch, feature by feature, member by member, joint by joint, sense by sense, leaving him to

[94] *Ibid.*, 1120.

cumber the earth, and tell the tale of a living death till there is nothing human left of him.[95]

Cholera, by comparison, is mercifully swift: 'in a few days, a night, an hour or two, its victims are at rest. They have no story to tell.'[96] The potential of leprosy for narrative is to become increasingly remarked and exploited from around this time.

Lambert's first article is a warning cry: 'leprosy has not ceased to be of living interest and concern to Englishmen ... with the expansion of England, it has been brought back to our very doors'.[97] John Seeley's *The Expansion of England* had been published the previous year, and taking her cue from this work Lambert ranges across the world describing the prevalence of leprosy in many of Britain's colonial territories. She argues that the 1867 Report's conclusion that the disease was non-contagious was contradicted by some of its own evidence, and she underlines Carter's subsequent publications on the need to segregate leprosy sufferers. Hansen's work is not mentioned, but she includes reports from Robben Island at the Cape about the infection of animals as well as humans, leprous pigeons, mice, pheasants and turkeys allegedly having been observed.[98]

Lambert's second article is a long and rather standard account of responses to leprosy in medieval Britain and Europe, but with glancing references to modern knowledge and practice. Among the ecclesiastical rites once performed for the segregation of lepers, Lambert describes the injunction to avoid the 'windward side' of a leper, and not to go down narrow streets 'where you might brush against anyone'. This prompts a rhetorical question: 'had the ecclesiastical authorities of those days lived in the full blaze of germ theories, and the most complete microscopic discovery and demonstration of bacilli and microbes, would it have been possible for them to have devised ... a more minute and searching law?'[99] Lambert concludes that the late nineteenth century should emulate the example of the medieval church in providing secure but compassionate isolation for lepers, this being 'the only sure means of really coping with the greatest and most mysterious of the maladies that afflict mankind'.[100]

Another popularising work, Henry Press Wright's *Leprosy and Segregation* (1885), tightened the screws of this argument. Wright warned

[95] Agnes Lambert, 'Leprosy: Present and Past', 1, *The Nineteenth Century*, 16 (1884), 211.
[96] *Ibid.*, 210.   [97] *Ibid.*, 212.   [98] *Ibid.*, 225–6.
[99] Lambert, 'Leprosy: Present and Past', 2, *The Nineteenth Century*, 16 (1884), 485.
[100] *Ibid.*, 488.

that Britain 'holds sway over regions and islands teeming with leprosy',[101] and was in no doubt that the disease was contagious: 'We know that leprosy is dependent on the invasion of the human body by a microscopic germ, which has the power to increase indefinitely in the tissues. Therefore we must look upon every single leper as a hot-bed of disease.'[102] Wright, an archdeacon, rector of Greatham, and formerly chaplain to the forces, became a leading proponent of segregation. In a letter to *The Times* prompted by Besnier's report to the French Academy of Medicine, he warned of the rapid spread of leprosy across the colonised world, drawing particular attention to Hawaii where 800 lepers were now segregated on the island of Molokai. He also struck a note that was to become increasingly familiar: 'The Chinese are swarming over the world, and living as they do, closely packed and careless of all sanitary protection, their huts are especially calculated to hasten the incubation of a disease, the germ of which was brought by them from China.' Leprosy, he warned, is coming home. He cites a recent case in an English village, and the presence of lepers in hospitals in London, Dublin and Glasgow. This 'new activity' of the disease demands action, first to ascertain the number of cases and then to secure their isolation.[103] Although the *British Medical Journal* thought Wright's letter unduly alarmist, it was by now supporting compulsory segregation in countries where leprosy was common, and warning that the very low official figures on leprosy in Britain were bound to be an underestimate: 'Lepers instinctively hide themselves.'[104]

The concern that leprosy was closer to home than previously suspected meant that its presence and movement within Europe was increasingly under scrutiny. The often-repeated assertion that leprosy had long since disappeared from the European mainland had always co-existed uneasily with its acknowledged persistence in isolated pockets of the continent. Norway could be presented as the exception that proved the rule, and a well-regulated exception at that, the apparent success of its public health policies offering reassurance. Reports of its prevalence in Spain, in Valencia, Alicante and Almeria, for example, were more disturbing, especially when a case brought from Spain ended fatally in a Paris hospital and led to the French government taking quarantine measures against Spanish vessels.[105] This prompted one Dr William Jelly to point out the he had warned the British Ambassador in Madrid of this 'leprous nursery-ground': 'Seeing that the lepers are the vine-raisin cultivators, harvesters, and packers, they have all the handling of the fruit . . . they are all packed in

[101] H. P. Wright, *Leprosy and Segregation* (London: Parker and Co., 1885), p. 104.
[102] *Ibid.*, p. 192.   [103] *The Times* (London), 8 November 1887.
[104] *British Medical Journal*, 2 (1887), 1055.   [105] *Ibid.*, 1 (1887), 685.

boxes *without stalks*, and are the raisins from which our best Christmas puddings are made.'[106] For Dr Jelly the threat was not just at the door, but inside the house and on the table.

Leprosy at home

An increasing number of leprosy cases were being reported in Britain during the 1880s. One of these attracted considerable attention in the medical press before becoming more public when the case ended up in the Court of Session in Glasgow. It was first recounted in the *British Medical Journal* in 1887 under the heading 'A Remarkable Experience Concerning Leprosy: Involving Certain Facts and Statements Bearing on the Question – Is Leprosy Communicable Through Vaccination?'[107] The writer was W. T. Gairdner, Professor of Medicine in the University of Glasgow, whom we have previously seen contributing to discussions of leprosy in Scotland in the 1850s. Gairdner's narrative was of a young boy brought to him six or seven years earlier suffering from a skin condition that was clearly leprosy. The boy came from an unnamed 'island in the tropics', and had been referred to Gairdner by his doctor on the island. Gairdner was puzzled that a practitioner with many years experience in 'a well-known endemic seat of leprosy' had not diagnosed the boy's condition himself. He advised that the boy should remain permanently in Britain, and following up the case several years later discovered him to be in a very poor state. At this stage Gairdner had learned that the island doctor's reluctance to diagnose leprosy had arisen from a desire to protect his own son whom he believed was leprous and had infected Gairdner's patient. This had occurred, he thought, through arm-to-arm smallpox vaccination. The doctor had first vaccinated his own son with virus from a native child, and then vaccinated Gairdner's patient directly from his own son. Subsequently he had discovered that the native child came from a leprous family.

The doctor's son had developed only very mild symptoms of leprosy, and following his father's death had been sent to boarding school in Britain, both the boy and the school in ignorance of his condition. Now in possession of these facts, Gairdner had consulted fellow specialists and decided to inform the school. The doctor's son was examined and a diagnosis of mild leprosy confirmed, but it was decided in the meantime not 'to disturb the boy's education'. Subsequently, following an attack of 'contagious eczema' in the school, this decision was reversed and the boy

---

[106] *Ibid.*, 1 (1887), 973.   [107] *Ibid.*, 1 (1887), 1269–70.

was asked to leave. The condition of Gairdner's initial patient had mean-while worsened, and the article implies that the recent death of this boy has freed Gairdner from any further professional obligation of silence.

Gairdner's story provoked a number of replies. William Jelly, no doubt reading this narrative as a confirmation of his fear of leprous raisins infecting the British Christmas pudding, thought it provided indisputable proof of the communicability of leprosy by inoculation and trusted it would prompt governments not to 'allow their leper-subjects to ramble among their healthy fellow men'.[108] C. Burgoyne Pasley, Acting Surgeon-General of Trinidad, was more focussed and sought further information: Were the island doctor and his wife European or native? If native, was there any constitutional taint of leprosy in their families? Was it blood or lymph that had been inoculated? Blood, he believed, could transmit 'constitu-tional diseases' such as leprosy and syphilis, but he doubted if these were communicable by lymph alone.[109] Beaven Rake, Medical Superintendent of the Leper Asylum in Trinidad, and later one of the Leprosy Commissioners to India, was interested in the racial background of both sets of parents. He argued that if infection by vaccine were to be proven it would need to be administered to a healthy child in a leprosy-free country. As it stood, Gairdner's story was explicable in the context of 'a tropical island in which leprosy is endemic'. Rake cited many failed attempts at introducing leprosy by vaccinating animals with lymph from lepers, and also a human experiment conducted by Eduard Arning in Hawaii, to be discussed later. Rake declared he would have 'no hesitation in vaccinating both my own children out here from native arms, Hindu and negro'.[110] A second letter from Rake, replying to Jelly's, carefully set out the problems with both contagious and heredity theories of the disease, and concluded that 'for the present I think very few will admit that anyone has "set at rest for ever all doubts on the subject"'.[111]

For all Rake's scepticism, however, the correspondence over Gairdner's story in the *British Medical Journal* showed there was widespread belief in the West Indies that vaccination spread leprosy. Another writer pointed out that as long ago as 1871 the Vaccinator-General for Trinidad, R. H. Bakewell, had given evidence to this effect before the Commons Committee of Inquiry into the working of the Vaccination Acts in Britain. This correspondent claimed that when medical men were vaccin-ating their own children, or those of patients in whom they were 'specially interested' (apparently a coding for European), they would use only English lymph in order to avoid the invaccination of leprosy.[112]

[108] *Ibid.*, 2 (1887), 176.   [109] *Ibid.*, 2 (1887), 270.   [110] *Ibid.*, 2 (1887), 433.
[111] *Ibid.*, 2 (1887), 647.   [112] *Ibid.*, 2 (1887), 335.

Gairdner eventually replied to all the correspondence, emphasising that in telling his story he had neither expressed opinions nor drawn conclusions. He made clear that both sets of parents and offspring were of 'unmixed European or British blood', and that although the doctor had vaccinated his child from a leprous family it was probably not from an actual leper. However, he also included a letter from another Trinidad practitioner claiming that the incidence of leprosy was increasing on that island, that arm-to-arm vaccination was definitely a factor in its spread, and that many 'respectable families' were tainted with the disease, particularly among the Portuguese. This correspondent believed that leprosy, like syphilis and tubercular phthisis, was both hereditary and contagious.[113]

Most of the letters came from Trinidad, which it seems to have been assumed was Gairdner's unnamed island, but other West Indies hands had their say. As John D. Hillis confirmed, it was believed throughout the West Indies that leprosy was communicated by vaccination, and that the 'white and coloured classes' would only use lymph imported from England. Like others, he used this debate to argue the increasingly popular case for segregation.[114]

A year after Gairdner's original article, the schoolboy, named as Michael Christison Piggott, brought an action against the governors of the school that had excluded him, now identified as Fettes College (Tony Blair's alma mater), for unlawful dismissal and breach of contract. The case was heard at the Court of Session in Glasgow, where it was argued that his removal from the school was illegal because he had been medically examined and declared healthy at the time of his admission in 1884. In defence the governors argued that Piggott had falsely answered the question: 'Is there any peculiarity of constitution which requires to be considered?' They pointed out that when Piggott's condition was diagnosed he had been allowed to remain at the school because the medical officers had decided that, 'Inasmuch ... as leprosy was not transmissible by mere personal contact ... [they] did not consider it imperative to disclose ... the nature of the disease, as such a disclosure would have a disastrous effect on the boy's prospects.' However, in 1887, with an outbreak of eczema at the school, Piggott's leg had suppurated and he was therefore asked to leave. The medical officers 'considered it no longer safe to keep the boy, because it was within the range of possibility that he might communicate the leprosy through the medium of the other disease'.[115] The judge found in favour of the school. He praised the governors for their humanity in keeping Piggott while his condition remained under

[113] *Ibid.*, 2 (1887), 799–800.   [114] *Ibid.*, 2 (1887), 1022–3.   [115] *Ibid.*, 1 (1888), 1398.

control, and ruled it had been correct to exclude him when his leprosy
re-emerged at the same time as the 'eczema' epidemic. At that point, 'it was
absolutely necessary to take action so as to prevent the whole of them
becoming lepers by contagion'. Acknowledging that Piggott's counsel had
argued that leprosy was not contagious, a point upon which the judge
contradictorily declared himself incapable of pronouncing an opinion, he
nevertheless declared that 'the existence of such a disease in the midst of a
community of boys like that of Fettes college, was calculated to create such
terror as to impair the usefulness of the institution'.[116] The case, therefore,
hinged on the question of contagion. While pronouncing himself unable to
decide on this matter, the judge at the same time used a presumption of the
contagion of leprosy to rule in favour of the school.

This whole episode illustrates the racialised fears of contracting leprosy
in tropical zones, and the impossibility in colonial settings of maintaining
the borders between Europeans and natives upon which colonial health
and authority was believed to depend. The distinction between tropical
colony and temperate metropole was fundamental. The only 'practical'
advice Gairdner could offer the first boy was that he should stay in Britain.
Behind this was a belief that the progress of leprosy would be slowed, if not
arrested, on European soil. This proved not to be so. When Gairdner
examined his patient a second time he found 'mutilation of the extremities ... external sores ... [and] internal lesions, which had reduced the
patient to the last stage of emaciation'. But the belief in home soil as a kind
of antidote to tropical disease was partly maintained by the story of the
other boy whose condition was invisible to the untrained eye. Indeed it is
remarkable how unalarmed Gairdner, the specialists he consulted, the
medical officers and the school itself, were at first. But the mildness of
the boy's condition and its virtual invisibility was unsettling as well as
reassuring. The decision to allow him to remain could not survive the
outbreak of 'eczema' and the fear that it would facilitate the spread of
leprosy, so Michael Christison Piggott was required to leave.

Gairdner's narrative raised a hornet's nest in Trinidad but it also intersected with concern in Britain about the spread of infectious diseases by
vaccination. The tightening of compulsory vaccination legislation in 1871
had produced an anti-vaccination movement with a journal and a national
association. This remained strong throughout the 1880s and 90s and
persisted until compulsory vaccination was ended in 1909, by which time
smallpox had virtually disappeared. This movement has often been represented as a defence of local liberties against metropolitan interference and

[116] *Ibid.*, 2 (1888), 1241.

state power, as no doubt it was,[117] but it had other specificities as well. It was widely believed that vaccination spread eczema, and there were fears that it could infect children with syphilis. The scars left by vaccination were commonly referred to as 'the mark of the beast',[118] a term often applied to leprosy as well. The extensively practised arm-to-arm method, in which lymph from an already vaccinated child was used for further vaccination, was thought to be contaminating. As Nadja Durbach has shown, there was a strong class element in this opposition to vaccination. Although seen on one hand as an imposition on the working classes, many respectable working-class parents also viewed it as enforced commingling with paupers.[119] As elsewhere in the empire, the contact of bodies and the penetration of skin, the body's defensive integument, was felt to threaten boundaries and the differences they marked, whether of class or race. And such connections were made. Compulsory vaccination was often likened to slavery, and anti-vaccination demonstrations sometimes included blacking up.[120]

The supposed danger of vaccination offers an example of the kind of shuttling and displacement between metropole and colony, especially in matters of health and disease, which helped constitute late nineteenth-century imperial culture. Gairdner's story of leprous infection by arm-to-arm vaccination on an unspecified island in the tropics took some of its meaning from the domestic context of anti-vaccination campaigns. Vaccination had become one focus of concern about the boundaries that operated between European settlers and the descendants of black slaves in the Caribbean, and at home within the class structure. Vaccination itself was a vivid example of boundary transgression, involving as it did the exchange of bodily fluids and the mingling of bodies that the social and political structures of imperial culture were intended to keep apart. The transgression of these boundaries, and the threat of infection that followed, was of increasing concern to both metropole and colony by the late nineteenth century.

The death of Father Damien

By the mid-1880s Hawaii had become an especial focus of concern. The rapid spread of leprosy in a relatively short time among a small population seemed to offer the best proof yet that the disease was contagious, and

---

[117] See, for example, F. B. Smith, *The People's Health, 1830–1910* (London: Croom Helm, 1979) pp. 166–8.
[118] Nadja Durbach, '"They Might As Well Brand Us": Working-Class Resistance to Compulsory Vaccination in Victorian England', *Social History of Medicine*, 13: 1 (2000), 47.
[119] *Ibid.*, 46.   [120] *Ibid.*, 57–8.

Hawaii was coming to be seen as the imperial world's leprosy laboratory. One experiment in particular had drawn attention to these islands. Beaven Rake had referred to Eduard Arning's human experiment and this episode hovered over most discussions about the communicability of leprosy in the late 1880s. Arning's work for the Hawaiian Board of Health involved cultivation and inoculation experiments, using specimens of leprous tissue from the bodies of patients to try and grow the lepra bacillus and solve the problem of communicability that had become so urgent in Hawaii. In 1884 he was given the opportunity of trying to implant the disease in a living human body. A Hawaiian man and convicted murderer, Keanu, agreed to exchange his death sentence for life imprisonment on the condition that Arning could experiment on him. A leproma about the size of a hen's egg was surtured into an incision on his arm. Within several years Keanu was showing signs of the disease and eventually he was removed to the leper colony on Molokai where he died in 1892.[121] Rake had written of the failure of Arning's experiment but this must have been before he knew of Keanu's infection. For a while it seemed that Arning had performed the first successful implant of leprous tissue in a human subject, but then doubts were cast on the conclusiveness of the experiment. In a setting where leprosy was epidemic it was clearly possible for Keanu to have caught the disease in some other way, and this became highly probable when it was discovered that several of his family, including his own son, were lepers. In 1890 the *British Medical Journal* gave a detailed report, including a pedigree of leprosy in Keanu's family and illustrations of Keanu and his diseased son and nephew. It also cited the Resident Physician on Molokai, Dr Swift, observing that if Keanu's leprosy had been caused by Arning's implant it had developed at unparalleled speed. It is interesting that this report and the illustrations in the *British Medical Journal* were immediately preceded by an illustrated history of the so-called Elephant Man, John Merrick, who had recently died. The juxtaposition of these two graphic accounts of startling bodily deformation, one at home, the other in an American colony, one manifesting abnormal outcrops and extensions of the body, the other its erosion, reverberates.[122] This uneasy mingling of science with fascination, horror and compassion when faced with unexplained manifestations of the monstrous is another instance of the overlapping of the domestic with the imperial in matters of health and disease at this period.

Hawaii also gave the imperial world its modern leper martyr. The Belgian Catholic priest Father Damien had worked among the lepers

---

[121] Gavan Daws, *Holy Man: Father Damien of Molokai* (Honolulu: University of Hawaii Press, 1984), pp. 138, 141–2, 234–5.
[122] *British Medical Journal*, 1 (1890), 916–18.

compulsorily segregated at the Kalawao settlement on the island of Molokai since 1873, transforming a neglected dumping ground for the diseased into an ordered community that had become a showpiece for the compassionate treatment of the victims of leprosy. By the mid-1880s it was known that Damien had contracted the disease himself, and as his death approached Molokai attracted increasing attention worldwide, and concern about leprosy intensified. The announcement of Damien's imminent death in the *British Medical Journal* in January 1889, for example, was followed by a leading article titled 'Leprosy in the United Kingdom'. This argued that although leprosy was demonstrably spread by contagion in other parts of the world, there was no evidence of this in England.[123] The telluric explanation that leprosy was contagious only in tropical climates, and that it was attached to locality as much as to the individual, was now often asserted. Among other things, this allowed Britain's status as the healthy centre of a disease-prone empire to be maintained.

Nevertheless, concern about Britain's susceptibility was also frequently raised and not always discounted. In 1889, the year of Damien's death, there was another volume from Henry Press Wright, *Leprosy: An Imperial Danger* (1889), which was explicit about the danger of leprosy returning to Britain from its tropical colonies and infecting the British people. Even those reviews that were sceptical about the alarmist aspects of Wright's book welcomed it as timely. Damien's death no doubt helped in its promotion. In the same year a leading British doctor, Sir Morrell Mackenzie, published a similar warning in a widely noticed essay in *The Nineteenth Century*: 'Leprosy has before now overrun Europe and invaded England, without respecting the "silver streak" which keeps off other enemies; and it is perfectly conceivable . . . it might do so again.' Mackenzie also dismissed the 1867 Report as a 'vast edifice of error'.[124]

Damien died in April 1889, the news reached the London newspapers on 11 May, and within a month a memorial fund had been set up under the auspices of the Prince of Wales. Leprosy had, as the *British Medical Journal* put it, become 'one of the questions of the day'.[125] The *Pall Mall Gazette* reported Damien's 'final words' and described how after his death all marks of leprosy had vanished from his face and the wounds in his hands had dried.[126] A deathbed photograph of Damien was bought by thousands of Londoners, and when the same photograph was displayed in a shop window in Birmingham a crowd gathered so quickly that the police

---

[123] *Ibid.*, 1 (1889), 721–2.
[124] Morrell Mackenzie, 'The Dreadful Revival of Leprosy', *The Nineteenth Century*, 23 (1889), 931, 933.
[125] *British Medical Journal*, 1 (1889), 1364.   [126] *Pall Mall Gazette*, 14 June 1889.

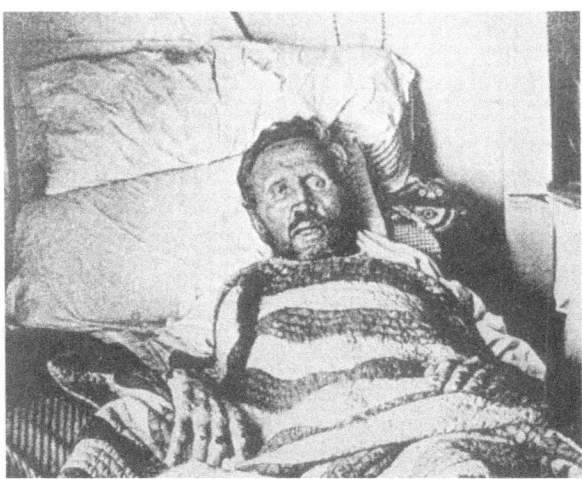

Figure 1. Father Damien on his deathbed. Photo by Sydney Bourne Swift, physician at the Kalaupapa leper colony on Molokai.

were called to clear the streets.[127] *The Times* memorialised Damien in a leading article. Leprosy, it declared, was at certain stages 'exceedingly infectious', especially in the South Seas because of 'the habits of the natives'. Damien, however, had made 'the brand of leprosy ... a cross of honour'. Furthermore, he had demonstrated that the leper settlement could be 'a model colony ... an ideal society, fitted to be a pattern and an example throughout the Pacific'.[128]

In June 1889 two lepers were exhibited at a widely reported meeting of the Epidemiological Society of London: 'One of the lepers introduced to the meeting was an old man who did not show any outward sign of disease, and who might have been passed in the street without any suspicion that he was a confirmed leper. He was, however, in a palsied state, and had lost the use of his hands, from which some of the fingers were missing.'[129] The same meeting heard a paper from Surgeon-Major Pringle, late of the Sanitary Department of the Bengal Army, warning that leprosy in India would spread to Britain unless segregation policies such as those implemented in Hawaii were introduced.[130] A suggestion that a leprosy ward should be established in London was publicly opposed by a doctor at the

---

[127] Daws, *Holy Man*, p. 10.   [128] *The Times* (London), 13 May 1889.
[129] *Pall Mall Gazette*, 13 June 1889.
[130] *The Times* (London), 13 June 1889. Pringle had written a letter in similar vein to *The Times* the preceding day.

Central Skin Hospital, King's Cross, on the grounds that it would attract lepers from the colonies who would then have 'free intercourse with fellow men' in London: 'The disease being infectious, the danger to the community is obvious.'[131]

There was growing alarm at the prospect of the invisible danger of leprosy stalking the streets of London. Germ theory implied that we lived surrounded by invisible enemies, and the German bacteriologist Koch had formulated the idea of the healthy carrier, which rendered everyone potentially suspect.[132] Leprosy had always been thought of as a highly visible disease, its horrifying physical symptoms a warning to others. Now it seemed otherwise. The man exhibited to the Epidemiological Society, like Michael Piggott at Fettes College, was an invisible carrier and therefore impossible to guard against. But there was also a significant difference between the two cases. London was the spatial antithesis of the boarding school, its open streets a potential conduit for secret agents of disease. No longer boarded up, leprosy was starting to cause a panic.

The inaugural meeting of the Father Damien Memorial Committee on 17 June was just several days after the two lepers had been exhibited at the Epidemiological Society. At this meeting the Prince of Wales claimed there was a leper working in the London meat market. There were alarmed calls for the man to be identified, and the accuracy of the claim was questioned.[133] London's sanitary authority, the City Commission of Sewers, discussed the matter and decided it was probably a case of eczema or some other skin disease brought about by handling diseased meat, rather than actual leprosy.[134] Briefly the disease was shifted from a human agent to dead meat. But next day *The Times* revealed that the man in question was one of the two recently exhibited at the Epidemiological Society. He was a salesman in the London meat market who had lost several fingers and had maimed feet as a result of leprosy.[135]

The story continued to develop. The following day *The Times* carried a letter from Dr Herbert Larder, medical superintendent of Whitechapel Infirmary where the man had been treated. Larder reported that the man was sixty-four years old, and that when not in the Infirmary he sold ox tails, sheep's heads and offal from Smithfield to the poor of Hoxton. He had ulcerated hands and feet, and in Larder's opinion it was 'a serious

---

[131] *Pall Mall Gazette*, 15 June 1889.

[132] Laura Otis, *Membranes: Metaphors of Invasion in Nineteenth-Century Literature, Science and Politics* (Baltimore and London: Johns Hopkins University Press, 1999), pp. 34–5.

[133] *Pall Mall Gazette*, 18 and 19 June 1889.   [134] *The Times* (London), 19 June 1889.

[135] *Ibid.*, 20 June 1889.

danger to the public that this man should be allowed to handle and sell meat'. *The Times* now reported that the man's hands and feet had been affected 'in so horrible a manner as to render it almost incredible that he should be able to do any kind of work'. It also disclosed that although the leprous meat-seller had travelled the world as a sailor as a young man, it had taken thirty years after coming ashore for his symptoms to develop. *The Times* also carried a reassurance from Dr P. S. Abraham that no one had yet been infected by the man, nor by a boy with leprosy who was currently in the Whitechapel Infirmary. Abraham, who had also spoken at the Epidemiological Society, insisted that the contagious nature of leprosy remained an inference rather than established fact.[136]

Although it reported the case very closely, *The Times* was also concerned to allay fears. It was sceptical of Pringle's claims that leprosy might spread in Britain, and a leading article emphasised the disease's obscure mode of transmission, and the unreliability of inoculation experiments in Hawaii and at the Cape (which had been on animals):

One thing is quite certain – namely, that the handful of lepers who exist in this country, mostly people in easy circumstances who have contracted the disease in India, are scarcely at all liable to impart it to those around them, even to their wives and children. In this climate, at least, and among a well-nourished population, the quality of contagiousness must be extremely feeble.[137]

The *Pall Mall Gazette*, however, highlighted Abrahams' potentially worrying observation that the incubation period in this case was unprecedented: 'The bacillus must have been asleep for nearly forty years, the germ dormant, like the "mummy" wheat!'[138] Damien's death had ended any lingering belief in European immunity to leprosy. The meat man, eventually named as Edward Yoxall, had almost certainly contracted the disease on his travels but it had, after a very long time, germinated in London's soil. Belief in climatic immunity had also been shaken, though not dispelled, and the unprecedented length of incubation contributed to the accumulating evidence of the inexplicable and worrying caprice of the disease.

The fear of leprosy as a paradoxically invisible disease was common to both metropolitan and colonial settings. Two days after the Epidemiological Society meeting, and two days before the Prince of Wales's startling disclosure, the *Pall Mall Gazette* carried a long interview with the superintendent of a leper colony in British Guiana who emphasised that leprosy was not only increasing but that it was spreading to 'white families of high standing':

The members of these white families never marry; and should a stranger to the colony begin to show attentions to any of the daughters, some one is always sure to

---

[136] *Ibid.*, 21 June 1889.   [137] *Ibid.*, 13 June 1889,   [138] *Pall Mall Gazette*, 20 June 1889.

(a)

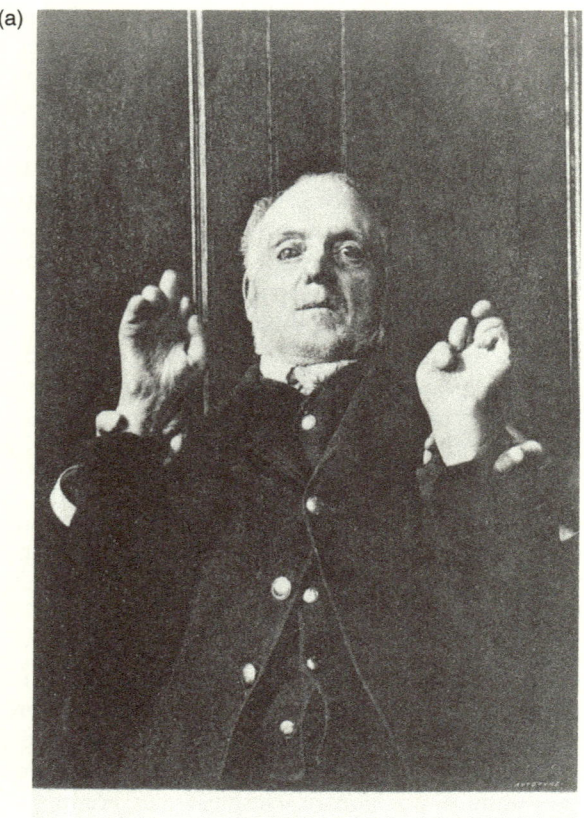

NERVE LEPROSY.

Figure 2. (a) Patient with nerve leprosy (probably Edward Yoxall). From George Thin, *Leprosy* (1891). Wellcome Library, London.

warn him ... It may not show itself in one generation, but the taint is there, and comes out in the next. These families have to hide the family skeleton the best way they can.[139]

This familiar colonial inflection suggests the lunacy of Bertha Mason in *Jane Eyre* and Jean Rhys's deconstructive treatment of the colonial theme of

---

[139] *Ibid.*, 15 June 1889.

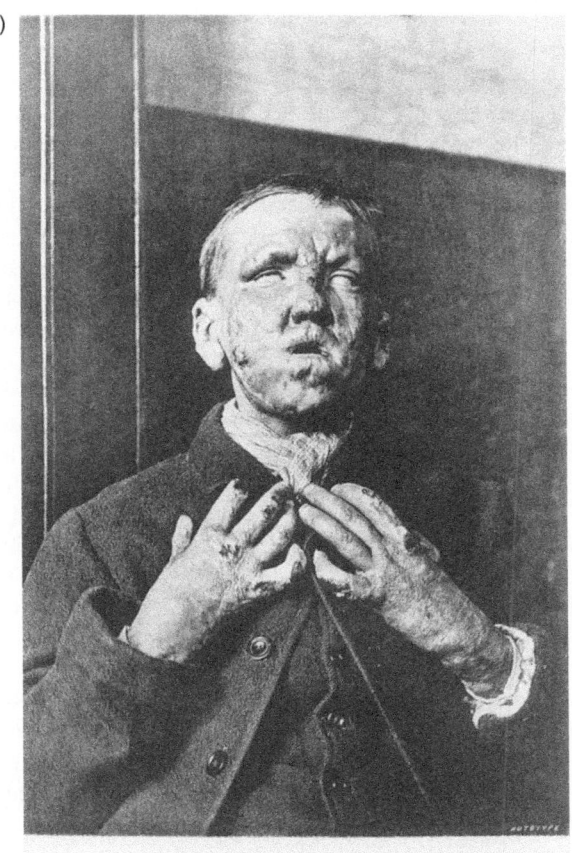

TUBERCULAR LEPROSY.

Figure 2. (b) Patient with tubercular leprosy. From George Thin, *Leprosy* (1891). Wellcome Library, London.

miscegenation in *Wide Sargasso Sea*.[140] Leprosy lines up with syphilis, madness, and other congenital traits associated with the tropics and with the sexual transgression of racial barriers. Although it is different, therefore, from the specific threat it brings in London, it has the same potential in both settings for protracted invisibility before sudden irruption.

[140] See Peter Hulme, 'The Locked Heart: The Creole Family Romance of *Wide Sargasso Sea*', in Francis Barker, Peter Hulme and Margaret Iversen (eds.), *Colonial Discourse/ Postcolonial Theory* (Manchester and New York: Manchester University Press, 1994), pp. 72–88.

Edward Yoxall was very soon secured in Whitechapel Infirmary and anxiety abated. Even the alarmist *Pall Mall Gazette* now implied that the affair had been needlessly exaggerated. The Prince of Wales sent Yoxall a cheque to take care of his immediate necessities, and Mrs Yoxall received assistance from the poor box.[141] Nevertheless, scattered reports of leprosy cases in the capital continued. One at St George's Hospital only came to light when the patient had died, suggesting that the stir over Yoxall had not resulted in the disclosure of other cases: 'the fact of there being a patient suffering from leprosy in the hospital appears to have been kept an absolute secret til his death'.[142] The cases of both Michael Piggott and Edward Yoxall resurfaced from time to time over the next decade. The Fettes College episode remained grist for the mill of the prominent anti-vaccination campaigner William Tebb who was quick to exploit the alleged link between the spread of leprosy and state-enforced smallpox vaccination; leprosy, he claimed, was being spread 'by the lancet of the public vaccinator'.[143] And nine years later there was a footnote to the meat market story at a meeting of the London Epidemiological Society where the spread of leprosy by Chinese coolie labour was being discussed. Dr Pringle now claimed that Yoxall had caught the disease from a leprous prostitute in India who had fled from her hill tribe to escape the normal fate of such women of being flung into a mountain torrent.[144]

Damien's death had drawn public attention to leprosy as a modern imperial problem. *Longman's Magazine* attacked the Hawaiian government for its failure to support Damien's work on Molokai, and the Hawaiian consul in London wrote to *The Times* in defence of his government.[145] In the same month *Blackwood's Edinburgh Magazine* carried a long article 'Lepers at the Cape: Wanted, a Father Damien', exposing the dreadful conditions of the leper colony on Robben Island.[146] *Cornhill Magazine* used the example of Damien as the starting point for a history of the disease in the Middle Ages.[147] Meanwhile the National Leprosy Fund was raising money for several projects. One of these, the establishment of a leprosy ward in London, was abandoned as too controversial, and by the start of 1890 the

---

141 *The Times* (London), 24 June and 1 July 1889.
142 Identical report in *The Times* and *Pall Mall Gazette*, 14 August 1889.
143 William Tebb, *The Public Health: Leprosy and Vaccination* (London: E. W. Allen, 1891), p. 10.
144 *British Medical Journal*, 1 (1898), 23.
145 *The Times* (London), 17 and 26 September, 1889.
146 *Blackwood's Edinburgh Magazine*, 146 (1889).
147 *Cornhill Magazine*, 13 (new series) (1889).

Fund's attention had shifted firmly towards leprosy in the colonies. A subscription dinner in January, chaired by the Prince of Wales, with the Archbishop of Canterbury, the Bishop of London, Prince David Kawananakoa of Hawaii, and Damien's brother Father Pamphile de Veuster among the guests, raised £2,500; the Queen, whose 'deep interest' in leprosy was reported by her son, contributed 50 guineas. One of the speakers, Sir Andrew Clark, caught the mood of the meeting and the time: 'not only did leprosy exist in larger measure than in recent years, but ... new germ centres were springing up in various quarters and the old centres were widening, and before England and the civilised world there was looming a condition of affairs which might, by growth, threaten civilisation'.[148]

India, where the scale of the problem was greatest, had become the centre of attention. With pro-segregation feeling increasing, and India believed to be the place where lepers were most permitted 'unbridled liberty',[149] it was here that research and action seemed most urgent. The executive committee of the National Leprosy Fund secured the co-operation of the Viceroy and by the end of 1890 an official Leprosy Commission had arrived in India to begin its investigations.[150] Its work was followed with interest around the world; the Japanese authorities, for example, were reported as waiting on the Leprosy Commission's findings before deciding their policy on segregation.[151] Yet publication of the report was repeatedly delayed. Sixteen months passed between the submission of the draft report to the executive committee of the National Leprosy Fund and its eventual publication in April 1893, during which time it was reviewed by a special committee and returned to the executive committee for individual comment by each of its members.

As the National Leprosy Fund and its committees pondered, concern at the spread of the disease around the world continued. The British newspaper and medical press carried frequent stories of leprosy in South Africa, Australia, New Zealand, Hong Kong, the Caribbean, Mauritius, Cyprus and elsewhere. It was reported that 5,000 out of 40,000 'kanakas' on New Caledonia were infected, along with a few Europeans as well.[152] Those contagionists who for years had argued against the findings of the 1867 Commission were now defiantly vocal. W. Munro reminded readers of the *British Medical Journal* that he had 'stood alone against the great authority of the Royal College of Physicians', that he had 'proved ... that leprosy

[148] *The Times* (London), 14 January 1890.
[149] *British Medical Journal*, 1 (1889), 1491; letter from Frederick Simms.
[150] *The Times* (London), 11 October, 22 October, 26 November, 8 December, 29 December 1890 and 2 February 1891.
[151] *Ibid.*, 17 September 1891.   [152] *British Medical Journal*, 1 (1890), 816.

had been carried to the Western Hemisphere by Negroes', and that Jews and North American Indians had been involved in the history of its transmission.[153] The pro-segregation climate was hospitable to the racial arguments that were so often at the heart of the contagionist case.

Leprosy scares continued at home. In July 1890 a Swedish woman suffering from the disease was reported to be in the Liverpool Workhouse Hospital. It was said that even photographs of the woman were causing anxiety, as if people were 'half-fearing contagion from their proximity to them',[154] an interesting contrast with the queues that formed in a Birmingham street to look at the photograph of the distant, dead and martyred Damien. The Pathological Society of London investigated an alleged case of indigenous leprosy but no leprosy bacilli were discovered.[155] In Belfast a young man born in Rangoon and suffering from leprosy escaped from a detached building in the workhouse grounds where he was being kept in isolation, causing 'considerable excitement in the locality'.[156]

Against this background the delay in publishing the report became worrying. Differences between the Commissioners and a majority of members of both the executive and special committees over the question of contagion and segregation became public. A parliamentary question was raised,[157] and the anti-vaccination lobby became convinced the report was being suppressed because of the Commissioners' refusal to concede that leprosy was spread by vaccination.[158] In 1893, with the report still to appear, the anti-vaccinator William Tebb brought out *The Recrudescence of Leprosy and its Causation* in which he repeated his argument that leprosy was being spread by smallpox vaccination. For Tebb the debate about leprosy had opened a new front in his unremitting campaign against smallpox vaccination, and during the early 1890s concern about leprosy in the empire and its possible return to Britain unfolded against the background of outbreaks of smallpox in various parts of England and public discussion over further compulsory vaccination legislation.[159] The intersections between imperial and national disease, already noted in the Fettes College case, continued.

---

[153] *Ibid.*, 2 (1889), 43.   [154] *Ibid.*, 2 (1890), 20–1.   [155] *Ibid.*, 2 (1890), 1067–8.
[156] *Ibid.*, 2 (1891), 138, 275, 662.   [157] *The Times* (London), 17 February 1893.
[158] See *British Medical Journal*, 1 (1893), 378–9, 489, 549, 608, 818 for correspondence between William Tebb and A. A. Kanthack, Royal College of Surgeons member on the Leprosy Commission for India, Beaven Rake, Royal College of Physicians member, and P. S. Abrahams, Hon. Sec. to the Special Committee of the National Leprosy Fund, on this matter. At the same time one of Tebb's supporters, Arthur Lovell, was writing to the daily press on the subject: see, for example, *Star*, 6 February 1893.
[159] See, for example, *British Medical Journal*, 1 (1893), 818, 912–13, 1065.

When the Leprosy Commission report finally appeared at the end of April 1893 it satisfied almost no one. Its rebuttal of the central finding of the 1867 Report, that leprosy was a hereditary disease, pleased contagionists less than might have been expected because it also concluded that 'the amount of contagion which exists is so small that it may be disregarded, and no legislation is called for on the lines either of segregation, or of interdiction of marriage with lepers'.[160] The Report also rejected the idea that leprosy originated from any particular food (explicitly refuting Jonathan Hutchinson's fish theory), or from any climatic or telluric conditions, or that it peculiarly affected any particular race or caste. While establishing that leprosy was of micro-biological origin, its aetiology and transmission was left vague: 'Leprosy in the great majority of cases originates ... from a sequence or concurrence of causes and conditions ... which are related to each other in ways at present imperfectly known.'[161] In other words, the Commission endorsed none of the existing schools of thought. Only *The Times* was satisfied. The Commission's conclusion that leprosy was, if anything, declining rather than increasing was taken to confirm its long-held conviction that leprosy was not an imperial danger, and that 'any fear of its extensive importation into this country must be regarded as absolutely visionary ... popular terrors about leprosy ... are simply groundless superstition'.[162]

The division over the Report within the Executive Committee of the National Leprosy Fund was mainly between its medical and lay members, with the latter endorsing segregation and the former being more cautious. However, this was not entirely clear-cut, and although most of its medical members agreed with the Commissioners that evidence of the spread of the disease by contagion was insufficient to justify the compulsory segregation of lepers, several drew the opposite conclusion and made public their disagreement. The *British Medical Journal* was sympathetic to their position. The Commissioners, it pointed out, had accepted that leprosy was a 'microbic' disease and admitted that in a few cases the microbe was conveyed by contagion, that is by contact with a leprous individual: 'What practical difference does it make', the *British Medical Journal* asked, 'if we assume, as they do – a perfectly gratuitous assumption, of which they give no proof – that the microbes first get into space, and thence in some unexplained way into a human being?' It was no surprise, the journal concluded, if 'men of the world' like Mr Curzon (Under-Secretary for India) should want steps taken to segregate lepers: 'for so far as we yet know, the sole habitat and manufactory of the leprosy microbe is the body

[160] *Leprosy in India: Report of the Leprosy Commission in India 1890–1891* (Calcutta: Superintendent of Government Printing, 1892), pp. 289–90.
[161] *Ibid.*, p. 416.   [162] *The Times* (London), 1 May 1893; see also 14 April 1893.

of the leper, and if we can segregate the leper and disinfect the discharges from his ulcers, we diminish the possibility of the spread of leprosy'.[163]

This same article drew attention to 'the diametrically opposite opinions' held by commissioners inquiring into the disease at the Cape. These commissioners had concluded that leprosy was decidedly contagious and that isolation on Robben Island should be vigorously pursued.[164] The work of the Cape Commissioners, conducted at the same time, became an alternative to the Indian Commissioners' findings and helped sustain the high-contagion argument and its corollary of segregation. The final element in the *British Medical Journal's* probing of the Indian Commissioners' report was to compare their inquiries with the investigations of Norwegian physicians over many years. However assiduously the Indian Commissioners had gone about their task, and valuable as the facts they had gathered might be, their findings were 'not to be compared' with those of Hansen, 'who has been able to devote continuous work to the subject over a long period of years, with ample material and every assistance from his Government, and with a knowledge of the habits and idiosyncrasies of the population which it is impossible for Europeans to obtain in a country like India'. Like Hansen, the Commissioners have concluded that leprosy is not hereditary, but unlike him they 'have been able to suggest no tangible theory which might take the place of contagion in explaining the undoubted existence of leper families'.[165]

The Report might have allayed fears in Britain but it caused consternation in its colonies. John D. Hillis reported from British Guiana that the Surgeon-General was using the Report to oppose segregation, and remarked that 'if it is to be quoted against segregation in colonies where segregation is not only necessary but practicable, it is painful to think of all the harm that must result'.[166] The Cape Leprosy Commission's final report to the Cape Parliament in 1895 insisted that leprosy was steadily increasing, that the disease was contagious, and that compulsory segregation was the only practicable way of arresting its spread.[167] Yet even in the colonies there was not complete unanimity. Dr Ashburton Thompson, Chief Medical Officer for New South Wales, denied that leprosy was spreading by contagion and argued that strict isolation policies were a contemporary revival of medieval ignorance.[168] This view, however, was not to prevail in the Australian colonies for much longer.

---

[163] *British Medical Journal*, 2 (1893), 137.   [164] *Ibid.*, 136.   [165] *Ibid.*, 137.
[166] *Ibid.*, 281–2.   [167] *The Times* (London), 19 June 1895.
[168] *British Medical Journal*, 2 (1895), 1514.

The Berlin International Leprosy Conference, 1897

This was the background against which the first International Leprosy Conference was convened in Berlin in 1897, a gathering that included most of the great names in European pathology and bacteriology. Under the presidency of Virchow, the speakers included Koch and Hansen, discoverers of the tuberculosis and leprosy bacilli, together with other prominent medical investigators of leprosy such as Neisser, Lasser and Arning. Although P. S. Abraham of the National Leprosy Fund attended and presented a paper on leprosy in the British Empire, the British government sent no official representative. *The Times* found this strange in view of the fact that the British empire was 'interested above all other States in the question of the treatment of leprosy'. Britain's absence, *The Times* felt, gave the unfortunate impression it was not doing all it could to combat the spread of the disease and improve the condition of lepers.[169] The aim of the conference was to establish whether or not the leprosy bacillus was the cause of the disease, if so how it was conveyed, and to set up 'international parallel action' to reduce its spread.[170] Opening the conference, the Prussian Minister of Public Instruction spoke of the special interest of the conference for Prussia, leprosy having crossed the Prussian frontier with forty-one cases recently reported from the district of Memel.[171]

Hansen's paper was the centrepiece of the conference, and British reports gave particular attention to his argument that isolation was the key to preventing the spread of leprosy and eventually eliminating it. Norway, where it was predicted that the disease would have been eradicated by the turn of the century, offered the paradigm for control.[172] The conference adopted Hansen's position, with Abraham registering mild dissent at the strong emphasis on segregation, partly because the experience of Hawaii and the Cape suggested that compulsory segregation forced many lepers into hiding. He also argued the need to take account of the varying social and political conditions between colonies. The Indian Commissioners had concluded it would be impossible to impose segregation in a country as large and diverse as India,[173] and Abraham was anxious about a strong conference resolution in favour of segregation. He was also uneasy about coercion.

---

[169] *The Times* (London), 14 October 1897.

[170] *British Medical Journal*, 2 (1897), 49; *The Times* (London), 12 October 1897.

[171] *The Times* (London), 12 October 1897; *British Medical Journal*, 2 (1897), 1122, made it thirty-four cases.

[172] *The Times* (London), 16 October 1897; *British Medical Journal*, 2 (1897), 1122.

[173] *Leprosy in India: Report of the Leprosy Commission*, p. 419.

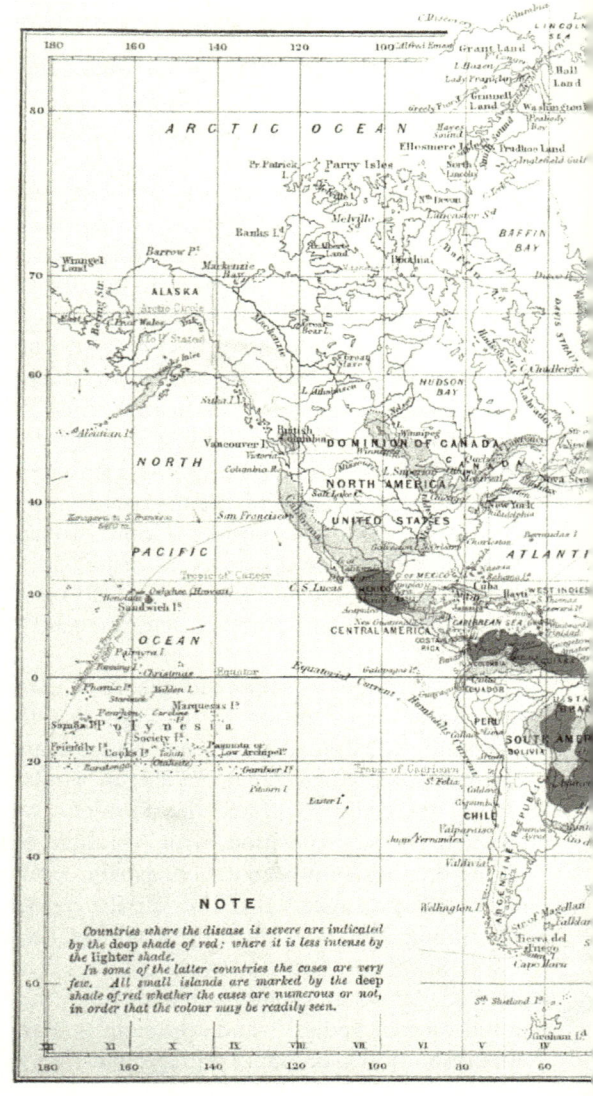

Figure 3. Map showing the distribution of leprosy around the world in 1891. From George Thin, *Leprosy* (1891). Wellcome Library, London.

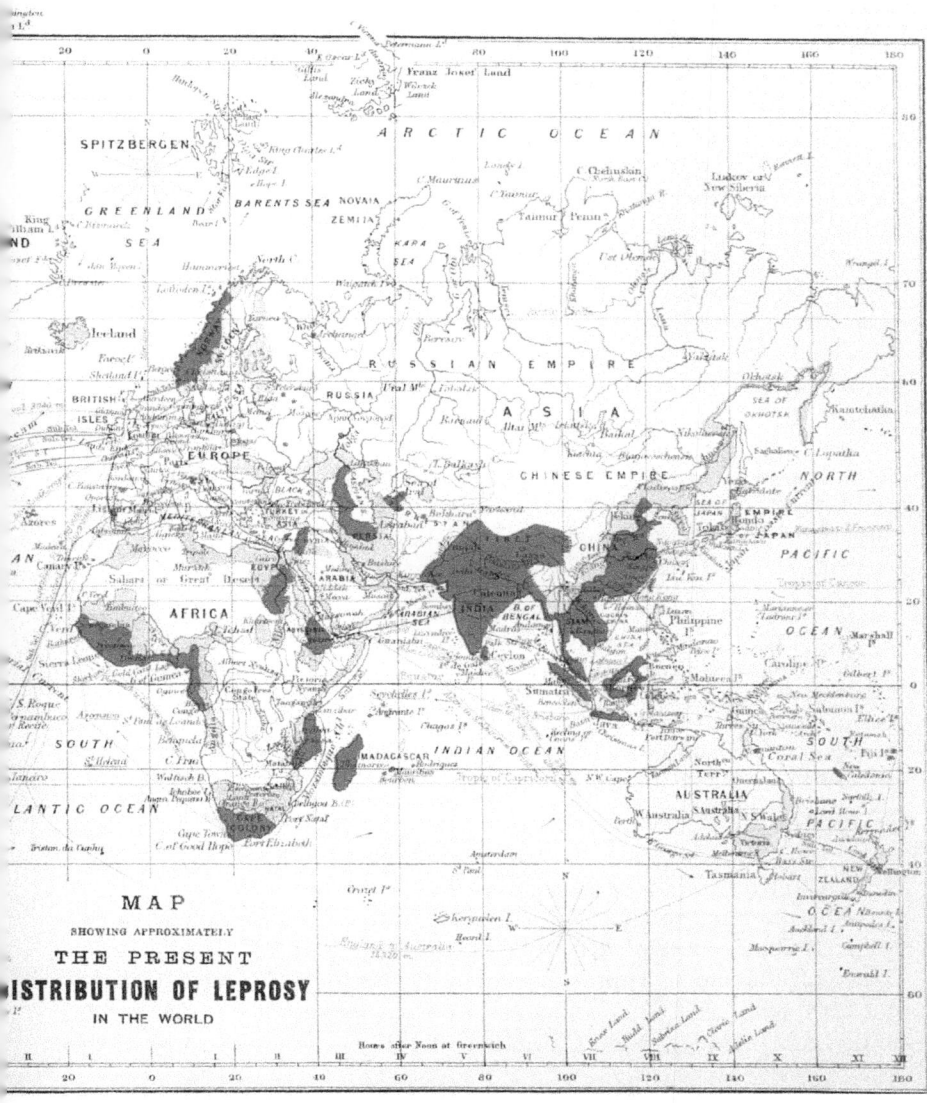

MAP

SHOWING APPROXIMATELY

THE PRESENT

DISTRIBUTION OF LEPROSY

IN THE WORLD

As he told the conference: 'Law-abiding though they be, British subjects do not tamely submit to what they may regard, rightly or wrongly, as unnecessary coercion.'[174] A diluted form of Milroy's concern with the individual liberties of British subjects had persisted.

Abraham's own paper to the conference was an extensive survey of the incidence of leprosy in Britain and the empire. In Britain, he concluded, there had been less than 100 cases in the previous decade, with most, probably all, of these having been contracted abroad. There was, nevertheless, a real need for a specialist institution to deal with these cases. Poorer patients often ended up in Poor Law infirmaries, and several had been forced to seek asylum in the dedicated St Louis hospital in Paris. Abraham's survey of the rest of the empire made clear the high degree of concern about the disease in recent years. Apart from India and the Cape, official inquiries had been set up in Mauritius (1888), Cyprus (1890) and the Straits (1893), and other colonies such as Australia, Jamaica and St Kitts had passed legislation aimed at controlling the movements of lepers – the 'vagrant leper' was seen as an especial menace in Jamaica – or checking the health of imported 'coolie labour'.[175]

At the end of the Conference *The Times* was upbeat:

> The first task of early civilization was to kill the wild beasts that prowled about man's dwellings ... The next task is to exterminate those enemies which walk in darkness and kill, maim, mutilate and enfeeble far more than wolves ever destroyed. We are but at the outset of the contest with malaria, diphtheria, typhoid, and a dozen other enemies equally deadly. But if the temper of the Berlin congress is justified, we have hard-pressed and driven into his last stronghold one of the oldest and worst of man's foes.[176]

Canon Knox Little's recent life of St Francis of Assisi, and Tennyson's late poem 'The Leper's Bride' were taken as evidence of a newly humane attitude to a disease previously regarded as 'typical of sin'.[177]

Evidence of the spread of leprosy around the world continued to be gathered. James Cantlie warned a meeting of the London Epidemiological Society of the infection spreading across the Pacific as 'coolies' from the southern part of China emigrated to the plantations of the Straits Settlements, Hawaii, New Caledonia and Fiji: 'with the coolie came

---

[174] *British Medical Journal*, 2 (1897), 414.   [175] *Ibid.*, 1409–14.
[176] *The Times* (London), 19 October 1897.
[177] Tennyson's poem had also been cited by the *Pall Mall Gazette*, 17 January 1890, on the occasion of the departure of a young woman from Bath, Sister Rose Gertrude, who was inspired by the example of Damien to go and nurse the lepers of Molokai. The paper supposed that 'The Leper's Bride' had been prompted by Damien's death, though in fact Tennyson had completed it the previous year.

leprosy and the dirt of the savage'.[178] Cantile's remedy was deportation, not segregation: 'segregation of Chinese lepers in an asylum ... will in time render that country a fresh focus of leprous infection'.[179] In fact, several of the Australian state governments were already deporting Chinese victims of the disease. Concern about leprosy in the United States was also increasing.[180] Although by the turn of the century heredity had virtually disappeared from the leprosy debate, the argument as to whether or not the bacillus was spread by personal contact continued. Tetanus, for example, although an infective disease was seldom if ever communicated by those suffering from it to the healthy. Dr Ashburton Thompson's pamphlet 'Leprosy in Hawaii: A Critical Study' (1898) argued for the telluric origin of leprosy and against segregation of the infected.[181] The recent spread of leprosy that for many was proof of contagion, was for Thompson more likely to be 'recrudescent activity in a localised virus'.[182] The Berlin conference had finally discredited the hereditary explanation of the disease, and, catching the mood of the time, had encouraged 'international parallel action', particularly worldwide segregation. It had not, however, established how the disease was communicated or suggested any effective treatment or cure. Nor was there even complete consensus on segregation, although this was to be the dominant policy in the early twentieth century.

The Royal College of Physicians

During the 1880s and 90s the Colonial Office would still occasionally consult the College of Physicians for advice on leprosy. Milroy died in 1886 after several years of illness, and the College of Physicians' responses became increasingly uncertain as the evidence for contagion seemed to accumulate.

In 1887, with compulsory segregation being introduced or discussed in several colonies, the College of Physicians was asked if it still maintained that the disease was hereditary. As the Colonial Secretary of the day wrote:

This opinion ... has never been accepted by the general public of those colonies where leprosy is endemic. A section of the local medical practitioners has held persistently the opposite view, and of late years the prevalence of this contrary opinion has decidedly increased, while it is supported by a growing desire of the

---

[178] *British Medical Journal*, 1 (1898), 23.
[179] James Cantlie, *Report on the Conditions Under Which Leprosy Occurs in China, Indo-China, Malaya, The Archipelago and Oceania* (London: Macmillan and Co., 1897), p. 12.
[180] *British Medical Journal*, 1 (1898), 841–2.   [181] *Ibid.*, 1215.   [182] *Ibid.*, 2 (1898), 1199.

community generally to guard themselves against danger from so loathsome a disease.[183]

A new Leprosy Committee was convened to consider this. It acknowledged that many colonial practitioners and inhabitants did not concur with the 1867 Report, spoke of the need for more investigation into the pathology of the disease, and suggested that the government set up such research for the College to direct and report upon.[184] Matters seemed back where they had started in the early 1860s.

But the context in which this question was now being asked was very different. Concern about the spread of leprosy in the empire had been augmented by the fear of its return to Europe, and the spectacular example of Hawaii had been highlighted by the work of Damien who was known to be dying of the disease. After receiving further material on the communicability of leprosy from the Colonial Office, the reconvened Leprosy Committee conceded that the evidence in favour of contagion was 'increasingly weighty' and expressed its willingness to explore the question further.[185] This was a month before the announcement of Damien's death. By its next meeting, in July, the Damien Memorial Committee had been set up and was now in the driving seat. The College of Physicians was content to work with the new committee in its plan for an empire-wide inquiry and seemed to accept that it would play only a supporting role in any such investigation. At the same meeting the Leprosy Committee declined to advise the Vice-Consul at Vera Cruz on how to deal with the problem: 'the whole subject of Leprosy, and how it can best be dealt with, is at the present time under the consideration of the College ... [which] is not prepared at this stage of their proceedings to give any particular direction as to its treatment'.[186]

The last stage of the saga was reached in 1898 when the Colonial Secretary Joseph Chamberlain asked the College whether, following the report from the Berlin conference of the previous year, they now had reason 'to change their previously expressed opinion ... on the question of segregating lepers or on any other point of importance in regulating the disease in the Colonies'. Yet another Leprosy Committee was convened

[183] Edward Wingfield, on behalf of Sir Henry Holland, to Royal College of Physicians, 19 February 1887, Correspondence Relating to the Contagious Nature of Leprosy 1876–9, 4119/264 (this letter of 1887 is included in the 1876–9 folder), Wellcome Library.

[184] Leprosy Committee Report, 15 July 1887, Leprosy Committee 1887–1898, 2248/7, Wellcome Library.

[185] Report of Leprosy Committee No. 2, April 1889, Leprosy Committee 1887–1898, 2248/8, Wellcome Library.

[186] Report of Leprosy Committee No. 3, 30 July 1889, Leprosy Committee 1887–1898, 2248/9, Wellcome Library.

and it conceded that the 1867 Report was ill-founded: 'That the communicability of Leprosy, by direct or indirect means, from Lepers to the healthy, must now be accepted as an established fact, the evidence in support of this belief being conclusive; and that there is no evidence of the disease arising or spreading in any other way.'[187]

---

[187] Leprosy Committee Report, 6 December 1898, Leprosy Committee 1887–1898, 2248/10, Wellcome Library.

3 The fear of degeneration: leprosy in the tropics and the metropolis at the *fin de siècle*

The tropics and disease

Tropical medicine was a late nineteenth-century construction. Before this, medical geography provided the dominant model of explanation, and doctors examined and treated 'diseases in the tropics' rather than practising 'tropical medicine'. Very few diseases were regarded as specific and most were explained in terms of the effects of climatic extremes on the ill-adapted constitutions of European bodies.[1] The main concern of medicine in the tropics was with Europeans although, as we have seen, the health of native subjects became increasingly entangled with this. At the same time, declining mortality levels in Europe and North America highlighted the far worse disease and mortality levels in tropical regions. In fact this contrast applied more to indigenes than Europeans, whose mortality rates in the tropics were actually declining in the later nineteenth century,[2] but pessimism about the ability of the white races to settle in equatorial regions nevertheless intensified. So too did the distinction between tropical and temperate zones.

Although the distinctiveness of the tropical environment and its maladies was a commonplace in the eighteenth century, there was optimism about the ability of Europeans to acclimatise through residence, a process referred to as 'seasoning'.[3] From the early nineteenth century, however, climatic theories of racial difference began to be reinforced by more essentialising biological ones. Mark Harrison cites James Thomson's *A Treatise on the Diseases of the Negro as they occur in the Island of Jamaica* (1820) as a significant marker of this shift, whose corollary was

---

[1] Michael Worboys, 'Tropical Diseases', in W. F. Bynum and Roy Porter (eds.), *Companion Encyclopedia of the History of Medicine*, 2 vols. (London and New York: Routledge, 1993), vol. I, p. 515.

[2] *Ibid.*, p. 518.

[3] Mark Harrisson, ' "The Tender Frame of Man": Disease, Climate, and Racial Difference in India and the West Indies, 1760–1860', *Bulletin of the History of Medicine*, 70 (1996), 70–5.

an increasing pessimism about the chances of European acclimatisation. Harrison also points to the influence of pathological anatomy on increasingly naturalistic conceptions of race and gender, categories that had previously been seen as more mutable and environmentally influenced.[4] As medical investigation of the interaction between racial constitutions and particular environments became inflected by emergent race theory and new kinds of pathology, acclimatisation was increasingly seen as very difficult, if not impossible.

Warwick Anderson has argued that whereas confidence in acclimatisation was based on the monogenist assumption that races could adapt to changed circumstances, by the middle of the nineteenth century the influence of polygenist ideas of racial fixity meant that existence outside a race's ancestral environment came to be seen as problematic. Anderson further argues that the loss of belief in acclimatisation eventually became part of 'the degenerationist narrative' of the late nineteenth century.[5] The influence of Cuvier's theory of the fixity of biological types, and the polygenist ideas of Knox and Hunt in the 1850s and 60s can certainly be seen in mid-century medical texts and doubtless contributed to scepticism about acclimatisation.[6] However, it was not necessary to be a polygenist in order to wonder if Europeans could survive in the tropics. Although Darwin had demonstrated that species adapted and evolved, the time-span required for this was such as to render acclimatisation an almost indefinitely long, as well as chancy, process. Charles Pearson's influential *National Life and Character* (1893), although convinced that the tropics 'cannot possibly be the homes of . . . the Aryan race, or indeed of any higher race whatsoever', does not rule out the possibility of eventual adaptation but sees this as so long-term as to be meaningless. The 'higher races' will have been 'elbowed out of the way' long before any significant adaptation has occurred.[7]

The tropics, therefore, came to present the colonial powers with a dilemma; although no place for the white man himself, they were where he exercised power over other races.[8] European bodies were becoming understood as constitutionally different from those of their subjects, with residence in tropical zones more likely to bring illness and death than acclimatisation. Optimistic readings of this essential difference were possible as well. Europeans were relatively immune to a range of 'non-tropical'

---

[4] *Ibid.*, 82–4.
[5] Warwick Anderson, 'Disease, Race, and Empire', *Bulletin of the History of Medicine* 70 (1996), 62–7.
[6] Harrisson, ' "The Tender Frame of Man" ', 87–8.
[7] Charles H. Pearson, *National Life and Character: A Forecast* (London: Macmillan, 1893), pp. 63, 85.
[8] Anderson, 'Disease, Race, and Empire', 63.

diseases such as measles or influenza that made terrible inroads into many indigenous populations but were never to be designated as 'tropical'. As European sanitary reforming practice was imported into many colonies the distinction between the clean white man and the filthy native became part of the grammar of difference upon which colonial hierarchies were based. In this way, native peoples could be represented as the source of their own sufferings, and their intrinsic susceptibility to certain diseases could be extended to include the idea that such peoples passively surrendered rather than actively resisted death. This melancholy fatalism was then, in turn, incorporated into a broader figuring of difference. The underlying point, however, is that health and disease were central to the process of establishing the difference upon which empire was founded and yet which would always haunt it. Alternative kinds of difference were established according to the types of disease chosen. Either immunity or susceptibility could figure as markers of superiority when attached to the white races, the former a sign of inherent robustness, the latter of a degree of civilisation and refinement too advanced for existence in tropical zones.

Nancy Stepan has shown how the ascendancy of medical environmentalism for much of the nineteenth century involved a 'darkening' in representations of the tropics.[9] Disease and race became intertwined as the world was divided into two major zones, the temperate and the tropical, in which the former was 'the silent norm against which the medical deviancy of the tropics was measured'.[10] With the discovery of microbes, however, medical geography was replaced by parasitology, and disease maps gave way to disease portraits and illustrations of pathogens and vectors.[11] Latour describes how rapidly European contagionists shifted their attention to the tropics, and Otis pictures Koch the microbe hunter assisting the spread of empire through his medical research in German-occupied parts of Africa.[12] Otis also makes clear a relation between imperial and bacterial worlds so close that they shared each other's language. 'Colonial dreamers' were described as having fallen victim to a 'colonial fever bacillus', while a new culture of bacilli was announced in Paris as 'the new French colonies'.[13]

---

[9] Nancy Leys Stepan, *Picturing Tropical Nature* (London: Reaktion Books, 2001), p. 48.
[10] *Ibid.*, p. 157.   [11] *Ibid.*, pp. 165–71.
[12] Bruno Latour, *The Pasteurization of France* (Cambridge, Mass. and London: Harvard University Press, 1988), p. 116. Laura Otis, *Membranes: Metaphors of Invasion in Nineteenth-Century Literature, Science, and Politics* (Baltimore and London: Johns Hopkins University Press, 1999), p. 31.
[13] Otis, *Membranes*, p. 31. See also Roy MacLeod and Milton Lewis (eds.), *Disease, Medicine and Empire: Perspectives on Western Medicine and the Experience of European Expansion* (London and New York: Routledge, 1988), p. 7.

The germ theory of disease, therefore, was a decisive factor in the erosion of a medical-geographical explanation of pathology and aetiology, and in establishing specific and unified concepts of disease that shifted attention away from place to person. Contagionism resulted in attaching disease to 'tropical people' rather than to the tropics per se, and attention became focused on the native subject as disease-carrier.[14] This, in turn, threatened the distinction between healthy temperate and diseased tropical regions. People were mobile, and even if their movements could to some extent be controlled, the transfer of invisible pathogens from donor to host was impossible to check. Even in the new context of germ theory, however, the influence of medical-geographic and climatic-determinist ideas persisted. Native peoples continued to be thought of in terms of the tropical places they inhabited, and these places in turn reinforced the belief that European bodies were very different from those of their subjects. As Warwick Anderson points out, the supposition that racial difference shaped disease expression in some way or another was continuous throughout the nineteenth century. Assumptions about the hereditary predisposition of different races persisted into the microbe era even if the understanding of that term was affected by new theories of disease aetiology. Racial typologies inflected modern tropical medicine and continued to provide contours for new disease maps and photographs.[15]

A comparison of Hirsch's *Handbook of Geography and Historical Pathology*, a three-volume work published in Germany in the 1860s and translated into English between 1883 and 1886, with Manson's *Tropical Diseases* (1898) will make clearer both the differences and continuities between medical geography and the new tropical medicine. Hirsch was Professor of Medicine at the University of Berlin. His preface to the English translation confidently described the scope and authority of medical geography just as it was about to be seriously undermined by germ theory. According to Hirsch, medical geography over the last thirty years has 'acquired finish to an extraordinary degree': 'Nowadays we can estimate the health-conditions of many of the most remote parts of the world, in regard to morbid anatomy and etiology, with as much exactness as we were privileged to do not so very long ago, for none but the most civilised States of Europe and North America.'[16] Deriving from Hippocrates, and with immediate antecedents in the work of Finke at the end of the

---

[14] Worboys, 'Tropical Diseases', vol. I, pp. 518, 523. Warwick Anderson, 'Immunities of Empire: Race, Disease, and the New Tropical Medicine', *Bulletin of the History of Medicine*, 70 (1996), 111.

[15] Anderson, 'Immunities of Empire', 96, 118.

[16] A. Hirsch, *Handbook of Geography and Historical Pathology*, trans. C. Creighton, 2 vols. (London: New Sydenham Society, 1883), vol. I, pp. vii–viii.

eighteenth century, and Boudin and Lombard in the nineteenth, this science of 'the influence of climate, soil, and manner of life upon the habit of the human body' is now equipped to deliver a unified 'historico-geographical pathology'.[17]

Hirsch dealt with leprosy in the opening chapter of his second volume under the general heading of 'Chronic Infective Diseases', alongside syphilis, yaws, endemic goitre and cretinism. In discussing leprosy he sounded a warning: 'superficiality or inacuracy [sic] in observing facts, and onesidedness or bias in judging of them, have nowhere obtruded themselves so much as to swell the doctrine of morbific causes with empty hypotheses as in the etiology of leprosy'.[18] If this sounds rather like Milroy it is because much of Hirsch's evidence about the nature of leprosy comes from the 1867 College of Physicians' Report. Although Hirsch goes much further than Milroy in conceding that for the production of the disease (as opposed to a predisposition) there must be 'a definite and specific noxious agent, a peculiar infective substance', he denies that leprosy is contagious. Hansen and Neisser have claimed it is an 'authenticated bacterial disease' and this is 'highly probable – I will not say proved', but the idea that leprosy is contagious is a medieval belief based on confusing it with syphilis.[19] Indeed, the apparent concession to germ theory apart, Hirsch discusses the disease in terms that are entirely familiar from the hereditarianism of Milroy and others in the 1860s and 70s. Leprosy is not caused by climate, soil or diet but these factors contribute to the disease when there is a prior disposition: 'its proper cause is to be sought rather in conditions which exert a *specific* effect, which are bound up with the locality or the manner of life, and very materially also with the racial characters of the inhabitants of the tropics'.[20]

For Hirsch, inheritance was the one kind of conveyance of leprosy 'which cannot be questioned'. The only debate concerns 'how high[ly] this pathogenetic factor is to be rated for the spreading of the disease, and whether the disease is inherited as such, or whether it is only a predisposition thereto ... a morbid diathesis which inclines the individual to fall into the sickness, or makes him specifically susceptible to the morbid poison'.[21] The susceptibility of particular races and nationalities is explained by hereditary predisposition, although their manner of life is also a factor. There is universal agreement that leprosy is commonest among negroes and those of 'mixed blood', and very rare among Europeans. Its varying frequency among Jews in different parts of the

[17] *Ibid.*, vol. I, pp. 2, 6.   [18] *Ibid.*, vol. II, p. 31.   [19] *Ibid.*, vol. II, pp. 43–4.
[20] *Ibid.*, vol. II, p. 33.   [21] *Ibid.*, vol. II, pp. 51–2.

world is 'very remarkable', one of those persisting 'puzzles' about the disease (its 'spontaneous origin' in places where leprosy has been extinct for centuries is another).[22] Hirsch's affinity with Milroy is most apparent in his scepticism about the supposedly rapid spread of leprosy in Hawaii. This test case for anti-contagionists finds Hirsch endorsing Milroy's scepticism and suggesting that the reports involved confusion between leprosy and syphilis.[23]

Patrick Manson's *Tropical Diseases* (1898) was the founding text of the new specialism of tropical medicine as it emerged and became institutionalised at the turn of the twentieth century. Manson had been the first to demonstrate the insect-borne transmission of disease when, in 1883, he had shown that elephantiasis was caused by a filarial worm that was transmitted by mosquitoes. This was to become the normative aetiological model of tropical medicine; it was at Manson's suggestion, for example, that Ronald Ross later pursued the research that established malaria as a mosquito-borne disease. Manson became medical adviser to the Colonial Office in 1897 and first head of the new London School of Tropical Medicine in 1899.[24] *Tropical Diseases* was reprinted twice in 1898, again the following year, and has continued to be revised, breaking free entirely of its original authorship. The twentieth edition that appeared in 1996 was by many hands but the work continues to be known as 'Manson'.[25]

Michael Worboys points out that 'tropical medicine' was, at first, a residual category involving those diseases met by medical practioners in tropical colonies that were not well covered in the European medical curriculum.[26] By the turn of the twentieth century, however, it had become institutionalised as a distinct branch of medicine in its own right, and it contributed significantly to the wider distinction between temperate and tropical zones that was structuring colonial discourse at this period. Manson conceded that his title was 'more convenient than accurate', excluding as it did many diseases found in the tropics while including some that were not confined to these regions. His uneasy attempt to explain the coherence and integrity of the category of tropical medicine is partly defined against Hirsch: 'I employ the term "tropical" in a meteorological rather than in a geographical sense, meaning by it sustained

---

[22] *Ibid.*, vol. II, pp. 55–7.   [23] *Ibid.*, vol. II, p. 19.

[24] Michael Worboys, 'Manson, Ross and Colonial Medical Policy: Tropical Medicine in London and Liverpool, 1899–1914', in MacLeod and Lewis, *Disease, Medicine and Empire*, pp. 21–3.

[25] *Manson's Tropical Diseases*, ed. Gordon C. Cook (London: W. B. Saunders, 1996).

[26] Worboys, 'Tropical Diseases', p. 512.

high atmospheric temperature; and by the term "tropical diseases", I wish to indicate diseases occurring only, or which from one circumstance or another are specially prevalent, in warm climates.'[27] Manson's break with the medico-geographical tradition are underlined by his insistence that, 'Modern science has clearly shown that nearly all diseases, directly or indirectly, are caused by germs': 'In the tropics, as in temperate climates, in the European and in the native alike, nearly all disease is of specific origin. It is in their specific causes that the difference between the diseases of temperate climates and those of tropical climates principally lies.'[28] This attempts to dismiss the pre-germ basis of distinguishing between the diseases of temperate and tropical zones while establishing modern scientific grounds for retaining the distinction.

As Manson concedes, his classification immediately runs into problems with leprosy. Tropical medicine includes:

certain cosmopolitan diseases, such as leprosy and plague ... which, properly speaking, do not depend in any very special way, or necessarily, on climatic conditions. They have been practically ousted from Europe and the temperate parts of America by the spread of civilisation, and the improved hygiene that has followed in its train; and are now practically confined to tropical and sub-tropical countries, where they still survive under those backward social and unsanitary conditions which are necessary for their successful propagation, and which are more or less an indirect outcome of tropical climate.[29]

As the qualifications proliferate – 'practically', 'more or less', 'indirect' – the reason for including leprosy as a tropical disease becomes less and less clear. Leprosy is once again a boundary disease, in this case neither really tropical nor temperate. It is *hors classe* in other senses as well. Manson has no doubt that leprosy is caused by the lepra bacillus, and that infection comes from another leper.[30] Unlike many other tropical diseases, however, no one has succeeded in cultivating it or conveying it by inoculation.[31] Also unlike most tropical diseases, there was no evidence of transmission by insect vector (this was occasionally suggested but never seriously entertained).[32]

There were other ways in which leprosy failed to conform to the emerging type of a tropical disease. It differed in developing very slowly and being, at first, difficult to diagnose. Manson's attempts to describe

---

[27] Patrick Manson, *Tropical Diseases: A Manual of the Diseases of Warm Climates* (London: Cassell, 1898), p. xi.
[28] *Ibid.*, p. xii.   [29] *Ibid.*, p. xvi.   [30] *Ibid.*, pp. 383, 390.   [31] *Ibid.*, p. 412.
[32] Worboys, 'Tropical Diseases', p. 531.

the initial skin eruptions are as laborious and unhelpful as those in Leviticus:

> They may be no larger than a millet seed, or they may occupy surfaces many inches in diameter; they may be numerous, or they may be only two or three. The earlier spots are usually ... darkest in the centre and shading off towards the periphery. But in some cases they may be pigmented from the outset ... In not a few lepers what ... was an erythematous patch may in time become pigmented, or it may become pale ... Or it may be that the centre of an erythematous patch clears up, the periphery of the patch remaining red and perhaps becoming pigmented.[33]

This catch-all account is an unhelpful guide to early diagnosis, and provides a marked contrast with classic tropical diseases where the onset is rapid and the symptoms vivid and unmistakable.

Yet for all this, Manson has no doubt that leprosy is a tropical disease, 'an element, and often an important element in the pathology of nearly all warm countries'.[34] His account of the later stages of leprosy emphasises and illustrates the atrophy and deformation wrought by the disease. This disfiguring is fundamental in designating leprosy as 'tropical'. Like many other so-called tropical diseases, leprosy was in fact a disease of poverty, malnutrition and unsanitary conditions, but the category served the ideological function of associating these diseases with natural rather than social, economic or political factors.[35] The bodily deformations of native subjects, copiously illustrated in Manson and subsequent textbooks of tropical medicine, reinforced this. The new genre of the tropical medical photograph featured visually horrifying diseases such as leprosy and elephantiasis. Europeans were not immune to leprosy, and elephantiasis affected both West Indian plantation owners and Pacific missionaries, but it was natives who normally provided the photographic evidence of these conditions.[36] Such images implied that native bodies were more susceptible to deforming diseases, and perhaps inherently debased. Leprosy, in particular, could be seen as a kind of X-ray of the native body, making visible the corruption that festered within.

Stepan argues that visual representation of this kind exemplifies the displacement involved in the constitution of tropical medicine as a distinct category and discipline.[37] As Europe slowly freed itself from an epidemiological past of cholera, malaria, leprosy and plague, these and other

---

[33] Manson, *Tropical Diseases*, pp. 392–3.   [34] *Ibid.*, p. 386.
[35] Worboys, 'Tropical Diseases', p. 513.
[36] Stepan, *Picturing Tropical Nature*, pp. 171–3. For a more detailed discussion of this point see Rod Edmond, 'Returning Fears: Tropical Disease and the Metropolis', in Felix Driver and Luciana Martins (eds.), *Tropical Visions in an Age of Empire* (Chicago: University of Chicago Press, 2005), pp. 279–81.
[37] Stepan, *Picturing Tropical Nature*, p. 172.

diseases were banished to the tropics where they became a primary signifier of native otherness.[38] Michael Worboys has emphasised the exceptionalist assumptions on which tropical medicine was constructed, ignoring as it did not only the persistence of many so-called tropical diseases in Europe but also worldwide scourges such as pneumonia and tuberculosis that were a major cause of death in European colonies.[39] The epidemiological criteria of tropical medicine were inseparable from contemporary ideas of the tropics and of race. Tropical medicine found its place at the heart of Europe's imperial mission. Intended to combat the virulent forms of disease often encountered in colonial settings, it also conceptualized the difference between Europe and its others in ways that underwrote the expansion of empires.[40]

Tropical medicine, however, was an inherently unstable discourse. Although the contrast between European health and native susceptibility was one of its ideological mainstays, it was often those very diseases labelled 'tropical' that most threatened the coloniser and from which the indigene seemed relatively immune. A French scientist described tropical diseases as 'the "generals" that defend hot countries against our excursions [sic] and prevent us from replacing the aborigines that we have to make use of'.[41] From this point of view tropical medicine was needed to compensate for the natural advantages of the native. Laura Otis has used the 'membrane model' to describe the process of constructing borders and boundaries to protect the health and integrity of imperial bodies from contact with native populations. The category of tropical medicine was itself a membrane, a way of distinguishing the temperate from the tropical, European from native, metropole from colony. It was also a classic example of the failure of this model. Microbes were indifferent to boundaries. Europeans were prone to disease in tropical settings and so-called tropical diseases such as leprosy threatened to return to temperate metropolitan centres, invisible agents whose effects would become disturbingly visible. This fear of return would ultimately come to haunt bacteriology itself, as diseases whose disappearance had been announced became resistant to the very means that bacteriology had devised for eliminating them.[42]

The category of 'tropical medicine', and its institutionalisation in the Schools founded in London, Liverpool, Paris and several other European

---

[38] David Arnold (ed.), *Imperial Medicine and Indigenous Societies* (Delhi: Oxford University Press, 1989), p. 7.

[39] Michael Worboys, 'The Discovery of Colonial Malnutrition Between the Wars', in Arnold, *Imperial Medicine and Indigenous Societies*, p. 211.

[40] McLeod and Lewis, *Disease, Medicine and Empire*, p. 7.

[41] Latour, *The Pasteurization of France*, p. 141.

[42] *Ibid.*, pp. 112–14. Stepan, *Picturing Tropical Nature*, pp. 166–7.

cities at the turn of the twentieth century, can be understood as a metropolitan imposition on the equatorial regions of the world at a time when
the relation between the cherished zones of temperate and tropical had
become troubled. Germ theory had made the disease maps of medical
geography untenable. A new kind of mapping was needed which could
take account of the ubiquity of germs without relinquishing the temperate/
tropical divide. A germ-based medicine in which the tropics lost some of
the traditional taint associated with their ecology, but were repathologised
in modern scientific terms as the natural home of deadly microbes, was
well adapted to this need. It followed from this that native bodies should be
similarly pathologised. It is easy to see how older forms of typifying the
tropics would carry forward into the new tropical medicine, supplementing
it as well as being replaced by it. New theories and constructions are
at their most persuasive when they incorporate part of what they replace.
In like manner Manson was prepared to concede that 'certain physio-
pathological qualities predisposing to the disease may be inherited',
while insisting that the leprosy bacillus and the disease it causes cannot
be hereditary 'in the scientific sense of the word'.[43] Tropical medicine,
therefore, was never simply the substitution of a germ-based colonial
medicine for a discredited medical geography. In Hirsch's concession to
emergent germ theory, and in Manson's continuing dependence on an idea
of the tropics derived from medical geography, can be seen a process of
overlapping and intersection analogous to, though different in detail and
outcome from, the accommodation in France between hygienists and
Pasteurians that has been analysed by Latour.

The tropics and the metropolis

Tropical medicine needs to be understood in the wider context of debate
over the relation between temperate and tropical zones at the end of the
nineteenth century. As we have seen, the relation between these two
defining zones of the globe was increasingly understood as difficult, even
antagonistic. The tropics were becoming Europe's other, a thick belt
around the middle of the earth that white men inhabited at their peril.
A number of influential works at the end of the nineteenth century
addressed the dilemma this posed for imperial and sub-imperial powers.
One of these was the previously mentioned Charles Pearson's *National Life
and Character: A Forecast* (1893). Pearson had been Professor of History
at King's College London before emigrating to Australia where he became

---

[43] Manson, *Tropical Diseases*, pp. 413–14.

Minister of Public Instruction in the Victoria State Parliament and a profound influence on the generation of politicians who oversaw the introduction of Federation in 1901.[44] Pearson argued that because the population of tropical zones increased more rapidly than that of temperate ones, the 'higher races' would become hemmed in, prevented by constitutional incapacity from living in tropical regions, and threatened at home as the inhabitants of the tropics swarmed across the world. Australia offered a telling example. On the one hand it seemed to provide a solution to the increasing lack of space in temperate zones: 'The natives have died out as we approached; there have been no complications with foreign powers; and the climate of the South is magnificent.'[45] Pearson divides 'the lower races' into two categories: the Chinese, Japanese, Hindus and negroes who are 'too numerous and sturdy to be extirpated', and the 'evanescent races' (the 'red man', Carib, Kanaka and Aboriginal) who 'seem to wither away at mere contact with the European'.[46] In this gently naturalised version of the extinction of certain native populations the Aboriginal people obligingly anticipate their inevitable fate. But if Australia did not have a native problem, it was acquiring an immigrant one through the influx of Chinese immigrants:

We know that coloured and white labour cannot exist side by side; we are well aware that China can swamp us with a single year's surplus of population; and we know that if national existence is sacrificed to the working of a few mines and sugar plantations, it is not the Englishman in Australia alone, but the whole civilised world, that will be the losers ... We are guarding the last part of the world, in which the higher races can live and increase freely, for the higher civilisation.[47]

When the Australian Prime Minister Edmund Barton introduced the Immigration Restriction Bill to the recently constituted Federal Parliament in 1901 he read out several passages from *National Life and Character*.[48] Pearson had argued that it was unlikely that 'the white race' could acclimatise to the northern parts of Australia, those closest to the tropical zone.[49] Australia, therefore, far from being a last chance for the white races threatened to become yet another example of an inexorable process: 'the black and yellow belt, which always encircles the globe between the Tropics, will extend its area, and deepen its colour with

---

[44] John Tregenza, *Professor of Democracy: The Life of Charles Henry Pearson, 1830–1894: Oxford Don and Australian Radical* (Melbourne: Melbourne University Press, 1968), pp. 2–3.

[45] Pearson, *National Life and Character*, p. 16.   [46] *Ibid.*, pp. 31–2.   [47] *Ibid.*, p. 16.

[48] Tregenza, *Professor of Democracy*, p. 234.

[49] Pearson, *National Life and Character*, p. 16.

time'.[50] The civilised and temperate races who value comfort will always increase more slowly than those that content themselves with 'bare existence'; 'in the long run the lower civilisation has a more vigorous life than the higher, the unprivileged gains upon the privileged caste, and the conquered people absorbs the conqueror'.[51] Imperial expansion, in fact, contains the seeds of its own destruction. By half-civilising native peoples, improving their health and introducing them to European technology, 'the races that are now our subjects ... will one day be our rivals':

The day will come, and perhaps is not far distant, when the European observer will look round to see the globe girdled with a continuous zone of the black and yellow races, no longer too weak for aggression or under tutelage, but independent ... in government, monopolising the trade of their own regions, and circumscribing the industry of the European.[52]

Pearson foresaw 'Chinamen and the natives of Hindostan ... African nations of the Congo and the Zambesi', with fleets in the European seas, participating in international conferences, and intermarrying with the white races: 'We shall wake to find ourselves elbowed and hustled, and perhaps even thrust aside by peoples whom we looked down upon as servile, and thought of as bound always to minister to our needs.'[53] The entanglement of the temperate world with the tropical threatens the end of those races 'that have taken their faith from Palestine, their laws of beauty from Greece, and their civil law from Rome'.[54] This imperial version of involution theory, with the worst driving out the best, had parallels with the contemporary fear in Britain of a degraded urban working class contaminating metropolitan society from below.[55] Common to both was a fear of rampant breeding, with a differential birth rate working to the detriment of civilised society at home and in the empire.

Another influential contribution to this distinctive two-world theory was Benjamin Kidd's *The Control of the Tropics* (1898). Kidd's *Social Evolution* (1894), which argued that the subjugation and even eradication of inferior races by the Anglo-Saxon peoples was inevitable, had been widely read and translated. *The Control of the Tropics* originally appeared as a series of articles in *The Times* in 1897 and was extensively noticed.[56] For Kidd, the 'great rivalry of the past' has been won by 'the English-speaking peoples', but the great rivalry of the future, which is already upon

---

[50] *Ibid.*, p. 64.   [51] *Ibid.*, pp. 68, 70.   [52] *Ibid.*, p. 84.   [53] *Ibid.*, p. 85.   [54] *Ibid.*, p. 14.
[55] See Gareth Stedman Jones, *Outcast London: A Study in the Relationship Between Classes in Victorian Society* (Oxford: Clarendon Press, 1971), especially Part 3.
[56] Sven Lindqvist, *'Exterminate All the Brutes'* (London: Granta Books, 2002), pp. 78, 138–9.

us, 'is for the inheritance of the tropics'.[57] Kidd emphasised the economic significance of the tropics for Britain and the United States, whose combined trade with these regions was almost half their total trade with the rest of the world. Modern life, therefore, depended heavily on the labour and products of tropical zones.[58] However, political and administrative relations with these backward regions upon which modern life so depended were 'either indefinite or entirely casual'.[59] This was because Kidd, like Pearson, did not think that the tropics could be settled by Europeans: 'in the tropics the white man lives and works only as a diver lives and works under water'.[60] This inability to acclimatise was, for Kidd, a result of evolution. The human race had developed northwards from the tropics. The 'natural inhabitants' of the tropics had remained like children and were incapable of developing the tropical world themselves. He cites the example of the West Indies which since the end of slavery has become like a former civilisation: 'Decaying harbours ... stately buildings falling to ruin ... deserted mines and advancing forests.'[61] In this Kidd is different from Pearson. The ascendancy of Western peoples and civilisation is beyond doubt because it is underwritten by evolution, and he questions Pearson's view of Europeans being elbowed out of the way.[62] Rather than a vigorous and expanding tropical world, Kidd fears a sedentary and regressive one. Both, however, see the relation between temperate and tropical worlds as the most pressing question of their time, and both agree there is an acute problem of managing the tropics because of the European inability to live there.

Charles Woodruff's *The Effects of Tropical Light on White Men* (1905) offered another evolutionary take on the relation between Europe and the tropics. Woodruff had been a United States army doctor in the Philippines. He rejected the idea that the human race had evolved in the tropics: 'That process required a cold severe environment which killed off all except the most intelligent in every generation ... and thus caused an evolution of the human brain.' This drives an even sharper wedge between temperate and tropical zones. Tropical peoples are permanently fixed at an inferior level of development but, by the same token, they inhabit a world the white man is unable to share: 'A species is sharply limited in its northern and southern extensions and though it may be found over longer distances east and west it is never found out of its zone. Migration would be followed by extinction sooner or later for acclimatisation is not

---

[57] Benjamin Kidd, *The Control of the Tropics* (New York and London: Macmillan, 1893), p. 3.
[58] *Ibid.*, pp. 8–11, 14.   [59] *Ibid.*, p. 6.   [60] *Ibid.*, p. 54.   [61] *Ibid.*, p. 73.
[62] *Ibid.*, pp. 78–80.

possible.' The tropics, therefore, were a distinct 'zoological zone' inhabited by an equally distinct 'anthropoid type'.[63] Life outside one's zone was unsustainable. According to Woodruff, there were no third-generation Europeans in India. Rudyard Kipling's *Kim* (1901) offers a version of this in the narrator's remark on Kim's initially rapid progress at his school: 'at St. Xavier's they knew the first rush of minds developed by sun and surroundings, as they knew the half-collapse that sets in at twenty-two or twenty-three'.[64] Prolonged exposure to tropical light caused the European to 'break down', a recurring phrase in Woodruff that comes to mean something almost as literal as physical decomposition.

By the end of the nineteenth century, therefore, the tropics were becoming troubling; difficult to manage and difficult to manage without. The expansion of empires, and the increased movement of trade, peoples and germs that accompanied this, demanded that the relation between temperate and tropical regions should be reconceptualised in terms that took account of the greater activity between the two zones. The static and polarised opposition that emerged in mid-century had broken down under this pressure in the high imperial era. At the same time, however, the mid-century loss of belief in acclimatisation persisted and if anything hardened. By the closing decades of the century the failure of acclimatisation was being extended to include sections of the metropolitan population as well, and a discourse of the tropics was increasingly applied to urban slums. In this way the problem of acclimatisation became part of the broader degenerationist narrative of the later nineteenth century.

The intersection of concern about tropical and urban degeneration was voiced in a discussion in the *British Medical Journal* in 1897. This centred on a long article by Luigi Sambon addressing the problem outlined by Pearson, Kidd and others. European states have come to 'look upon the development of the Dark Continent as the means of relief of the over-crowding of their populations, and of securing new markets for the produce of their industries'. At the same time, however, there is 'almost universal agreement ... that complete acclimatisation of Europeans in the tropics is impossible'.[65] Sambon then considers the parallel argument about the impossibility of permanent acclimatisation to the modern city. It is frequently claimed that 'the strongest blood cannot endure continuous city life for more than three generations, but must be kept alive by the

[63] Charles E. Woodruff, *The Effects of Tropical Light on White Men* (New York and London: Rebman, 1905), pp. 1–3.

[64] Rudyard Kipling, *Kim* (Harmondsworth: Penguin, 1987), p. 173.

[65] Luigi Sambon, 'Remarks on the Possibility of the Acclimatisation of Europeans in Tropical Regions', *British Medical Journal*, 1 (1897), 61.

infusion of country blood, or by return in some degree to country life'. Boudin, he reports, could not find any 'pure Parisians who could trace the residence of their ancestors in the city back for more than three generations'.[66]

The parallels between non-continuance and degeneration in the tropics and the modern metropolis were becoming commonplace by the time Sambon discussed them. James Cantlie's *Degeneration Amongst Londoners* (1885) described London as a city lacking ozone, which the author believed to be the source of all vital powers. The city's 'outer circle' of human beings absorbs all the fresh air and adds 'pollutions' to it, so that 'the air breathed within a given area, centred around ... Charing Cross, or the Bank, has not had fresh air supplied to it for, say, 50 or 100 years'.[67] Londoners, Cantlie suggests, are like someone returning from the tropics, 'blanched and pale ... suffering from Asiatic diarrhoea or dysentery.'[68] Those whose parents were also born in London grow up physically under-developed, of scrofulous aspect, with squints and misshapen jaws.[69] Suffering from 'urbomorbus' or 'city disease', their bones fail to develop, becoming soft and spongy and unable to support the body.[70] Cantlie contrasts the ozone-deprived inhabitants of inner London with the strong and vigorous offspring of those whose fathers emigrated to Canada or Australia.[71] The only note of comfort is that these people cannot repro-duce: 'Nature steps in and denies the continuance of such; and weakness of brain power gives such a being but little chance in this struggling world.'[72] In this they are like third-generation Anglo-Indians for whom the 'attain-ing of adult years is impossible'. The colonial problem of 'non-continuance' has now come home: 'It is beyond prophecy to guess even what the rising degeneration will grow into, what this Empire will become.'[73] Significant sections of the British population are not even acclimatised to their own environment. Cantlie's recommended solution of cycling and lawn tennis hardly seemed to meet the problem he described.

Cantlie was a doctor who had become concerned with the physical condition of the urban poor while working at London's Charing Cross Hospital. He had then worked in Egypt and become interested in tropical diseases. In 1887 he had taken over Manson's practice in Hong Kong where he remained for a decade before returning home and assisting Manson to establish the London School of Tropical Medicine in 1899.

---

[66] *Ibid.*, 62. Sambon himself was trying to counter these ideas, arguing that Europeans could reproduce in tropical regions and survive tropical disease.

[67] James Cantlie, *Degeneration Amongst Londoners* (London: Field and Tuer, Leadenhall Press, 1885), pp. 8–13.

[68] *Ibid.*, pp. 13–16.   [69] *Ibid.*, pp. 20–3.   [70] *Ibid.*, pp. 24, 34.   [71] *Ibid.*, p. 31.

[72] *Ibid.*, p. 23.   [73] *Ibid.*, pp. 45, 52.

He was an original member of the staff of that School and founder editor of the *Journal of Tropical Medicine and Hygiene*.[74] Cantlie's writing exemplified the close relation between fears of disease and degeneration in nation and empire. In 1890 he published *Leprosy in Hong Kong*, a vivid expression of the contemporary fear of the migrant leper, in which the free port of Hong Kong was described as being overrun by Chinese lepers. In 1897 the British National Leprosy Fund published Cantlie's *Report on the Conditions Under Which Leprosy Occurs in China, Indo-China, Malaya, The Archipelago and Oceania*, which opened with a parallel between the contemporary world and 'the dim centuries' of the past; once again, 'civilised and uncivilised man confront each other with the canker of incurable leprosy in their midst'.[75] Cantlie urged the need for the medical inspection of Chinese migrants using European shipping lines, and for the deportation rather than segregation of all migrant Chinese lepers. Segregation, he argued, merely produced new centres of infection. Cantlie concluded with a picture of leprous Chinese spreading out across the Pacific and 'tainting the world'.[76] Back in Britain, where there was widespread concern about the physical deterioration of the nation prompted by the poor condition of recruits for the South African war, Cantlie returned to the degeneration theme. In *Physical Efficiency* (1906) he once again diagnosed a single problem connecting empire and metropolis: that of 'the wastage of life . . . in the cities of our own country . . . [and] the loss of health and life attaching to the governing and commercial development of our Crown colonies, of the great Empire of India, and of many countries lying within the tropics'.[77]

Although alarm at the physical condition of the metropolitan poor peaked at the beginning of the twentieth century with the government of the day setting up a Committee on Physical Deterioration, it had been a growing concern through the 1880s and 90s. J. Milner Fothergill, member of the College of Physicians and another at this time who was combining medicine with a kind of urban sociology, claimed that the inhabitants of inner-city London constituted a separate species. In *The Town*

---

[74] For biographical material on Cantlie see Mark Harrison's entry in H. C. G. Matthew and Brian Harrison (eds.), *Oxford Dictionary of National Biography, From Earliest Times to the Year 2000* (Oxford: Oxford University Press, 2004), vol. IX, pp. 962–64. On Cantlie and the London School of Tropical Medicine see also G. C. Cook, *From the Greenwich Hulks to Old St. Pancras: A History of Tropical Disease in London* (London: Athlone Press, 1992).

[75] James Cantlie, *Report on the Conditions under which Leprosy Occurs in China, Indo-China, Malaya, the Archipelago and Oceania* (London: Macmillan, 1897), p. 9.

[76] *Ibid.*, p. 125.

[77] James Cantlie, *Physical Efficiency: A Review of the Deleterious Effects of Town Life Upon the Population of Britain, With Suggestions for their Arrest* (London and New York: G. P. Putnam's Sons, 1906), p. 19.

Dweller: His Needs and Wants (1889) Fothergill argued that the city dweller had regressed from the 'Anglo-Dane' to the 'smaller and darker … Celto-Iberian race'. And in the case of 'the true bred cockney of the East End, the most degenerate cockney', reversion had gone ever further. Citing Cantlie's observations and measurements of this group, Fothergill discerned an 'earlier archaic type of man', a pre-Aryan race which had been dispossessed by the Celto-Iberians. This was 'the small and ugly Erse', remnants of which were still to be found in the poorer districts of Ireland.[78] The belief that city dwellers degenerated to older racial types intersected with the contemporary mapping of Africa on to London. William Booth's *In Darkest England and the Way Out* (1890) had signalled this in its title, and in a sustained comparison between H. M. Stanley's account of an African jungle and the modern city. Stanley's equatorial forest, 'where the rays of the sun never penetrate, where in the dark, dank air, filled with the steam of the heated morass, human beings dwarfed into pygmies and brutalized into cannibals lurk and live and die', suggested to Booth the cities of darkest England with their own 'barbarians' and 'pygmies'. The only difference, Booth claims, is that in Britain 'the ghastly devastation is covered, corpselike, with the artificialities and hypocrisies of modern civilization'.[79]

The tropicalising of London, the failure of its inhabitants to acclimatise to the contemporary metropolis, and the concern with degeneration this prompted are frequently linked in late nineteenth-century fiction. George Gissing's *The Nether World* (1889) represents working-class life as nasty, brutal and short. One of its dominant images is of the city as a jungle in which the struggle for survival is never-ending, and in which the strongest and cruellest prevail. Exemplifying this is the character of Clementina Peckover, whose 'forehead was low and of great width', and whose nose 'had large sensual apertures'. She is the 'embodiment of fierce life independent of morality', and her rapacious cruelty, captured in her name, is compared with that of a savage running wild: 'Civilisation could bring no charge against this young woman; it and she had no common criterion.'[80] Even her apparently robust physical condition is somehow debased: 'Her health was probably less sound than it seemed to be; one would have compared her, not to some piece of exuberant normal vegetation, but

---

[78] In Robert Louis Stevenson, *The Strange Case of Dr. Jekyll and Mr. Hyde*, ed. Martin A. Danahay (Peterborough, Ontario: Broadview Press, 2001), Appendix 1, pp. 176–7.

[79] William Booth, *In Darkest England and the Way Out* (London: Charles Knight and Co., 1970), pp. 9–10, 13.

[80] George Gissing, *The Nether World* (London: Dent, 1973), pp. 6, 8.

rather to a rank, evilly-fostered growth. The putrid soil of that nether world yields other forms besides the obviously blighted and sapless.'[81]

Most denizens of Gissing's nether world, however, are of the blighted and sapless kind. Like Cantlie's description of the Spitalfield weavers as 'a stunted puny race, who become prematurely old',[82] they are physically and morally degraded by the squalor, poverty and disease of their environment. The overwhelmingly physical modes of description, used by commentator and novelist alike, focus the degeneration theme. The inhabitants of the imperial centre are increasingly similar to those of tropical colonies and this is most legible in their bodies. Sometimes the comparison is between working-class and native bodies, and sometimes between sickly European bodies at home and abroad. Such interchangeability is characteristic of discussions of degeneration, which once perceived is then seen everywhere.

The standard point of reference for this theme is Max Nordau's *Degeneration*, translated into English in 1895. For Nordau, degeneration expresses itself physically in terms of what he calls 'stigmata':

[D]eformities, multiple and stunted growths in the first line of asymmetry, the unequal development of the two halves of the face and cranium; then imperfection in the development of the external ear, which is conspicuous for its enormous size, or protrudes from the head, like a handle, and the lobe of which is either lacking or adhering to the head ... squint-eyes, hare-lips ... pointed or flat palates, webbed or supernumerary fingers.[83]

The emphasis on facial and cranial deformity suggests how readily the face of the leper could serve as a way of figuring degeneration, a correspondence that is also encouraged by the disease model that Nordau consistently uses. Degeneration is ubiquitous, and is to be found in the 'mental physiognomy' of modern writers and painters, those 'borderland dwellers' between reason and madness, as well as in the distorted bodies of the inhabitants of the modern city.[84] The various maladies threatening civilisation are likened to micro-organisms such as the bacilli of cholera and influenza: 'We stand now in the midst of a ... sort of black death of degeneration and hysteria.'[85] As with Cantlie, however, natural selection is progressive as well as regressive. Although, on the one hand, the black death of modernity seems irresistible, on the other its virulence is bound to abate: 'Degenerates must succumb ... They can neither adapt themselves

[81] *Ibid.*, p. 8.   [82] Cantlie, *Degeneration Amongst Londoners*, p. 39.
[83] Max Nordau, *Degeneration* (London: William Heinemann, 1895), pp. 16–17.
[84] *Ibid.*, pp. 17–18.   [85] *Ibid.*, p. 537.

to the conditions of Nature and civilisation, nor maintain themselves in the struggle for existence against the healthy.'[86]

In like manner, Gissing's *The Unclassed* (1884) presents a striking example of involution in the character of Slimy: 'a very tall creature, with bent shoulders, and head seeming to grow straight out of its chest; thick, grizzled hair hiding almost every vestige of feature, with the exception of one dreadful red eye, its fellow being dead and sightless. He had laid on the counter, with palms downwards as if concealing something, two huge hairy paws.'[87] This evolutionary throwback is at once threatening – he inhabits Litany Lane which is the centre of pollution in the novel – and harmless, in that the sightless eye and other repellent physical features imply there is little possibility that Slimy will reproduce. The degeneration he represents is both deeply disturbing and a dead end.

Degeneration was invariably pathologised, and leprosy, in its gradual, at first invisible, destruction of the body offered a vivid way of figuring this, providing an image with which to fix a culture's fears. Oscar Wilde's *The Picture of Dorian Gray* (1891) is a striking and subtle fictional treatment of the degeneration theme at the end of the century that draws on the figure of leprosy in dramatising the relation between body and portrait. This relation involves a form of othering analogous to that of coloniser and colonised, with the depredations of the former being displaced on to the latter. It also represents the invisible and, therefore, even more disturbing process of degeneration. The contrast between outer and inner, civilisation and vice, beauty and disfigurement, apparent health and festering disease are among the oppositions established by the relation of Dorian's social body in the drawing room to his picture in the attic. As the portrait begins to degenerate Dorian wraps it a Venetian coverlet that is likened to 'a pall for the dead'. The portrait, however, 'had a corruption of its own, worse than the corruption of death itself – something that would breed horrors and yet would never die. What the worm was to the corpse, his sins would be to the painted image on the canvas . . . They would defile it and make it shameful. And yet the thing would still live on. It would be always alive.'[88]

This condition between life and death, grotesquely partaking of both, parallels the manner in which leprosy has often been conceived. Dorian considers with horror the prospect of his cheeks becoming 'hollow or flaccid', of how his mouth 'would gape or droop', of 'the wrinkled

[86] *Ibid.*, p. 541.
[87] George Gissing, *The Unclassed* (Hassocks: Harvester Press, 1976), p. 66.
[88] Oscar Wilde, *The Picture of Dorian Gray*, ed. Norman Page (Peterborough, Ontario: Broadview Press, 2002), p. 153.

throat . . . the twisted body'.[89] This image of degeneration is a caricature of the body's prolonged corruption as it ages towards death.

Dorian is, at first, able to relish the contrast between the perfection of his own body and the corruption of the portrait, placing 'his white hands beside the coarse bloated hands of the picture', mocking 'the misshapen body and the failing limbs'.[90] The self that is represented by the decomposing portrait is repeatedly associated with those diseased parts of outcast London that were felt to threaten the health and integrity of the city. Like Sherlock Holmes, Dorian disguises himself in order to become his alter ego in 'the sordid room of the ill-famed tavern near the Docks',[91] in 'dreadful places near Blue Gate Fields',[92] in the opium-den of Malays, half-castes and syphilitic women of the novel's night-town sequence in chapter 16. Unlike Holmes, however, Dorian dresses as his other to become himself rather than to rescue London from its diseased and outcast quarters (which is not to deny Holmes's fascination with the disorder he cures). The orientalising of the opium-den is familiar and insistent (even one of the haggard prostitutes has 'a crooked smile, like a Malay creese'[93]) but it also undermines the aestheticising of other eastern references that has been central to Dorian's attempt to embroider his life. The 'dainty Delhi muslins', 'Dacca gauzes', 'elaborate yellow Chinese hangings', and 'Japanese Foukousas with their green-toned golds and their marvellously-plumaged birds'[94] that Dorian collects in the West End, lose their decorative power in the East End, that ground zero of the late nineteenth-century cultural imaginary.

Other kinds of relation between Dorian and his portrait, apart from the draping of degeneration with beauty, are explored. Dorian, a proto-modernist, rejects the idea of the ego as 'simple, permanent, reliable, and of one essence', for one in which the self is 'a complex multiform creature . . . whose very flesh was tainted with the monstrous maladies of the dead'.[95] One recalls that, for Nordau, painters and writers were the epitome of contemporary degeneration. In constructing a variety of imagined versions of himself, Dorian consults the portraits of familial ancestors and the narratives of literary and historical antecedents with whom he feels an affinity. Among the ancestors and analogues Dorian considers is Charles VI, 'who had so wildly adored his brother's wife that a leper had warned him of the insanity that was coming on him'.[96] Whatever aesthetic or psychological excursus it explores, the novel always returns to disease, disfiguring and degeneration. The unveiling of the corrupted portrait to the artist who had painted it, Basil Hallward, is the climactic instance.

---

[89] *Ibid.*, p. 156. [90] *Ibid.*, p. 162. [91] *Ibid.* [92] *Ibid.*, p. 173. [93] *Ibid.*, p. 218.
[94] *Ibid.*, pp. 171–2. [95] *Ibid.*, p. 175. [96] *Ibid.*, p. 178.

Although the image is barely recognisable to its creator, the brush-strokes are: 'It was from within, apparently, that the foulness and horror had come. Through some strange quickening of inner life the leprosies of sin were slowly eating the thing away. The rotting of a corpse in a watery grave was not so fearful.'[97] The exposure of the painting is also the exhumation of a living corpse, and leprosy is the chosen image with which to fix the various associations of disease and degeneration that have accrued round it. Dorian must now kill Basil in order to preserve himself intact. The price of this is that the portrait will continue to decompose.

Ultimately the compound of otherness and sameness of the picture becomes intolerable to its subject, and the knife that Dorian has used to kill Basil becomes the weapon of his inadvertent suicide. As Dorian stabs the painting that has been his preserver, determined to expunge that other that is also himself, he unwittingly takes back everything he has projected on to the canvas. The attempt to keep separate body and soul, beauty and decay, health and disease, life and death has failed. The portrait strikes back leaving Dorian dead on the floor with a knife in his heart, 'withered, wrinkled and loathsome of visage'.[98] This conclusion satisfies as well as horrifies. The painting is restored and the threat of degeneration is dispelled. Cantlie and Nordau, for all the pessimism of their cultural diagnosis, had argued that degeneration was unable to perpetuate itself and would therefore die out. In like manner, the end of *The Picture of Dorian Gray* implies that degeneration bears within it the germs of its own destruction. The threat it represents has been overcome and both the painting and the social order are restored. In this respect, Robert Louis Stevenson's *The Strange Case of Dr. Jekyll and Mr. Hyde* (1886) is more troubling. Jekyll is not restored in death. Instead it is the ape-like Hyde, 'in clothes far too large for him',[99] who lies stretched out on the floor of Jekyll's study.

Behind the relative comfort of the ending of Wilde's novel, however, is the failure of Dorian's attempt to keep degeneration at bay. The two worlds of the novel are shown to be one as its polarities of beauty and corruption, and health and disease, collapse. It is not so much that the boundaries between these two worlds are porous as that they are non-existent. Degeneration is not really located in the slums at all, as Cantlie and Gissing suggest, but at the heart of metropolitan culture. And 'non-continuance' extends beyond the tropics and the East End to the cultured world of upper-class London, marked by suicide and seemingly unable to reproduce itself: 'Fin de siècle' murmurs Lord Henry, only to be trumped

---

[97] *Ibid.*, p. 188.   [98] *Ibid.*, p. 251.
[99] Stevenson, *The Strange Case of Dr. Jekyll and Mr. Hyde*, p. 66.

by Lady Narborough's 'Fin du globe.'[100] The corruption of Dorian's soul expresses the degeneration of the social world he charms. This sham world of masks and surfaces is itself diseased and, wealth apart, there is no essential difference between London's West and East End. The attempt to wall one from the other, whether on the personal or social level, is futile.

Leprosy and literature in the Victorian period

Throughout the nineteenth century leprosy had retained its traditional figurative power to express decay and disgust. In *Past and Present* (1843), Thomas Carlyle had used it to express his angry conviction that neglect of the soul was the defining sign of his time. The loss of soul and the misguided belief in the remedies of the 'Body-politic' was a 'plague-spot . . . center of the universal Social Gangrene, threatening all modern things with frightful death'. French Revolutions, Reform Bills and other political remedies – elsewhere dismissed as mere 'Morrison's pills' – are simply analgesics: 'The foul elephantine leprosy, alleviated for an hour, reappears in new force and desperateness next hour.'[101] The 'Body-politic's' belief that it can cure itself is fatal; in the absence of soul, the body must rot. This is a traditional use of leprosy linking the human with the social body in order to express disgust or disquiet at the condition of the world.

Equally traditional, but more personal, is George Eliot's striking use of the disease to express Maggie Tulliver's complicated psychology of guilt in *The Mill on the Floss* (1860). When Stephen Guest passionately kisses Maggie at the dance at Park House, her happiness at his company is 'smitten with a blight – a leprosy'.[102] The intense pleasure she briefly enjoys involves 'treachery' to both her cousin Lucy and her friend Philip, and leprosy is a proleptic figure of the retribution that will follow, anticipating Maggie's ostracism by the town of St Ogg's when she returns after her aborted elopement with Stephen and is shunned as if indeed she were a leper. In associating leprosy with a kiss, Eliot is also drawing on the traditional use of the disease as a consequence of sexual transgression, after the manner of Donne's Elegy IV, 'The Perfume': 'By thee the silly amorous sucks his death / By drawing in a leprous harlot's breath'.

Compared with these traditional uses of the disease, Elizabeth Gaskell's story 'An Accursed Race' (1855) strikes a contemporary note. Its narrator illustrates in vivid and disturbing detail the superstition and fear that

---

[100] Wilde, *The Picture of Dorian Gray*, p. 209.
[101] Thomas Carlyle, *Past and Present* (London: Ward, Lock and Bowden, 1897), pp. 190, 32–3.
[102] George Eliot, *The Mill on the Floss* (Harmondsworth: Penguin, 2003), p. 461.

has prompted the virtual genocide of the Cagot people of western France, who were thought to be lepers. Describing the story as 'a catalogue of persecution', Jenny Uglow sees it as a further example of the sympathy Gaskell had already expressed in her first novel, *Mary Barton* (1848) for 'the leper, the outcast'.[103] However, 'An Accursed Race' is also precisely of its time and derives from the same understanding of leprosy as hereditary and non-infectious that Milroy was to expound and the Royal College of Physicians to defend. Its narrator shares Milroy's distaste for stigmatising the disease and segregating those who were believed to have contracted it. The story reveals the arbitrariness of identifying the leper, describing with heavy irony how although it is self-evident that all Cagots are lepers, they are actually so difficult to distinguish from other people that an identifying mark such as a piece of red or yellow cloth, or the foot of a duck or goose sewn prominently on their dress, is needed. In fact, the narrator continues, 'there are two kinds of leprosy, one perceptible and the other imperceptible, even to the person suffering from it'.[104] 'An Accursed Race' is narrated as if it were a lecture, but irony consistently undermines its apparently reasonable tone and makes clear the ignorance and prejudice, encouraged by church and state, that produces and sustains exclusion and stigma. Science is helpless in the face of politically and religiously sanctioned prejudice. A medical report establishing there was no physical reason why Cagots should be kept apart merely intensified the insistence on difference and exclusion. Milroy was to feel that he experienced something similar throughout the 1870s. Gaskell's story, therefore, is a developed literary expression of the mid-century hereditarian understanding of leprosy. Its corollary was a liberal critique of exclusion and segregation.

Subsequent nineteenth-century imaginative writing was to remain preoccupied with boundaries and their transgression, though with an increasing concern to reinforce rather than remove the leper line. Swinburne's poem 'The Leper', first published in *Poems and Ballads* (1865), purports to come from an early sixteenth-century French text, telling the story of a lascivious noble Lady cursed with leprosy, cast out by her family and former lovers, and tended until her death by a clerk, her servant. Like 'An Accursed Race' it takes us back into a late medieval world in which leprosy was rife, sexualised and rigorously segregated, but Swinburne's poem is radical and transgressive rather than liberal and humanitarian.

---

[103] Jenny Uglow, *Elizabeth Gaskell: A Habit of Stories* (London: Faber and Faber, 1993), p. 472.

[104] Elizabeth Gaskell, 'An Accursed Race', in *My Lady Ludlow and Other Stories*, ed. Edgar Wright (Oxford: World's Classics, 1989), pp. 217–18.

'The Leper' takes its place in a tradition running from Browning's 'Porphyria's Lover' and Tennyson's *Maud* to John Fowles' novel *The Collector*, in which obsessive love becomes diseased and necrotic. According to the prose note that Swinburne attached to the poem, the clerk, 'remembering this woman's former great beauty, [now] ravaged, often delighted in kissing her foul and leprous mouth and in caressing her gently with his loving hands'. In the poem itself, which is spoken by the clerk, the leprous woman becomes a figure for the morbid love of the monologist. When the Lady was in health the clerk was fixated on particular parts of her body: the space 'between her brows', 'Her curled-up lips and amorous hair', and her feet. These repeated descriptions suggest the displaced or transposed objects of the fetishist. Her feet, both of which 'could lie into my hand', are imaginatively transposed into breasts, and the fixation on her brows becomes vaginal. As the Lady decomposes and dies the clerk continues 'For joy to kiss between her brows', and to hold 'In two cold palms her cold two feet':

> Love bites and stings me through, to see
> Her keen face made of sunken bones.
> Her worn-off eyelids madden me,
> That were shot through with purple once.

The speaker is sexually excited by the Lady's purulent state: 'keen' compresses emaciation, fervour, coldness and death into one packed adjective; the toe-curling 'worn-off eyelids', once adjacent to that space between her brows, are simultaneously arousing and frustrating. The horror of the poem lies in the lack of horror felt by its speaker.

'The Leper', therefore, is a poem about transgression. The most obvious form this takes is the transgression of social rank, that stock feature of romance. But overwhelmingly, and in total contrast to the romance plot, is the transgression of the fundamental boundary separating life from death. I have earlier referred to Julia Kristeva's category of the 'abject body' and suggested that the body of the leper can be understood as the most disturbing variant of this category. Alive but putrefying, decomposing while still able to reproduce, even more than the corpse it challenges the distinction between life and death. This is a fundamental reason why leprosy has horrified and fascinated Judeo-Christian cultures since biblical times, and the segregation practised by these cultures can be understood as akin to the rituals surrounding the treatment of the dead.

Swinburne's clerk accompanies the Lady 'without the camp', defying the rule of segregation, but the most disturbing of his transgressions is the lascivious pleasure in her wasting, rotting body. He delights in her incompleteness, scorning the idea of wholeness upon which, Mary Douglas has argued, our fundamental ideas of purity and order are based.[105] The integrity of the body, and its importance as an expression of cherished, fundamental distinctions and categories, is challenged and undermined by the clerk's pleasure in the Lady's imperfections. She is no longer the perfect container. As a 'syphilitic leper' her body is turning inside out, revealing its contents as another fundamental boundary, that between the visceral self and the world, erodes. Swinburne's poem lays all this bare. Rather than concealing or displacing the source of our fear of leprosy, the clerk makes it visible by transforming fascinated horror into perverse pleasure, by revelling in danger, not purity. In doing this, the poem confronts and mocks the Judeo-Christian response to the figure of the leper. It also anticipates, shadows and parodies the sacrifices of Father Damien, Albert Schweitzer, Graham Greene's Dr Colin and other modern saints. Morally 'burnt out', the clerk is perversely attentive, meticulous and scrupulous, a diseased saint whose necrotic fantasies and obsessions dissolve yet another cherished distinction, and ironise one of the stock redeeming types of the modern colonial period.

By the late nineteenth century leprosy was being used figuratively in many different situations and settings. In Bram Stoker's *Dracula* (1897), for example, Mina Harker sobs 'Unclean, unclean!' after her neck has been pierced by the Count and declares that she must no longer touch or kiss her husband.[106] When Van Helsing tries to protect her from further contamination by touching her forehead with a sacred wafer it burns and brands her flesh, causing Mina to pull her hair over her face 'as the leper of old his mantle', while she repeats the cry of 'Unclean! Unclean!'[107] Somewhat later as the corruption becomes visible in her features – 'the characteristics of the vampire coming in her face'[108] – the description is reminiscent of how the emerging features of the leper, such as thickened forehead and elongated ears, were frequently depicted.

Other treatments of leprosy in the writing of the high imperialist era are more explicit. Two such stories are Kipling's 'The Mark of the Beast' published in the collection *Life's Handicap* (1900), and Conan Doyle's 'The Adventure of the Blanched Soldier', a late Sherlock Holmes story published in 1926 but set in 1903 in the aftermath of the South African war. These stories are, above all, concerned to maintain boundaries. In both, the border between health and illness, purity and danger, coloniser and

---

[105] Mary Douglas, *Purity and Danger: An Analysis of Concepts of Pollution and Taboo* (Harmondsworth: Penguin, 1970), pp. 65–70.
[106] Bram Stoker, *Dracula* (Oxford: World's Classics, 1996), p. 284.
[107] *Ibid.*, p. 296.   [108] *Ibid.*, p. 323.

colonised is threatened but survives, and is strengthened as a result. Kipling's treatment of this is altogether more edgy than Doyle's. 'The Mark of the Beast' opens at the liminal moment of New Year's Eve. The setting is a station club, somewhere in the Himalayas. As the anonymous narrator puts it: 'When men foregather from the uttermost ends of the Empire they have a right to be riotous.'[109] After a night of heavy drinking, revels and maudlin nostalgia, the main protagonist, Fleete, 'gorgeously drunk',[110] is helped home by the narrator and by Strickland of the Police (who figures in other Kipling stories). Passing the temple of Hanuman, the monkey-god, Fleete rushes inside and stubs out his cigar on the forehead of the image of the god, declaring; 'Mark of the B-beasht! I made it. Ishn't it fine?' In response, a Silver Man appears from a recess behind the image: 'He was perfectly naked ... and his body shone like frosted silver, for he was what the Bible calls "a leper as white as snow." Also he had no face, because he was a leper of some years' standing, and his disease was heavy upon him.' The Silver Man holds Fleete and 'nuzzles' his head on the Englishman's breast, mewing like an otter.[111]

Fleete is immediately taken with shivering fits, sweating, and repeated scratching of his left breast. Next morning he is strangely marked, keeps demanding underdone chops that he eats like an animal, and his proximity to the horses drives them into a frenzy. His increasingly bestial actions are set against the civilised behaviour of the other two as they ponder Fleete's transformation. As they pass the temple the Silver Man comes out and mews at them. Fleete has begun rolling in the garden and howling like a wolf. The black leopard-rosette mark on his breast has blistered, and mewing is now heard outside the house. Fleete (now 'it', the personal pronoun is temporarily dropped) is tied up and gagged, and a doctor is summoned who diagnoses hydrophobia. However Strickland and the narrator know that this case is beyond medicine. Desperate situations require desperate measures.

Armed with polo sticks they capture the Silver Man, now described as 'the leper', and tie him down. The problem is how to assault something you cannot touch. When the narrator places his foot on the leper's neck, 'even through my riding-boots I could feel that his flesh was not the flesh of a

[109] Rudyard Kipling, 'The Mark of the Beast', in *Life's Handicap* (London: Macmillan, 1900), p. 241.
[110] *Ibid.*, p. 244.
[111] *Ibid.*, p. 243. Another striking use of leprosy in Kipling's *oeuvre* is the poem 'Gehazi' (1915), a distasteful attack on Rufus Issacs: 'What means the risen whiteness / Of the skin between thy brows? / The boils that shine and burrow, / The sores that slough and bleed – / The leprosy of Naaman / On thee and all thy seed?' The poem ends: 'Gehazi, Judge in Israel, / A leper white as snow!'

clean man'.[112] Strickland has had the barrels of his shotgun heating in the fire, and the leper is tortured into removing 'the evil spirit' from Fleete. In assisting with this, the narrator comes to understand how it must have been to see a witch burnt alive: 'though the Silver Man had no face, you could see the horrible feelings passing through the slab that took its place, exactly as waves of heat play across red-hot iron – gun-barrels for instance'.[113] Fleete's mark disappears, the leper departs no longer mewing, Strickland has a fit of hysterics and the narrator, struck that we 'had fought for Fleete's soul ... and had disgraced ourselves as Englishmen for ever ... laughed and gasped and gurgled just as shamefully as Strickland'.[114] The story's resolution is both sadistic and guilty. Fleete's plight justifies the savage attack on the leper but leaves the assailants feeling they have crossed the divide separating the Englishman from the native. The infected other can only be defeated by letting go of one's Englishness and becoming a version of that other. Fear of the invisible or the unknown, whether in the form of disease, religion or, more broadly, that region 'East of Suez' (the story's opening words) provokes a desire for revenge in the mind of the coloniser. However, this in turn is brought up against the impossible task of destroying what cannot be understood or even touched. In Kipling's story the Silver Man capitulates but his power remains, indeed is confirmed by the touch of his hands that cures Fleete and renders the Englishmen's victory pyrrhic. Strickland's suggestion, years after the event, that the incident should now be put before the public suggests, not unlike the ancient mariner's tale, the guilt of the witness and the survivor.

Like most leprosy stories, 'The Mark of the Beast' is sexualised. It is a story without women in which, nevertheless, masculinity is identified with imperialism and femininity is seen as inimical to it. There is a long, well-documented tradition of representing colonised peoples, and Hindus in particular, as feminine. Typically, this is understood as a way of representing the docility of the indigene. The Silver Man in Kipling's story is conspicuously feminised, though to opposite effect. The Biblical leper 'white as snow' was Miriam (Numbers 12), and the Silver Man's action of taking Fleete 'round the body' and dropping his head on his victim's breast underlines this feminisation.[115] It is also reinforced by the repeated mewing sound uttered by the leper, which is compared to that of a she-otter, and the feline leopard-markings that disfigure Fleete. Leprosy, therefore, comes from the temple in the form of a feminised native, and this diseased femininity prompts Fleete's animalistic behaviour. It also

---

[112] Kipling, 'The Mark of the Beast', p. 255.   [113] *Ibid.*, p. 256.   [114] *Ibid.*, p. 258.
[115] *Ibid.*, p. 243.

seems to be a coded expression of anxieties about miscegenation. The antidote to all this comes from a pair of male friends, apparently bachelors who, in the narrator's words, fight for Fleete's soul with the Silver Man. Clearly there is more than the soul of one man at stake.

Conan Doyle's 'The Adventure of the Blanched Soldier' is set just after the end of the 'Boer War'. James Dodd, late of the Imperial Yeomanry, has been seeking his former comrade-in-arms Godfrey Emsworth, shot in action outside Pretoria and now disappeared, said by his family to have gone on a voyage round the world. While visiting the Emsworths' country house, Dodd sees his friend's face pressed against the window, a 'ghastly face glimmering as white as cheese in the darkness ... [with] something slinking, something furtive, something guilty – something very unlike the frank, manly lad that I had known' about it.[116] This leads him to a building in the garden where he catches a rear view of his friend, sitting in the company of a man in a black coat. Caught spying by Emsworth's father, a Crimean VC, Dodd is expelled from the house and comes straight to Holmes.

In this story Holmes is for once on his own: 'The good Watson had deserted me for a wife, the only selfish action which I can recall in our association. I was alone.'[117] Without his amanuensis Holmes is obliged to tell his own story, and in trying to avoid what he describes as Watson's 'meretricious finales',[118] he concentrates instead on the inner narrative related by Emsworth once the secret (leprosy, of course) has been exposed. Shot through the shoulder with an elephant bullet and left for dead, Emsworth had staggered into a remote house and collapsed into an empty, unmade bed. He woke to find himself in a bare, whitewashed dormitory with 'a small dwarf-like man with a huge, bulbous head ... waving two horrible hands which looked ... like brown sponges' standing over him. Arrayed round him was a group of laughing people: 'Not one of them was a normal human being. Every one was twisted or swollen or disfigured in some strange way. The laughter of these strange monstrosities was a dreadful thing to hear.'[119] Emsworth had strayed into a Leper Hospital and, still bleeding from his wounds, had spent the night in a leper's bed.[120]

This nightmare scene of waking in an infected bed surrounded by the diseased suggests a related upper-class male horror of waking after a night

---

[116] Arthur Conan Doyle, 'The Adventure of the Blanched Soldier', in *The Complete Sherlock Holmes* (Harmondsworth: Penguin, 1981), p. 1004.
[117] *Ibid.*, p. 1000.   [118] *Ibid.*, p. 1008.   [119] *Ibid.*, p. 1009.
[120] Doyle had visited a leper hospital on a visit to Norway in 1892. See Martin Booth, *The Doctor, the Detective and Arthur Conan Doyle: A Biography* (London: Hodder and Stoughton, 1998), p. 173.

on the town to discover a syphilitic prostitute alongside.[121] It has several other interesting features. The 'creature with the big head', whose sheets Emsworth has been sleeping in, makes furious attempts to drag the intruder from his bed, 'uttering wild-beast cries',[122] before Emsworth is rescued by the hospital doctor, an anticipation of the story's denouement. As in 'The Mark of the Beast' leprosy is animalistic, grotesquely violent rather than abjectly passive; the detail of the elephant gun also gains resonance in this context. Unlike Kipling's story, however, the infecting agent seems to be Dutch rather than native. This is a war between competing colonising powers, and although disease thrives in warm latitudes and colonial terrains (Holmes's knowledge that leprosy is common in South Africa helps him to solve the mystery), in this particular setting the main problem is not with native subjects but colonial rivals.

When Holmes forces Emsworth to come out of hiding, leprosy seems self-evident: 'One could see that he had indeed been a handsome man with clear-cut features sunburned by an African sun, but mottled in patches over this darker surface were curious whitish patches which had bleached his skin.'[123] Not for the first time, however, Emsworth is to be rescued by a doctor. An unnamed third person has travelled with Holmes and Dodd from London, and remained outside in the carriage while Holmes confronts the family. He proves to be Sir James Saunders, 'the great dermatologist', of 'austere figure ... [and] sphinx-like features', who is able to diagnose the affliction as 'pseudo-leprosy or ichthyosis ... unsightly, obstinate, but possibly curable, and certainly noninfective'.[124]

Doctors are particularly significant in this story. Emsworth is rescued by one, guarded by another, and saved from a living death by a third. The first, in the Leper Hospital, offers help and some comfort; the second maintains the cordon sanitaire placed around Emsworth by his family; the third is able to dispel the horror through his specialised knowledge and expertise. The ordinary doctor provides comfort and assistance, but the specialist in the carriage waiting to be called upon to resolve the mystery is, for Doyle at least, a modern deus ex machina. The figure of the detective is

---

[121] In particular it recalls Frank Harris's account of Randolph Churchill waking up in an unfamiliar room. 'The paper on the walls was hideous – dirty – and ... there was an old woman lying beside me; one thin strand of dirty grey hair was on the pillow ... She had one long yellow tooth in her top jaw that waggled as she spoke.' Churchill rushed straight to the doctor terrified that he had contracted syphilis. Frank Harris, *My Life and Loves*, ed. John F. Gallagher (London: W. H. Allen, 1964), pp. 483–4. Although R. F. Foster describes Harris's account of how Churchill contracted syphilis as 'unlikely' it has representative if not particular truth. R. F. Forster, *Lord Randolph Churchill: A Political Life* (Oxford: Oxford University Press, 1981), p. 389.
[122] Doyle, 'The Adventure of the Blanched Soldier', p. 1010.   [123] *Ibid.*, p. 1009.
[124] *Ibid.*, p. 1012.

another. Several critics have drawn attention to the ways in which Holmes's ability to decipher the human body is crucial to the defence of the social body.[125] This was understood by G. K. Chesterton at the time:

[T]he romance of police activity keeps ... before the mind the fact that civilisation itself is the most sensational of departures and the most romantic of rebellions. By dealing with the unsleeping sentinels who guard the outposts of society, it tends to remind us that we live in an armed camp, making war with a chaotic world, and that the criminals, the children of chaos, are nothing but the traitors within our gates.[126]

The threat from without is at least as great and probably harder to contain. Holmes's cases often involve characters that have lived abroad in colonial settings, and leprosy figures in at least one other story. In 'The Yellow Face' (1893) the secret offspring of a remarried widow is disguised and hidden in a picturesque cottage close to her mother's new home, a villa at Norbury, on the edge of London. The startling face of this child – first described as 'a livid chalky white', later as 'yellow livid'[127] – leads to Holmes being called in to perform his ritual unmasking. Significantly perhaps, this is one of the few cases Holmes gets wrong. He surmises that the face is of the woman's first husband who must have 'contracted some loathsome disease and become a leper or an imbecile'. When he peels off the literal mask of this story, however, he reveals 'a little coal-black negress, with all her white teeth flashing'.[128] As in 'The Blanched Soldier', the threat of leprosy is dispelled but the resolution is uneasy. Although the second husband accepts his responsibility as a step-parent, the black face behind the yellow mask discovered in this 'pretty two-storied place, with an old-fashioned porch and a honeysuckle about it'[129] continues to disturb. In both these stories the country house, or the house in the country, acts as a last line of defence, aided by the vigilance of the detective and, where necessary, the expertise of the medical specialist. Although in both cases the threat of leprosy is imaginary, it serves nevertheless as a reminder that the arbitrary and invisible menace of disease is the hardest of all foreign bodies to guard against and detect. If it were to get beyond the country house into the teeming modern city it would cause untold damage at the heart of empire.

---

[125] Rosemary Jann, 'Sherlock Holmes Codes the Social Body', *ELH*, 57 (1990), 685–705; Ronald R. Thomas, 'The Fingerprint of the Foreigner: Colonising the Criminal Body in 1890s Detective Fiction and Criminal Anthropology', *ELH*, 61 (1994), 655–83.

[126] G. K. Chesterton, *The Defendant* (London: Dent, 1901), p. 161.

[127] Arthur Conan Doyle, 'The Yellow Face', in *The Complete Sherlock Holmes* (Harmondsworth: Penguin, 1981), pp. 355, 357.

[128] *Ibid.*, p. 361.   [129] *Ibid.*, p. 354.

Kipling's story, set at the frontier of empire, must do without the protection of the detective and the specialist, and has none of Doyle's faith in medicine. The doctor in 'The Mark of the Beast', Dr Dumoise, is mistaken in his diagnosis and rather put out when Fleete recovers, feeling that his professional reputation had been injured. Medical science, especially when practised by a Frenchman, is found wanting; instead we have the rough medicine and justice of the English colonists. Only the Silver Man has the power to lift the curse, even if colonial torture provides the incentive. But the confidence in science which Doyle's story seems to express is also shakily founded. If it really were leprosy that Emsworth had contracted then modern medicine would have been helpless. According to contemporary medical opinion, Emsworth should have been infected, believes he was, but has actually had a miraculous escape. The doctor in the Leper Hospital, who considers himself immune to the disease by now, nevertheless makes clear he would still not lie in a leper's sheets. In the closing paragraph the great dermatologist suggests a psychological basis for Emsworth's infection. Fear of contagion has resulted in a simulation of its symptoms. If this is so, then although medical science can allay some of the phobias of colonialism it is helpless when faced with real infection. The story, therefore, dramatises the modern colonial horror of leprosy, the mystery of its transmission, and the absence of treatment or cure rather than the conquest of leprosy by medical science.

A final point of comparison underlines this. In Kipling's story the infection of Fleete is provoked and therefore, in a sense, justified. Sacrilege is committed, even though it is presented as a drunken prank and quickly forgotten as the story comes to focus on saving the Englishman. Revenge stories only make sense within some kind of moral scheme. In Doyle's story, however, infection is arbitrary and inadvertent. Emsworth is fighting valiantly for the British empire and does nothing to disgrace himself as an Englishman. His supposed infection is, within the terms and assumptions of the story, quite arbitrary, and his deliverance at the end of the story equally capricious. 'The Adventure of the Blanched Soldier' is more concerned than 'The Mark of the Beast' to dispel uncertainty and restore order, but remains visibly troubled by the disorder it seeks to contain.

Ultimately both stories are fantasies. Leprosy is understood as both an unavoidable imperial risk and an intolerable imperial burden. Kipling's story is concerned with its danger in a colonial setting; Doyle's with the danger it would present if brought back to the metropolitan centre. Its threat, however, is dispelled by violent retribution in one, and through the diagnostic authority of modern medicine in the other. Common to both is the importance of male friends in offering relief. Sir James Saunders clears up the mistake but this would never have happened without the loyal, loving friendship of Dodd. As he explains to Holmes (who is himself without his friend and chronicler Watson): 'We formed a friendship – the sort of friendship which can only be made when one lives the same life and shares the same joys and sorrows.'[130] A more complex version of this kind of relationship binds the narrator of Kipling's story to Strickland and Fleete. Based on the codes and practices of the public school, the army and the colonial service, and reinforced by the isolation and incipient paranoia of living as a dominant but minority group, both authors pit male comradeship against the invisible or unrecognised dangers of imperialism, calling it up to ease the anxieties and guilt of that project.

Summary

This chapter began by discussing tropical medicine as a response to the perceived inability of Europeans to acclimatise to the tropical regions of the modern colonial world, and to the accompanying fear of physical and moral corruption in these zones. It also viewed tropical medicine as a response to the increased contact between Westerners and indigenes in colonial settings, and between colony and metropole. The fears arising from this contact were, in turn, magnified by the emergent germ theory of disease. The common belief that the tropics were dangerous fever nests, uninhabitable by Europeans for any prolonged period, intensified at the moment when the tropics themselves were of increasing economic and imperial importance for European powers and the United States. Consequently there was a pressing need to redefine the relation between tropical and temperate zones, and between metropole and colony. Health and disease were an important element in this refashioned grammar of difference, and tropical medicine played a significant role in naturalising the basis upon which difference was constructed. In doing so, tropical medicine selected those diseases that threatened Europeans in tropical climates rather than including all diseases that presented a danger to tropical populations. It was also centred in the metropolis rather than the colony, becoming a laboratory-based study of the clinical treatment of these diseases rather than an epidemiological study of disease incidence, control and prevention.

The new science of tropical medicine was therefore one of several kinds of attempt to put a fence around Europe and around the European in the tropics. It was, in other words, what Laura Otis has called a membrane, an

---

[130] Doyle, 'The Adventure of the Blanched Soldier', p. 1001.

attempt to preserve identity by sealing the metropole and the coloniser from the world they were colonising. This membrane, however, mediating as it did between those two worlds, was necessarily of a semi-permeable kind, a filter rather than a wall. This, in turn, heightened the anxiety over boundaries and their transgression. The discovery that invisible germs spread by human contact could penetrate bodies and cause illness was transforming perceptions of inter-human and inter-cultural relations. Koch's notion of the 'healthy carrier', previously mentioned, which rendered all people potentially suspect, added to the feeling of being surrounded by invisible enemies. By the late nineteenth century it was feared that imperial bodies might be in danger from colonised ones even when they were at home. There was also the associated worry that degeneration was occurring in the metropole even when there was no direct contact with the outlying colonial world. The alarm over leprosy was one expression of this, and the invention of tropical medicine was an attempt to describe and control this process.

Another important function served by the category of tropical medicine was that it enabled and justified coercive forms of medical intervention in colonised territories. By assisting the capacity of settlers to survive in the tropics, and by pathologising native populations, it could be used to implement forms of segregation at times of epidemic disease.[131] By the end of the nineteenth century the imperial response to leprosy had become a distinctively punitive form of coercion in which segregation was very often for life. There was to be nothing permeable about this particular membrane. The next section of this book will examine the spread and institutionalisation of the leper colony in the later nineteenth century, which developed into an extreme example of the boundary thinking that had come to dominate relations between colony and metropole.

---

[131] Shula Marks, 'What is Colonial about Colonial Medicine?', *Social History of Medicine*, 10: 1 (1997), 213.

4 Segregation in the high imperial era: island leper colonies on Hawaii, at the Cape, in Australia and New Zealand

Total institutions

Isolation of one kind and another was a time-honoured way of dealing with leprosy. Compulsory segregation, however, only became widespread in the later nineteenth century, and even then there was variation across the imperial world. In most parts of Africa colonial governments lacked the resources to enforce segregation, and in India the scale of the problem defied any such policy. The most rigorous application of the compulsory segregation of lepers occurred in smaller colonies with a higher proportion of European settlers. Many of these were island colonies in the Caribbean, Pacific and Indian Oceans, or coastal ones such as the Cape Colony or around the fringe of the island continent of Australia. Such settlements typically had offshore or contiguous islands where lepers could be removed and detained. Although there were many inland leper colonies as well, island ones best typified the new forms of intervention and institutionalisation that marked the response to leprosy in this period. They were also an especially visible example of more general disease practice and related forms of control that were central to the repertoire of high imperialism.

In this section I shall consider and compare several island leper colonies from different parts of the late nineteenth- and early twentieth-century imperial world. Islands, because of their bounded geography, have frequently been used for detention and quarantine. They are natural sites of concentration, places where contaminants from the mainland can be dumped. Although Foucault argued that the madman replaced the leper as the liminal figure of early modernity, one of his prime markers of this change, the *Narrenschiff* or Ship of Fools, is curiously apt for the treatment of the leper in the modern colonial period.[1] In Hawaii, Cape Colony,

---

[1] Michel Foucault, *Madness and Civilisation: A History of Insanity in the Age of Reason* (London: Tavistock Publications, 1979), pp. 3–11.

Australia and New Zealand lepers, like Foucault's madmen, were expelled and delivered across the dividing and purifying element of water to a place of permanent exile. This, in effect, was the modern equivalent of the medieval ritual of separation in which as lepers stood in a grave the priest tossed three spadefuls of earth on their head, announcing they were dead to the world but would be reborn in God.[2] Islands were ideal sites for such death-in-life. They removed the visibly diseased leper from the sight of the healthy and isolated the threat of infection.

These island graveyards for the still-living, halfway houses on the road to eventual salvation, can usefully be understood in terms of Erving Goffman's theory of 'total institutions'. Goffman defines such institutions in terms of their encompassing character expressed through barriers to communication with the outside and to departure: 'locked doors, high walls, barbed wire, cliffs, water, forests or moors'.[3] Although he limits his discussion to metropolitan institutions it can readily be extended to many of the practices and techniques of colonialism. The island leper colony, in particular, is almost the caricature of a total institution. Whereas Goffman's total institution must sustain a controlled relationship between itself and the outside world that can then be used as 'strategic leverage' in managing its inmates,[4] the leper colony aims to sever that relationship entirely. Especially in leper colonies run by missionaries, mediation was not between the institutional world and the home world of the leper, but between the leper colony and the afterlife. The incommutable life sentence of leprosy in fact removed most of the sanctions that managers of less absolutely total institutions had at their disposal. S. P. Impey, Surgeon-Superintendent of the Robben Island leper colony off Cape Town in the early 1890s, remarked on how troublesome lepers were to deal with: 'You cannot starve them and you cannot flog them; all you can do is to deprive them of their liberty.'[5] And although the island seemed ideal for this purpose, allowing, as Impey remarked, control to be exerted without stirring public opinion, it also reinforced solidarity among inmates with absolutely nothing to lose. One leprosy worker in Nyasaland recalled that her patients referred to themselves as 'The Dead'.[6] Managing detainees was difficult when there were no sanctions left to impose.

[2] Megan Vaughan, *Curing their Ills: Colonial Power and African Illness* (Stanford, Calif.: Stanford University Press, 1991), p. 79.

[3] Erving Goffman, *Asylums: Essays on the Social Situation of Mental Patients and Other Inmates* (Harmondsworth: Penguin, 1975), pp. 15–16.

[4] *Ibid.*, p. 24.

[5] Harriet Deacon, 'A History of the Medical Institutions on Robben Island, Cape Colony 1846–1910' (unpublished PhD thesis, University of Cambridge, 1994), p. 227.

[6] Vaughan, *Curing their Ills*, p. 87.

Another characteristic of Goffman's total institution is that inmates undergo a mortification of the self. They are absorbed into their new environment in such a way as to strip them of their previous identity.[7] This process involves 'various forms of disfigurement and defilement through which the symbolic meaning of events ... fails to corroborate [the inmate's] prior conception of self'.[8] In the case of the leper, however, this mortification and disfigurement has quite literally begun prior to being detained; it is the very reason for their incarceration. In a sense, therefore, one of the defining practices of Goffman's total institution precedes admission, being performed by the disease itself. Then, with tragic irony, this becomes the limited ground of their severely circumscribed freedom within the most total of institutions.

The final stage in this process involves what Goffman terms a 'reassembly of the self' through 'institutional colonisation'.[9] This was especially prominent in mission-run leper colonies. Megan Vaughan, in her study of African leper colonies in this period, describes the missionary-led attempt to engineer a 'leper identity' through the projection of a powerful Christian disease symbolism. Only when lepers relinquished their previous social identities and allowed the disease to define them would they find 'peace'.[10] While 'peace' seems an unlikely outcome of their situation, many inmates of leper colonies were probably persuaded to redefine themselves as 'lepers', although as Megan Vaughan points out, the degree of this acceptance is difficult to assess, not least because of our heavy dependence on missionary sources for knowledge of the inhabitants themselves.[11] But, as we shall see, acceptance of the leper identity did not necessarily lead to quiescent subjects. The uncompromisingly total nature of leper colonies, particularly those situated on islands, removed the very basis for controlled negotiation upon which the successful management of a total institution depended.

Molokai

Robert Louis Stevenson visited the leper colony on Molokai a month after Damien's death. He described the 'gloomy and abrupt' windward coast of the island with its wall of cliff, between two and three thousand feet in height, at the base of which was a low flat volcanic peninsula, several miles wide and jutting a mile or so out into the ocean.[12] It was here, following the

---

[7] Goffman, *Asylums*, pp. 24–5, 32.   [8] *Ibid.*, p. 40.   [9] *Ibid.*, pp. 57, 62.
[10] Vaughan, *Curing their Ills*, pp. 77, 86.   [11] *Ibid.*, p. 85.
[12] Robert Louis Stevenson, *Travels in Hawaii*, ed. A. Grove Day (Honolulu: University of Hawaii Press, 1973), p. 46.

(a)

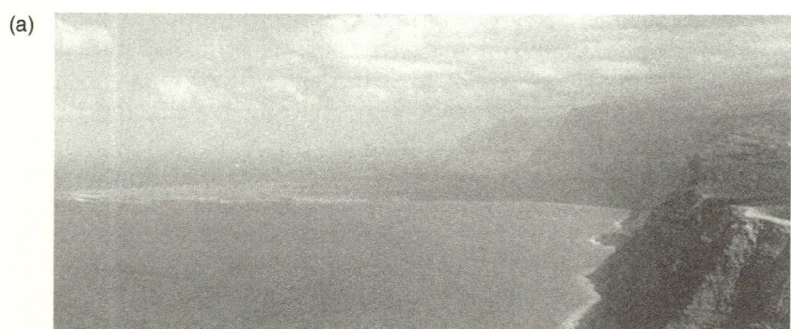

(b)

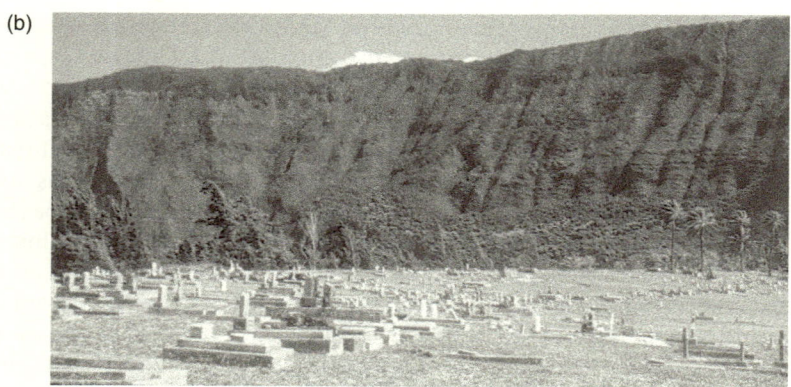

Figure 4. (a) Kalaupapa peninsula, Molokai. (National Park Service, Hawaii).
(b) Graveyard at Kalaupapa. Photo by author.

passing of an 'Act to Prevent the Spread of Leprosy' in 1865, that lepers
had been isolated and a rudimentary settlement established at Kalawao on
the eastern shore of the peninsula.

The first cases of leprosy in the Hawaiian group had been detected
around mid-century, and it was believed that the disease had been introduced by Chinese indentured labourers brought in to work on the newly
established sugar plantations; hence its original Hawaiian name of *mai
Pake*, the Chinese disease. By the 1860s, it had become a predominantly
native disease, although there were a few cases of European infection as
well. The continuing spread of leprosy caused particular alarm among the
white settler population of Honolulu and from the 1870s a rigorous
segregation policy was enforced. The islands were scoured for lepers, and
those detained were removed to Molokai. Infected Hawaiians often went

into hiding with their families to escape detention. The native name for the disease had now become *mai ho'okawale*, the separating sickness. The agency used to name the disease had shifted from the supposed source of infection, the Chinese, to the policy regulating its treatment. In many native eyes the so-called remedy was worse than the disease. Indeed, not only were Hawaiians normally prepared to shelter their afflicted, but some chose to live with them at the colony as *kokua*, or helpers.

Segregation, however, was not simply a Western imposition on a native population indifferent to its own health. Hawaii remained formally independent of the United States until 1898, and segregation had the support of the Hawaiian royal family alarmed at the depopulation of its people. Even one of its own members, Peter Kaeo, the part-European cousin of the Queen, spent three years on Molokai before being allowed to return to die in Honolulu.[13] But this was exceptional. Those sent to Molokai were overwhelmingly Hawaiian or part-Hawaiian commoners. Most of the small number of Europeans found to have the disease were able to buy their way out of the hands of the examining physician and leave the islands.[14] The segregation policy, then, was overwhelmingly but not exclusively racial. Class was a factor too, while the very small number of Europeans at the colony reflected the low incidence of leprosy among the white population as well as racially based distinctions between its victims.

Although segregation failed to stem the disease, by the 1880s its implementation had become even stricter. More than 5 per cent of the national budget was now being spent on efforts to control leprosy, an allocation without parallel elsewhere in the world.[15] In part this reflected the prosperity of the islands. A commercial treaty with the United States in the 1870s had guaranteed the Hawaiian sugar industry a market, white plantation owners were making large profits and government tax revenues were swelling. But it also reflected fear. Cases of European infection continued, although their proportion remained very low. The white Protestant establishment's insistence that leprosy was a native disease became as much a hope as a conviction. After the limitation of the powers of the Hawaiian King in 1887 (a prelude to the end of the monarchy in 1893 and United States annexation in 1898), enforcement of the segregation laws was unequivocally a matter of colonial power exerted by the United States government.

From the point of view of the settlers the leprous body of the Hawaiian threatened their own clean form with contamination and death. Their

[13] Gavan Daws, *Holy Man: Father Damien of Molokai* (Honolulu: University of Hawaii Press, 1973), pp. 79–82.
[14] *Ibid.*, p. 132.   [15] *Ibid.*, p. 71.

unease was intensified by the sexualisation of leprosy. At first this was a way of keeping leprosy at a distance, allowing it to be moralised as a just punishment for a diseased society, something rooted in the promiscuous sexuality of the indigenous culture. The old tradition of associating leprosy with syphilis was revived in the 1880s by a government physician who argued that the disease was the final stage in the course of syphilis. This association of leprosy with race, sex and dirt lay behind the unfounded charges that Damien had contracted the disease from having sexual intercourse with native patients on Molokai. The slander originated from a Protestant clergyman and schoolmaster in Honolulu, Charles McEwan Hyde, and produced in turn a blistering response from Robert Louis Stevenson in the form of his 'Open Letter to the Reverend Dr. Hyde of Honolulu'. Stevenson had picked up the story in a Sydney newspaper in 1890, and the name of Damien's accuser must have added spice to his passionate defence of the missionary. *The Strange Case of Dr Jekyll and Mr Hyde* had been published four years earlier and the spectacle of an apparently pious clergyman spreading malicious gossip about the saintly Damien must have been an irresistible invitation.

Hyde's opinion of Damien was expressed in a private letter to a fellow Protestant clergyman in California and had been published without his knowledge. He described Damien as 'a coarse, dirty man ... not a pure man in his relations with women', and suggested that 'the leprosy of which he died should be attributed to his own vices and carelessness'.[16] There was no evidence whatsoever for this accusation, but understanding what lay behind it gives a useful insight into the state of mind of the white population of the islands at this time. Hyde was generally appalled by what he saw as the lax state of Hawaiian culture. His letters home to the American Board of Commissioners for Foreign Missions are full of comments about the 'disgusting and degrading' behaviour he saw going on around him.[17] Many of his remarks on the specific problem of leprosy run seamlessly into a more general abhorrence of the unsanitary world in which he feels he is caught. He associates the disease with the lack of an adequate sewage system in Honolulu and with opium smoking.[18] Fearful of leprosy itself, it is clear that for Hyde the disease is a synecdoche for the whole culture: 'what are we to do with a nation of lepers? ... The loose living of the Hawaiians, the utter absence of privacy in their homes, the eating,

---

[16] *Ibid.*, p. 12.
[17] Hyde to Rev. Clark, 10 March 1883, Letters of Charles McEwan Hyde to American Board of Commissioners for Foreign Missions (ABCFM), Hawaiian Mission Children's Society Library, Honolulu.
[18] Hyde to Rev. J. Smith, 15 October 1884, and 31 August 1885, *ibid.*

smoking, and drinking together with hands ... and the taking and using everything in common has spread the disease dreadfully.'[19]

Hyde experienced direct contact with leprosy at the school he ran in Honolulu. In 1884 he had three cases of the disease among his students, one of which caused him especial grief. This concerned a young man Hyde described as being 'as pure minded and clean bodied, as kind hearted as whole souled a Christian as I ever saw'. This twenty-two-year-old student had been at the school for four years and it was intended he would soon take charge of a parish. Hyde agonised over the case: 'Must I give him over to a life of seclusion, a living death in the midst of loathsome suffering, debased humanity?' He could see no alternative, but described how he sobbed with grief over the fate of this exemplary 'disciple of Christ'. These cases in his school also made Hyde paranoid about the disease. In the same letter he spoke of the 'fearful risk' he was exposed to, and of the impossibility of diagnosing leprosy in its early stages: 'the incipient stages are of that no one [sic] would think of danger – a little place on the skin that is not sensitive to the touch. Is that leprosy?'[20]

Hyde, in fact, was already caught in a nightmare, convinced he had been infected:

Six weeks ago in putting on my stockings fresh from the wash, with a new pair of shoes sent from Boston, I noticed an irritation which I attributed to the tightness of the new shoes. The next week a rash came out. That disappeared leaving some pimples on the ankles, which I took to be flea bites ... These disappeared but left a discoloured spot. Last week in shaving I found that my skin was easily cut by the razor and that the blotches were spreading. I presume I have been poisoned, whether with syphilis or with leprosy remains to be seen. You will please say nothing about this, but I think it is right that you should know what risks a man runs in living among a people when such a malady is allowed to spread, the government making only a sham and a pretence of any segregation of infectious diseases. I am the more alarmed at these symptoms for I saw only last week at Dr. Arning's a leprous boy with matter exuding from his stockings which doubtless were sent to some Chinaman to wash. I have put myself at once in care of our family physician. He cannot tell how it will result, as syphilitic and leprous symptoms are so intermingled in this country.[21]

This tortured passage could only have been written by a Boston Puritan, although the kind of panic it captures is familiar enough. The minute self-examination, together with the moralising, terror and disgust are revealing. The 'new shoes from Boston', at first supposed to be the cause of the rash, soon become a contrast to a world of fleas, oozing socks, Chinese

[19] Hyde to Rev. Aldin, 31 January 1884, *ibid.*
[20] Hyde to Rev. Aldin, 31 January 1884, *ibid.*
[21] Hyde to Rev. Clark, 15 February 1884, *ibid.*

laundries and syphilitic lepers. Hyde's only defence against this world is his skin (the significance of his name multiplies), first undermined by rashes, pimples and blotches, and then breached while shaving. In such a world there is nowhere to hide. Infection is everywhere and all touch is potentially contaminating. Yet it is precisely the task of the missionary to touch and heal. The fear that by doing so Hyde is destroying himself rather than saving others captures, in miniature, the dilemma that leprosy provided for empires at large. In a subdued postscript six weeks later, Hyde wrote: 'I am almost entirely rid of my eczema. It has proved annoying and troublesome ... rather than dangerous and hopeless.'[22] The embarrassment of someone who has panicked needlessly retains nevertheless a defiant note of what might have been, or nearly was.

The key phrase in all this is Hyde's remark that the spread of leprosy is the result of 'taking and using everything in common'. The missionary attempt to privatise the Hawaiian body had met strong cultural resistance. New England domestic values had little purchase on Hawaiian family practices. In Bakhtinian terms, the closed-off and uptight Western body was confronted with an indigenous body that remained incorrigibly open to the world and flagrantly exceeded its own limits, in so doing endangering both itself and the world it inhabited.[23] For Hyde and his kind, this inability to recognise the limits of the self, and to contain it safely within the confines of the monogamous nuclear family, facilitated the spread of disease, leprosy in particular, and threatened the whole basis of social order. It was therefore necessary to counter the danger of leprosy by shutting it away totally. Hyde's remark about the sham of government segregation policies refers, in the first instance, to Walter Murray Gibson, Hawaiian premier in the mid-1880s, who was thought by many *haole* (Europeans) to be soft on segregation in order to win electoral support from indigenous Hawaiian voters.[24] But Hyde's anger at the government's failure to impose segregation with sufficient stringency was also a displaced expression of his sense of helplessness at the spread of the disease. Later in 1884 he wrote: 'To such an extent does leprosy prevail that the segregation of lepers is a physical impossibility.'[25] The hard line on segregation demanded by *haole* was always shadowed by the knowledge that it seemed to be making no impact on the disease. And Hyde, as we have seen, could be most uncomfortable with segregation when it applied to specific

---

[22] Hyde to Rev. Clark, 31 March 1884, *ibid.*
[23] Mikhail Bakhtin, *Rabelais and his World* (Bloomington: Indiana University Press, 1984), pp. 19–26.
[24] On Gibson and the politics of leprosy see Daws, *Holy Man*, pp. 126–30 and 171–2.
[25] Hyde to Rev. J. Smith, 15 October 1884, Letters of Charles McEwan Hyde to ABCFM.

individuals or groups known personally to him. Noting that the Kakaako shore hospital for lepers in Honolulu, intended as a way station for Kalawao, had forty children among its patients, he reflected that 'it seems insensate cruelty to send such little helpless ones to the festering mass of vile humanity on Molokai'.[26] Nevertheless, when festering humanity threatened wholesome humanity isolation of the former was imperative, no matter how cruel or ineffective.

And what about the leper colony itself? The standard narrative of Damien's work at Kalawao is one of creating order out of anarchy and replacing neglect with care. On his death *The Times* carried a leader in which Damien was said to have made the leper settlement 'nothing less than a model colony'.[27] Traveller-writers such as Charles Warren Stoddard and Robert Louis Stevenson who visited Molokai wrote eloquently of Damien's transformation of the wretched site. Jack London, visiting in 1906, reported that patients found to have been misdiagnosed, or whose cases had burnt out, were reluctant to leave.[28] And Arthur Mouritz, resident physician at the leper colony from 1884 to 1887, described *kokua* attempting to produce signs of leprosy on their body by rubbing and burning their skin in order to ensure 'a lazy, free from care existence ... [and] to get their daily food free'.[29] Such accounts, however, conform too closely to familiar European narratives of rescuing native peoples from themselves, and to European stereotypes of idle natives unable to cope with modern life, to be taken entirely at face value.

The story of Molokai has repeatedly been reduced to the story of Damien. But as Pennie Moblo has pointed out, Kalaupapa was not a deserted peninsula but already inhabited by taro and sweet-potato farmers working the adjacent Waikolu Valley; further, the colony was far more self-organising than the stock narrative suggests, and its official administrative structure normally involved a Hawaiian or part-Hawaiian patient as the superintendent. Damien was temporary superintendent for several years in the late 1870s but was removed from this post by the Hawaiian Board of Health after complaints about his arbitrary use of power.[30] Mythic histories of Molokai have emptied its landscape of all but Damien and the lepers, and greatly simplified a complex record of

[26] Hyde to Rev. Clark, 15 August 1884, *ibid.*   [27] The *Times*, 13 May, 1889.
[28] Jack London, *The Cruise of the Snark* (London and New York: KPI, 1968), p. 110.
[29] Arthur Mouritz, *The Path of the Destroyer: A History of Leprosy in the Hawaiian Islands and Thirty Years Research into the Means by Which It Has Spread* (Honolulu: Honolulu Star-Bulletin, 1916), pp. 79–82.
[30] Pennie Moblo, 'Blessed Damien of Molokai: The Critical Analysis of a Contemporary Myth', *Ethnohistory*, 44: 4 (1997), 692, 694, 704–5.

antagonism and negotiation between Damien's mission, the Hawaiian Board of Health and the leper population itself.[31]

The cult of Damien was enlisted in support of missions, and more generally of colonialism. The modern figure of the leper was partly a missionary construct, linking nineteenth-century colonialism with the example of Saint Francis and the teaching of Christ. Judeo-Christian abhorrence of the disease heightened the heroism and compassion of missionary work among lepers while ratifying the task of religious and cultural conversion. Megan Vaughan has argued that in Africa the lazaret became a 'colony within a colony', a place where the values of civilisation could be instilled in a setting insulated from other pressures. Within the leper settlement the truly powerless native subject could be isolated, reconstructed and incorporated into a community whose authority structure was a model of the ideal colony. The leper was therefore doubly colonised, disfigured and disempowered by disease, and controlled through the dispensation of material and spiritual aid. By learning to be 'a leper' and accepting the loss of all other identities, the patient became an ideal type of the colonial subject, marooned and dependent.[32] The accounts of Molokai after Damien's death were of this sort. His courage and humanity had produced a well-ordered and deferential colonial settlement, an island commonwealth with a missionary king, to update Gonzalo's contradictory vision of an island utopia.

The colony to which Damien came in 1874 had recently been described by the Hawaiian Board of Health as one in which social order had broken down, and according to Damien the colony's maxim was 'Aole kanawai ma keia wahi' (In this place there is no law).[33] There was, in fact, a formal rudimentary administration and many of the leper detainees had financed and built their own homes.[34] The mainly informal structures through which Damien came to establish some authority over the peninsula developed slowly, unevenly and were never total. Nor were they unchallenged. While it is clear that under Damien's influence, but also with greatly increased expenditure on the colony, a new form of European Christian order was established, this was often evaded or resisted. Prostitution and secret stills were common across the peninsula. One patient recalled 'women ... roariously drunk staggering about the village of Kalawao naked', and described how drinkers and dancers of the hula would meet at a place known as *ka pa pupule* (the crazy pen or the village of fools).

---

[31] *Ibid.*, 715.   [32] Vaughan, *Curing their Ills*, pp. 79–84.

[33] A. Johnstone, *Recollections of Robert Louis Stevenson in the Pacific* (London: Chatto and Windus, 1905), p. 323.

[34] Moblo, 'Blessed Damien of Molokai', 694, 704.

Damien would sometimes invade this place, driving out the dancers and overturning their drinking calabashes with his walking stick.[35] There was a riot at Kalawao in 1890 in which Catholic priests and sisters were threatened. A resident priest described Kalawao as gayer, lazier and more licentious than other Hawaiian villages. As Daws concludes: 'Damien never subdued the whole settlement to Christian obedience.'[36]

Charles Warren Stoddard's *Diary of a Visit to Molokai in 1884* has vivid evidence of the sexualisation of life in the settlement. The published version of the diary recorded that at the girl's home 'there were chalk frescoes on the walls – obscene cartoons probably done by the girls and certainly understood by them for they giggled excessively when they saw us looking at them'.[37] Stoddard's editor omits, without mention, the next paragraph of the original diary:

Dr. Fitch called two of the prettyiest [sic] girls – born of leprous parents but who do not yet show signs of leprosy – 10 to 12 years of age – and to show us that they were not scarred he draws them each to him, in turn, and raising their garments left them exposed from the shoulder blades to the heels. 'Ooueh – Awwah' cried Father Damien in dismay, and when the Dr. began to examine the ... [word indecipherable] sexual parts through the dress – the girls screamed with delight.[38]

Fitch was the Board of Health physician who had argued that leprosy was a late stage of syphilis. Stoddard describes him on this visit to Molokai, 'whooping through the villages, kicking up his heels and being in most cases received with laughter and with alohas', and later 'spanking one of the larger wretches with a shingle': 'Very disgusting', he concluded, 'and a mortification to the poor Father who has all his teaching knocked so out of tune by one single exhibition of the low, vulgar nature.'[39] The editor of Stoddard's diaries clearly did not want the discordant effect of Damien witnessing such scenes and apparently powerless to prevent them.

Megan Vaughan has shown that the attempt to engineer a new community and identity for lepers could be compromised by the need to retain the co-operation of patients and to maintain order. In African leper colonies this problem was often met by the recreation of a village community within the asylum and the selective reinforcement, indeed even invention, of ethnic identities and customs.[40] Something similar appears to have occurred on Molokai, or at least this was the impression received by

[35] Daws, *Holy Man*, pp. 111–12.   [36] *Ibid.*, pp. 243–5.
[37] Charles Warren Stoddard, *Diary of a Visit to Molokai in 1884*, ed. Oscar Lewis (San Francisco: Book Club of California, 1933), p. 10.
[38] Stoddard Diaries, 7 October 1884, Box 1, p. 9, Charles Warren Stoddard Papers, Hamilton Library, University of Hawaii, Manoa, Honolulu.
[39] *Ibid.*, pp. 8–9.   [40] Vaughan, *Curing their Ills*, p. 79.

Jack London and Charmian Kittredge when they visited the colony in 1906. Their accounts of the Fourth of July celebrations they witnessed describe a hybrid world of old and new. The leprous colonial subjects of Molokai are celebrating the culture of their colonisers but in terms that also recall a traditional indigenous culture no longer found elsewhere in the islands. To the visitors, the colony exemplified a productive intermingling of Hawaiian tradition and Western modernity, the best elements of old and new.[41] The Honolulu Board of Health had given permission for London and Kittredge to visit Molokai in the hope that they would write favourably of its segregation policy, and no doubt this influenced their accounts. Their visit also coincided with a moment of carnival. But their accounts capture well how the internal colony of the leper settlement could point up many of the tensions within the wider colonial context.[42] Nostalgia for a bygone world combines with admiration for the vigour of youthful United States democracy but is tempered by unease at the damaging consequences of its colonial expansion.

There were other forms of Hawaiian cultural practice at Molokai apart from those that were fashioned or staged. Jonathan Lamb has drawn attention to a cultic renaissance among the early inhabitants of the colony, described by Damien himself: 'The Hawaiian "hula" was organised after the pagan fashion, under the protection of the old deity Laka.'[43] Damien saw this as an expression of madness and despair. Lamb interprets it as a manifestation of 'millennial nostalgia' by a group of people cut off from the quotidian certainties of their previous existence.[44] Even if Damien was successful in replacing indigenous cults with orthodox Catholic religious observance, the evidence suggests that the image of Molokai as a model colony had as much to do with Damien's apotheosis as with the reality of the settlement. The leper settlement was an internal colony to which those felt to threaten the wellbeing of the colonised and soon-to-be annexed nation were expelled. As its numbers grew and the disease continued to spread, Molokai became a constant reminder of the human and cultural cost of colonisation. It was less a model colony than a monstrous reflection of the real thing.

Although the failure of segregation to affect the spread of leprosy made no difference to the policy of isolating its victims, it made more urgent the need for a cure. Removal to Molokai was an admission that, for the

---

[41] London, *The Cruise of the Snark*, pp. 99, 110; Charmian Kittredge London, *Jack London and Hawaii* (London: Mills and Boon, 1918), p. 123.

[42] Vaughan, *Curing their Ills*, p. 79.

[43] Johnstone, *Recollections of Robert Louis Stevenson in the Pacific*, p. 324.

[44] Jonathan Lamb, *Preserving the Self in the South Seas 1680–1940* (Chicago: University of Chicago Press, 2001), p. 160.

meantime, the disease was incurable and difficult to contain. This encouraged a proliferation of cures of one kind and another. Apart from the dietary prescriptions that leprosy had always seemed to prompt, there were an increasing variety of skin applications. Among *haole* concoctions, Daws lists solutions of beeswax and lard, tobacco and papaya juice, dog manure and molasses. Hawaiian *kahuna* (medical priests) resorted to traditional applications such as wild ginger and turmeric.[45] As we have seen in the case of Beaupethuy's cure, governments were ready to take seriously almost any claim to have found a remedy. King David Kalakaua had learned of one such, the so-called Goto method, when visiting Japan in 1881. This involved a holistic treatment involving diet, medication and hot baths, and its proponent Masanao Goto was invited by the Hawaiian Board of Health to work at the Kakaako shore hospital in Honolulu. He arrived in 1885 at the same time that Arning was conducting his laboratory experiment with Keanu. The Board of Health was now supporting two contrasting approaches to the problem of leprosy: the bacteriological investigations of Arning and the methods of Goto derived from traditional Japanese practice. Damien favoured the latter. Having undergone the Goto treatment himself at Kakaako, he planned a hospital complex based on its methods for Kalawao. The Board of Health rejected this as too expensive, but Damien managed to improvise a scaled-down version of the plan, installing bathhouses, tubs and a boiler room. For a while the treatment was incorporated into the daily life of the colony.[46]

Other remedies were introduced to Kalawao. Edward Clifford, a Protestant philanthropist and amateur artist, visited the colony at the end of 1888 with a supply of gurjun oil. Clifford had observed the use of this oil, both applied to the skin and taken internally, when visiting leper settlements in India. He was convinced of its efficacy but Damien, now in the last months of his life, was no more than politely interested, the oil having already been tried at the colony with no more success than other attempted remedies.[47] Daws points out that all these hopeful medications came from the East.[48] This practice of importing a cure from those regions from which the disease was commonly believed to derive persisted into the twentieth century, with chaulmoogra oil becoming the basis of most treatment before the development of dapsone in the 1940s.

The bacteriological approach of Arning continued as well, most notably after annexation in 1898 when the United States Public Health Service

---

[45] Daws, *Holy Man*, p. 138.   [46] *Ibid.*, pp. 162–5.
[47] Edward Clifford, 'With Father Damien and the Lepers', *The Nineteenth Century*, 25 (1889), 689–700; Daws, *Holy Man*, pp. 202–4.
[48] Daws, *Holy Man*, p. 238.

established a Leprosy Investigation Station at Kalawao. Patients on the island, however, disliked the idea of becoming subjects for experiment and kept away from the laboratory; it closed after only two years.[49] Not until dapsone became available was the laboratory-based investigation of leprosy brought into productive relation with its treatment and cure, and older remedies abandoned. Compulsory isolation on Molokai persisted until 1969 and a number of older patients still remain at the settlement today. The peninsula itself became part of the United States National Park System in 1980, although access remains restricted to protect the privacy of the remaining residents.

Robben Island

Robben Island has a long and notorious history as a place of custody. A low-lying island of rock and sand at the entrance to Table Bay, off the coast of Cape Town, it had been used as a prison for East Indian and indigenous African convicts in the first half of the nineteenth century. In 1846 the Cape government established a General Infirmary on the island for 'lepers, lunatics and the chronic sick', a change of use that reflected rapid social change at the Cape following the end of slavery in 1838. Fit and healthy convicts were required on the mainland to provide labour for new public work schemes, and they were replaced on the island by new figures of concern – the infectious leper, the dangerous lunatic and the sick pauper.[50] Leprosy at the Cape had a longer history but less spectacular development than in Hawaii. Although it was believed to have been widespread among 'Hottentots' (Khoisan) since the late eighteenth century, it was not the main worry at the time the Infirmary was established. At first the chronic sick predominated, but by the 1860s and 70s the balance of patients had shifted to the mentally ill, and it was only in the 1880s that lepers became the dominant group and the prime concern.[51] The sequence observed by Foucault in Europe, in which the asylum replaced the lazar house, was therefore reversed at the Cape.

The consolidation of white settler identity at the Cape following the granting of responsible government in 1872 was constructed around an intensified sense of racial difference. As race became the dominant

---

[49] Ibid., pp. 235–6.

[50] Deacon, 'A History of the Medical Institutions on Robben Island', pp. 38, 59.

[51] E. Burrows, A History of Medicine in South Africa up to the End of the Nineteenth Century (Cape Town and Amsterdam: Medical Association of South Africa, 1958), pp. 65–6; Harriet Deacon, 'Outside the Profession: Nursing Staff on Robben Island 1846–1910', in A. Rafferty, J. Robinson and R. Elkon (eds.), Nursing History and the Politics of Welfare (London: Routledge, 1997), pp. 85–6.

structuring force of Cape society it played a significant part in an increasing concern about leprosy. The traditional association of the disease with the 'idle, dirty, promiscuous, nomadic Hottentot' was now extended to include Africans, Malays and 'half-castes'.[52] As in Hawaii, the fear of leprosy was often focused on sexual behaviour. Voluntary segregation on Robben Island had been justified in mid-century on the grounds of protecting Cape society from the sexual promiscuity of the leprous. By late-century, when white opinion was strongly advocating compulsory segregation, there were fears that black female servants were transmitting leprosy and syphilis to young children, and a more general concern about white degeneration through lower-class racial intermixing.[53]

Compulsory segregation was finally introduced in 1892. This had been made both more urgent and more complicated by the spread of the disease among the white population. Previously the very few, mainly poor European lepers had been assimilated to the native pariah stereotype, but as the number of white lepers increased and their class base became more varied an alternative racially selective image of the leper was fashioned. Better-class white lepers, instead of carrying the negative stigma of the disease as dangerous and repellent, were seen as victims and martyrs. The 1892 legislation allowed home segregation for white lepers whose families could meet the cost of separate amenities. Seventy Cape Muslims, however, were refused a petition that they should have their own institution on the mainland. Not all white families, though, were comfortable with home segregation, and during the 1890s there was public concern for the situation of white lepers detained on Robben Island. As a result they were allowed better clothes and food, and Cecil Rhodes donated a bath chair for the use of female European lepers.[54]

The example of the Cape became one particular focus of the imperial debate over compulsory segregation in the last quarter of the century. At first it was used by anti-contagionists who contrasted the policy of voluntarily segregating pauper lepers with the much harsher compulsory segregation practised in Hawaii. (That said, Harriet Deacon has pointed out that many lepers detained on Robben Island before 1892 were unaware

---

[52] Deacon, 'A History of the Medical Institutions on Robben Island', pp. 208–10; Harriet Deacon, 'Racial Categories and Psychiatry in Africa: The Asylum on Robben Island in the Nineteenth Century', in W. Ernst and B. Harris (eds.), *Race, Science and Medicine 1700–1960* (London: Routledge, 1999), p. 116.

[53] Deacon, 'A History of the Medical Institutions on Robben Island', pp. 204, 211–12, 217–19.

[54] *Ibid.*, pp. 215, 223–4, 238–9.

that they were legally free to leave.[55]) At the same time, however, pressure was building at the Cape for much stricter measures. A smallpox epidemic in 1882, when Malays were believed to be the prime source of infection, helped precipitate legislation in 1884 making the segregation of lepers compulsory. This, however, was not promulgated. The Cape legislature was alarmed at the expense of implementing the measure, and was to some extent still constrained by the British government's official concern with the civil liberties of leprous subjects. Nevertheless, lepers on Robben Island were now subject to greater restrictions on their freedom, a policy vigorously implemented by a new Surgeon-Superintendent of the island, W. H. Ross, who had wanted the bill to become law. It finally became so in 1892, after a decade in which the number of recorded cases of leprosy had risen from around sixty to more than five hundred, and the British government had begun to review its policy on segregation.[56]

In the meantime, a scandal had broken over conditions on Robben Island. In 1889 *Blackwood's Edinburgh Magazine* printed an exposé of conditions there, titled 'Lepers at the Cape: Wanted, a Father Damien.' This was an account of a visit to Robben Island, with graphic descriptions of the physical state of the lepers and the squalid conditions in which they lived. The 'rough unpleasant transit' to the island on a 'dirty little tug', the freight comprising 'twenty sheep tied up by the legs and as cruelly piled on each other', struck all the keynotes of the article. It described both the lepers and the island as being in an advanced stage of degradation, with people 'disfigured ... almost beyond recognition', lying on 'foul rags and fouler mattresses' in huts with bare earth floors over which 'large loathsome snakes crawl at night in search of mice'. The writer asked: 'Is this disgraceful cabin a Cape Government hospital, or is it a lazar-house which even the pariahs of the East would scorn to inhabit?' His final reflections on quitting the island were: ' "All ye who enter here abandon hope;" and, "Wanted, a second Damien." '[57]

This article was headed with an editorial note expressing amazement that 'so inhuman and disgraceful a state of things could have been permitted ... in any British colony', and commending the account 'to those philanthropists at home who have lately been showing so benevolent an interest in the question of leprosy'. This was, of course, the year of Damien's death and the founding of the National Leprosy Fund. The *Blackwood's* story circulated in the press, with its still-anonymous author

[55] Harriet Deacon (ed.), *The Island: A History of Robben Island 1488–1990* (Cape Town and Johannesburg: Mayibuye Books and David Phillip, 1996), p. 66.
[56] Deacon, 'A History of the Medical Institutions on Robben Island', pp. 23, 67, 217–18.
[57] *Blackwood's Edinburgh Magazine*, 146: 887 (1889), 293–9.

contributing to a debate in *The Times* about the accuracy of his account.[58]
The October issue of *Blackwood's Edinburgh Magazine* included a series of
letters and newspaper extracts expressing horror and disgust at the conditions described. A year later the author of the account, by now known
to be one Colonel Knollys, contributed a follow-up piece, 'About the
Lepers – Once More'. This was headed with a further editorial note
reminding its readers of the 'painful revelations' of the previous article,
and announcing that reaction to it had resulted in the removal of 'a dark
blot upon the common humanity' of Britain and Cape Colony. Knollys'
sequel is a redemptive narrative. Revisiting the island a year later he
reported contented lepers living in a transformed environment. The
British contribution to this transformation was emphasised: 'best of all,
there are numerous parcels of books, newspapers, clothing, and eatable
luxuries strewing the beach, and bearing evidence of the thoughtfulness of
many quiet English homes for far-off sufferers'. These included 'a large
supply of Fortnum & Mason's bonbons, which the Princess of Wales had
desired me to deliver with messages of sympathy from her'.[59]

Knollys also discussed 'the heartrending but absolutely indispensable
Segregation Bill' that the Cape government was still hesitating to introduce. The reforms prompted by his original article, as a result of which 'an
Inferno ... has, in the space of a year, been transformed into a benevolent
institution which bids fair to become a model to other countries', were
presented as preparing the way for the compulsory but humane segregation that must necessarily follow. Robben Island has become another
Molokai, and can now serve alongside it as an example to the rest of
the imperial world. In a very short time the Robben Island leper colony
had shifted from providing a voluntary alternative to the Molokai model,
to being its degraded opposite, and finally to imitating its shining
example. By the mid-1890s, therefore, Robben Island had become the
strong alternative within the British empire to the liberal position on
segregation recommended by the India Leprosy Commission. As its own
Leprosy Commission reported to the Cape Parliament in 1895, leprosy
was on the increase, the disease was communicable to the healthy, and
compulsory segregation was the only practicable way of arresting its
spread.[60]

This helps make clear the significance of the figure of Damien as the
imperial world became convinced that compulsory segregation was the
only way of containing the spread of leprosy. His example, real enough but

---

[58] *The Times*, 21 October, 30 October, 29 November 1889.
[59] *Blackwood's Edinburgh Magazine*, 146: 889, (1890), 733–40.
[60] *The Times*, 19 June 1895.

increasingly mythologised, could be used to mitigate the disturbing implications of incarcerating the diseased, thereby salving the conscience of the
metropolitan world. This is not to deny that there was genuine concern
that leper colonies should be as humane as possible. Sympathy as well as
horror had often been characteristic of Judeo-Christian responses to the
disease. But the two *Blackwood's* articles were exemplary as much as
documentary. The trussed sheep piled one on another anticipated the
suffering that Knollys was to uncover. A year later this suffering had
been alleviated and a wilderness had become a garden. The shape and
trajectory of his two reports are familiar from many nineteenth-century
missionary narratives. The result is to reassure those donors at home about
the imperial civilising mission and to make them feel part of it. The
tortured ambivalence of Hyde, for whom enforced isolation was a terrible
necessity, has been eased. Molokai and Robben Island offered a benevolent and humane model for the alleviation of the plight of the leper. The
horror inspired by the first *Blackwood's* article is an essential prelude to the
absolution of the second.

The reality of life on Robben Island in the 1890s was rather different,
and the continuities with the previous decade were more striking than the
changes. The period between 1884 and 1890, when Ross was Surgeon-
Superintendent, had brought an intensifying racialisation and sexualisation of the disease. Leprosy, Ross wrote, was most prevalent among

the coloured paupers of the copper-tinted vagrants descended from Chinese and
Batavian bastards. The pure native races, like the Zulus and Kaffirs, are seldom
effected [sic] ... but among the Korennes and cross breeds between native women
and the nomadic Boers of the coast districts are to be found a large number of cases
with leonine countenances, sodden and leaden coloured features ... The popular
opinion here is ... that the spread of syphilis has been accessory to its wide
dissemination ever since South Africa was garrisoned by English troops, and the
native woman came more and more under the influence and operation of European
diseases and vices.[61]

This passage illustrates the need to pin the disease on particular groups,
and shows how readily leprosy became the focus of more general concern
about miscegenation and contamination.

Ross also gives an interesting example of a leper resisting his demands.
'The [lepers] would not do a stroke of work. I saw a coloured [leper]
working in the garden and I told him to come over to my garden and
I would pay him something to pull up the weeds in the path. He said he was
not in want of any pay, but would willingly pay me if I would come and

---

[61] *Journal of the Leprosy Investigation Committee*, 2 (1891), 78.

work in his garden.'[62] Ross's description of the lepers in his charge is characteristic of those of colonial administrators throughout European empires at this time. They are 'sulky idle people', 'habitually torpid in movement and impassive in gestures', and yet they are also 'turbulent subjects'.[63] The contradictions are immediately apparent. The idle leper who refuses to weed Ross's path is, in fact, working in his own garden at the time. Lepers as a group are both passive and restive. Contradictory stereotypes of the idle and the threatening leprous native result in a figure that lacks any middle ground, a temperate zone as it were. This is no doubly colonised model subject, but a type of the indigene that frustrated and angered colonial administrators around the world.

The 1892 legislation at the Cape went well beyond medical segregation, rendering those detained because of leprosy as dead people in law.[64] Sharpening racial and gender distinctions were reflected in the spatial management of the island, which now had separate quarters for black and white, male and female. A dog quarantine station was placed between the male and female settlements, and Boundary Road, which no leper was permitted to cross, protected the island village from the leprous.[65] These changes did not result in the grateful leper of Knollys' second *Blackwood's* article. Resistance to the regimen became more concerted, particularly after an attempt was made to cut off all communication between male and female lepers. The women refused institutional work, a ward was burnt down, six lepers escaped in a boat, and the Queen was petitioned. In response, police were brought to the island, a lock-up was built in the male quarters, and the organiser of the petition was removed to the mainland.[66]

Religion was another point of conflict. When lepers were prevented from attending the same church service as the staff they refused to attend church at all. And although medical missionaries might have been sustained by the example of Jesus curing Lazarus, the lepers of Robben Island refused to listen to readings about their biblical counterparts. As a European leper wrote to the Colonial Secretary in 1907: 'read the 13th chapter of Leviticus and you will see that I am not what God's Law describes'.[67] This discrepancy between biblical and modern forms of the disease had been noted by Knollys, who asked the doctor on the island: 'Where are the Miriams, the Naamans, and the Gehazis, lepers as white as snow?' He was told this was the Eastern form that did not exist at the

---

[62] Deacon, 'A History of the Medical Institutions on Robben Island', p. 219.
[63] *Ibid.*, p. 213.   [64] *Ibid.*, p. 221.   [65] *Ibid.*, pp. 236–7.
[66] *Ibid.*, pp. 226–7; Deacon, 'Outside the Profession', p. 95.
[67] Deacon, 'A History of the Medical Institutions on Robben Island', pp. 216, 219.

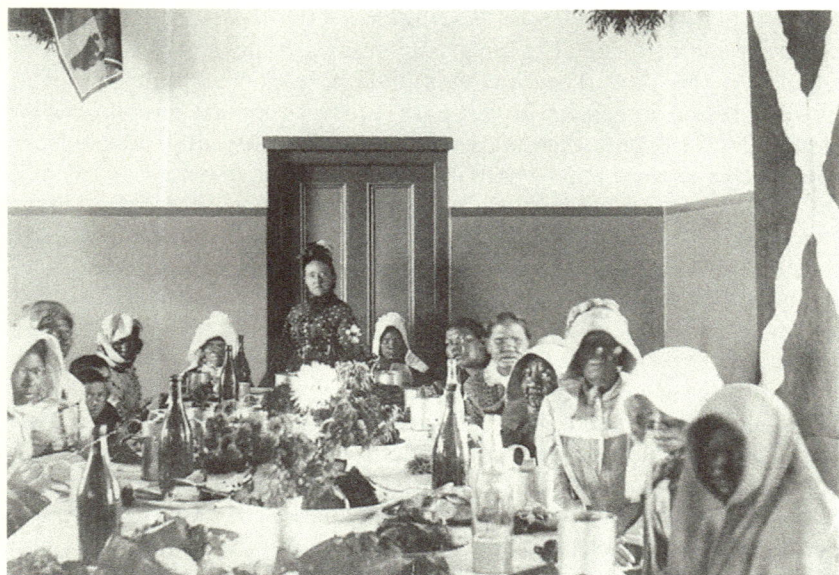

Figure 5. Christmas party for female lepers, Robben Island (early twentieth century). Cape Town Archives Repository (Ref. C16/4/3/2).

Cape.[68] It would be interesting to know how commonly this difference was remarked by lepers elsewhere who must also have been subjected to biblical accounts of their condition.

In the 1890s there was also a new scientific approach similar to that in Hawaii at the end of the century. This was influenced by increasing acceptance of the bacteriological causation of leprosy, and by the bad publicity of 1889 that made it important to present segregation as medically necessary and humane.[69] Before the 1892 Act Robben Island was emphatically a prison rather than a hospital. Treatment, such as it was, was mainly herbal and self-administered.[70] After 1892 some attempt was made to remodel the leper colony as a hospital. A group of trained nurses was brought in to administer more frequent washing and dressing of ulcers.[71] Under Impey, Surgeon-Superintendent from 1891 to 1895, new wards were built and new treatments sought. Bacteriologists were recruited from Europe and

[68] *Blackwood's Edinburgh Magazine*, 146: 887 (1889), 295.
[69] Deacon, 'A History of the Medical Institutions on Robben Island', p. 225.
[70] *Ibid.*, p. 76.   [71] Deacon, 'Outside the Profession', p. 96.

detailed patient records were kept of the family history, type of leprosy and progress of the disease.[72]

These measures had only mixed success. The more systematic nursing routine was resented by male patients in particular, and there was organised resistance to many of its new practices. Within a year most of the nurses had left, and the dressing of sores was resumed by untrained nurses and patients.[73] Very little laboratory work was actually undertaken, and many patients refused to give details of their family history or to be photographed.[74] Although there is no doubt that after 1892 lepers on Robben Island were given much closer attention, it is also clear that the more regulated existence they were compelled to lead was resented and opposed. Knollys' picture of grateful institutionalised lepers was a fantasy. Impey, upon leaving the island in 1895 became an opponent of compulsory segregation, arguing publicly for the non-contagiousness of anaesthetic leprosy and supporting agitation against the detention of such lepers.[75]

Australia

There are interesting comparisons between the response to leprosy in Hawaii, at the Cape, and in the settler colonies of the Pacific. European fears of contracting the disease had come relatively late at the Cape, mainly due to the lack of cross-cultural mixing. In Hawaii, where the intermixing of Europeans and the indigenous population was more widespread and accepted, there had been greater fear of cross-cultural infection and so compulsory segregation was introduced much earlier. On the other hand, the more open relations between the settler and native population meant there was less instinctive European horror at whites and natives sharing the same segregated environment than at the Cape. The most interesting differences between Hawaii and Australia concern attitudes to the Chinese. Although it was believed that Chinese indentured labourers had introduced the disease to Hawaii, the disease had spread most rapidly among the indigenous population. The Chinese, therefore, were never the main target of control. In Australia, where it was also believed that leprosy had been introduced by indentured labourers from China, they were intensively and enduringly stigmatised as the source of contagion. Whereas there was never any move to restrict Chinese immigration to Hawaii, this was a pressing subject in late nineteenth- and turn-of-the-century

[72] Deacon, 'A History of the Medical Institutions on Robben Island', pp. 229–32.
[73] Deacon, 'Outside the Profession', p. 96.
[74] Deacon, 'A History of the Medical Institutions on Robben Island', p. 232.
[75] *Ibid.*, p. 228.

Australian politics.[76] And in comparison with the Cape, the Australian states had less compunction about implementing compulsory segregation. Between 1885 and 1892 all the state governments introduced legislation that made leprosy compulsorily notifiable and empowered authorities to isolate those infected, and in 1908 the Commonwealth of Australia made leprosy a quarantinable disease. In doing so, as Alison Bashford notes, it was effectively declaring the disease to be infectious.[77]

This would hardly have been greeted as news, least of all in Queensland and the Northern Territory where anxiety about leprosy was most intense, the treatment of its sufferers harshest, and concern about its implications for this nation-in-the-making most blatantly expressed. Although there were a few instances of Europeans in the northern states of Australia being infected with leprosy, fear of the disease was as much concerned with its implications for the emerging nation as with the possibility of individual infection. As Warwick Anderson argues, 'medicine ... was as much a discourse of settlement as it was a means of knowing and mastering disease'.[78] More so than in Hawaii or at the Cape, leprosy was represented as a threat to racial integrity. Chinese, and to a lesser extent Pacific, indentured labourers were targeted as external contaminants threatening the health of the colony, in particular through sexual relations with Aboriginal women. In Australia it was less a question of whether or not to segregate lepers than where to put them. Most common was the practice of using small offshore islands to isolate lepers, frequently in appalling conditions.

In Queensland in 1889 a small group of Chinese lepers was taken from a quarantine station in Cookstown and left on Dayman Island in the Torres Strait. Several more were sent a few months later. By the end of the following year only two survived and it seems likely the others had starved to death. There was no legislative warrant for this removal and detention, and it was only when the New South Wales government introduced a leprosy bill that the Queensland authorities seem to have realised this omission. A temporary bill was pushed through with permanent legislation

---

[76] The association of the Chinese with leprosy was a persisting commonplace; see Captain W. E. Johns, *Biggles in the South Seas* (Leicester: Brockhampton Press, 1940), p. 39, where it is asserted as an unquestioned fact and a prime cause of Pacific depopulation.

[77] Alison Bashford, *Imperial Hygiene: A Critical History of Colonialism, Nationalism and Public Health* (Basingstoke and New York: Palgrave Macmillan, 2004), p. 94.

[78] Warwick Anderson, *The Cultivation of Whiteness: Science, Health and Racial Destiny in Australia* (New York: Basic Books, 2003), p. 4.

following in 1892.[79] The Act was also prompted by the case of James Quigley, a European discovered to have leprosy. The *Evening Observer* declared that 'a Chinese leper station is a horrible place to which to send a Queenslander', and the Colonial Secretary in Queensland agreed it would be 'little short of murder to send the unfortunate young man to Damien [sic] Island', an interesting slippage. On the other hand, a suggestion that he should be isolated with the elderly, inebriate and criminal on Stradbroke Island in Moreton Bay provoked strong opposition because of the fear of infection.[80] Leprosy was so intensely racialised in Queensland that there was no place for the white leper, an anomalous figure who nevertheless could not be ignored. The problem of accommodating the unassimilable white leper led to some island shuttling. Dayman Island was evacuated and Friday Island (how these names resonate), off the north Queensland coast, was established as a leper station for non-Europeans. Quigley was allowed to stay among the several detention-islands much closer to home in Moreton Bay, but was isolated from non-leprous detainees.[81]

Unlike the Cape, where separate quarters were established on Robben Island for white and non-white lepers, in Queensland it was felt necessary to place the white leper on an altogether separate island. More fine-tuning was required in the case of a young woman, Bella Clarke, diagnosed in 1895 as having leprosy. She had worked in a laundry and a grocery and was described by her employer as 'no better than a common prostitute'. Bella was typed as a promiscuous female leper associated with clothes and food, two recurring sites of anxiety in leprosy narratives, particularly in relation to the Chinese. It was therefore necessary to find yet another island for her, and in 1896 she was isolated on Peel Island, which later become a permanent lazaret.[82]

Pacific Islanders, also seen as a contaminating presence, were represented somewhat differently from the Chinese. *The Worker*, a virulently racist paper, explained both the differences and the common threat posed by these two immigrant groups: 'Used-up kanakas are as numerous in Bundaberg as mosquitos in a gully on a summer night and as malodorous as a procession of over-laden night-carts. They lie about, physical and moral wrecks as they are, filling the air with social disease germs more deadly than influenza or leprosy.'[83] These decaying Pacific bodies, like the more active and insidious Chinese presence, shared an underlying

---

[79] Jo Robertson, 'In a State of Corruption: Loathsome Disease and the Body Politic' (unpublished PhD thesis, University of Queensland, 1999), pp. 144–53.
[80] *Ibid.*, pp. 166–7.   [81] *Ibid.*, pp. 188–94.   [82] *Ibid.*, pp. 203–12.
[83] *The Worker*, 21 May 1892, in Robertson, 'In a State of Corruption', pp. 251–2.

similarity: 'Asiatics and kanakas are of a different civilisation to ours. They ... live in a much lower hygienic plan than the lowest member of our civilisation, and their peculiar susceptibility to dirt diseases makes their presence now a danger of greater gravity than ever.'[84]

Jo Robertson has analysed how the fear of disease was transferred from the body of the non-European immigrant worker to the state body itself, a move that political rhetoric has so often found irresistible. The physical symptoms of leprosy, of course, offered an especially potent metaphor in body/state discourse: 'Queensland is tainted ... Queensland is now as leprous in political mind as she is in actual body: she lies rotting in the lazarette which she has created for herself.' The characteristic feminisation of the state resulted in the inevitable figure of the diseased female, concealing 'beneath her white vesture – between her breasts – ... the mouldering leper's scab'.[85] Queensland had become like the beautiful lady Geraldine in Coleridge's 'Christabel', whose 'silken robe and inner vest' conceals that 'her bosom and half her side / Are lean and old and foul of hue'. The corrupted bosom signals the threat of disease transmission. Just as the innocent Christabel will awake from a night in the arms of Geraldine bearing 'This 'mark of [her] shame, this seal of [her] sorrow', so too the state of Queensland has been infected by welcoming strangers to its castle.

By the turn of the century the Aboriginal population was becoming the main target group. Most Chinese people with leprosy were now being deported, and as racially based immigration control was introduced after Federation in 1901 the spread of the disease among the indigenous population became the main concern. For many this was a short-term problem. Aboriginal people were commonly thought to be dying out, so, as one Australian official put it, 'this problem will probably solve itself'.[86] In the meantime, however, it was necessary to detain and incarcerate those with the disease. Treatment and care were not an issue, and the island lazarettes on which they were held were regarded as halfway houses to extinction.

One of these was Mud Island in Darwin harbour, also known as Living Hell Lazarette, where lepers were detained from 1884. Rev. W. Eddy of the Mission to Lepers described the conditions in which they existed: 'No one came to care for them, even to dress their wounds. No one fed or clothed them ... nine escaped to the mainland, swimming through water infested with sharks and crocodiles.'[87] Mud Island was abandoned in 1931 and the

---

[84] *The Worker*, 5 May 1900, *ibid.*, p. 252.

[85] *The Worker*, 25 March 1899, *Ibid.*, pp. 254–5.

[86] Suzanne Saunders, *A Suitable Island Site: Leprosy in the Northern Territory and the Channel Island Leprosarium 1880–1955* (Darwin: Historical Society of the Northern Territory, 1989), p. 10.

[87] *Ibid.*, p. 28.

lepers were transferred to Channel Island, further out in the harbour. This former quarantine station had no fresh water or cultivatable soil, and its trees were soon used up as firewood for the colony. Different quarters separated Aboriginal from part-Aboriginal detainees, a form of racial segregation parallel to that being practised on Aboriginal reservations at this time. When a European patient arrived in 1938 she was provided with a separate cottage. Patient numbers throughout the 1930s averaged between 100 and 130. Rudimentary nursing was provided by a group of Catholic sisters but there was no specialist leprosy care and patient records were almost non-existent. This was because Cecil Cook, who combined the posts of Chief Medical Officer, Chief Quarantine Officer and Chief Protector of Aborigines in the Northern Territory, believed that any information derived from Aboriginal people was too unreliable to be useful.[88]

In 1928 the Northern Territory passed legislation for the suppression of leprosy that authorised police and medical officers to arrest any leper suspect, in effect criminalising the disease. An eyewitness from the 1930s recalled seeing some twenty Aboriginal suspects 'with chains around their necks, under their legs and on to the next person and the next'. Those being brought to Channel Island travelled to Darwin on a 'leper van', a converted cattle truck with partly open sides. Gazing at caged lepers as they arrived at Darwin became a form of public entertainment.[89] There were many attempts at escaping from the island, and several were successful. The most spectacular of these was a mass escape in 1946 when twenty-three patients set off for Darwin to make known their complaints about conditions on the island. Intercepted by the police, they were forcibly returned. Their protest prompted an investigation that resulted in repairs to the buildings, the installation of a power plant, and the transfer of three European patients to other institutions on the mainland. The leprosarium remained little changed, however, until its closure in 1955.

Jo Robertson has argued that the concern with leprosy in Australia was part of a national imaginary in which it was imperative for Australia to be white, and Alison Bashford and Maria Nugent suggest that the question of a coherent settler identity was especially pressing at Australia's northern extremities. Here, in a tropical zone regarded as inimical to European health and identity, the emergent nation confronted

---

[88] *Ibid.*, p. 38.   [89] *Ibid.*, pp. 47–8.

its Asian neighbours.[90] Warwick Anderson has demonstrated how medical science and public health provided 'a rich vocabulary for social citizenship in an anxious nation'. In his words they were a means of 'bounding a territory, and of filling it in'.[91]

The geographical borders of the nation had to be secured, and the expulsion of contaminants that threatened the integrity of the mainland was part of this process. This involved a kind of racial sealing, with leprosy an especial focus of miscegenation fears. The occurrence of the disease among European males in the northern states was attributed to the lack of white women in these territories. Aboriginal women were said to be the conduit for leprosy, contracting it from the Chinese or Pacific Islanders and passing it on to white men. There was also a belief that leprosy became more virulent as it passsed through Aboriginal bodies.[92] Young white women were therefore encouraged to go north and stabilise the tropics, becoming, as Anne McClintock has shown elsewhere, markers of the nation's borders and symbols of the purity of its imagined community.[93] Chinese and Pacific immigrants were expelled, but Aboriginal people were concentrated. Inland reservations and island lazarets provided a means of containing this contamination threat from within, offering empty spaces where the indigenous population could be held while they awaited their inevitable extinction. A variant on this was the so-called 'leper line', created by the Western Australian government in 1941, which, to limit the spread of leprosy, prevented Aboriginal people from travelling south of the twentieth parallel.[94]

New Zealand

In July 1903 a Chinese fruiterer, Kim Lee, living in the Newtown suburb of Wellington, was diagnosed as having anaesthetic leprosy and was removed to Somes/Matiu Island, a quarantine island in the harbour. Those already on the island objected to the presence of a leper and Kim Lee was soon moved to an adjacent island, Nga Mokopuna, where he lived much of the time in a cave. Nga Mokopuna was little more than a rock, about fifteen

---

[90] Robertson, 'In a State of Corruption', p. 258; Alison Bashford and Maria Nugent, 'Leprosy and the Management of Race, Sexuality and Nation in Tropical Australia', in Alison Bashford and Claire Hooker (eds.), *Contagion: Historical and Cultural Studies* (London and New York: Routledge, 2001), p. 117.

[91] Anderson, *The Cultivation of Whiteness*, p. 4.

[92] Saunders, *A Suitable Island Site*, p. 13; Bashford, *Imperial Hygiene*, p. 96.

[93] Anne McClintock, *Imperial Leather: Race, Gender, and Sexuality in the Colonial Conquest* (New York and London: Routledge, 1995), p. 354; Bashford and Nugent, 'Leprosy and the Management of Race, Sexuality and Nation in Tropical Australia', pp. 118–20.

[94] Bashford, *Imperial Hygiene*, pp. 6, 106.

metres off Somes/Matiu. In good weather the lighthouse keeper on the main quarantine island would row across the narrow channel to deliver food and water, and a flying fox was rigged up so that Kim Lee could be provisioned when it was rough. He died in March 1904, according to his death certificate from anaesthetic leprosy, enlargement of the liver, interstitial nephritis and cardiac failure, although one imagines that severe depression must also have contributed to his rapid death. He was fifty-six and had been living in New Zealand for eighteen years. Mokopuna subsequently also became known as Leper Island.[95]

The Chinese had first come to New Zealand during the 1860s to work in the South Island gold diggings, and by the 1880s they were the largest non-British immigrant group. Between 1871 and 1920 15,500 Chinese entered New Zealand, although many of these went home again; the total population of Chinese in New Zealand during this period never exceeded 5,000 people at any one time.[96] A Select Committee of Inquiry into the Chinese Question in 1871 had decided they posed no risk to the morality and security of the country, and were no more likely to introduce infectious diseases than any other immigrant group.[97] By the end of the decade, however, there were demands for immigration restriction, former Governor and Premier Sir George Grey citing the threat of leprosy as a reason for this. The first in a series of Chinese immigration restriction acts was passed in 1881, and in the next couple of decades New Zealand experienced some of the anti-Chinese feeling also being generated in Australia. Much of this was led by Richard John Seddon, Prime Minister from 1893 to 1906, whose rhetoric echoed that being heard across the Tasman. Belich offers a couple of choice examples: 'I would rather a case of the plague here than see a hundred Chinese land'; 'The chow element in New Zealand is like a cancer eating into the vitals of our moral being and slowly and insidiously encompassing the doom of its victim.'[98] The language of disease was so constantly associated with the Chinese on both sides of the Tasman that it all but ceased to be metaphorical.

---

[95] For information on Kim Lee I am grateful to the Wellington historian Lynette Shum, and to an unpublished essay by Michael Lowe.

[96] James Belich, *Making Peoples: A History of the New Zealanders from Polynesian Settlement to the End of the Nineteenth Century* (Auckland: Allen Lane/Penguin, 1996), pp. 317–18; James Belich, *Paradise Reforged: A History of the New Zealanders from the 1880s to the Year 2000* (Honolulu: University of Hawaii Press, 2001), pp. 227–9.

[97] Ng Bickleen Fong, *The Chinese in New Zealand* (Hong Kong: Hong Kong University Press and Oxford University Press, 1959), pp. 17–18.

[98] Belich, *Paradise Reforged*, p. 228.

The year after Kim Lee's death an old and crippled Chinese man was shot dead in Wellington. His murderer, Lionel Terry, claimed to be resisting the 'yellow peril' and denied the killing was a crime. He was detained in a mental hospital for the rest of his life (he died in 1952), but Terry was acclaimed by many as a patriot and was freely given shelter on several occasions when he escaped from the relaxed custody in which he was held.[99] The public sympathy for Terry helps explain the social climate in which Kim Lee was detained on his rock.

New Zealand differed from Australia, however, in that there was little or no fear of Chinese immigrants contaminating the indigenous population, and this in spite of the almost total absence of Chinese women among the immigrant group in either country (in New Zealand in 1881 there were only nine women among the 5,004 Chinese in the country.[100]) In Australia it was believed that Aboriginal women were a bridge for the transmission of leprosy from the Chinese to the white population. This was never an element in New Zealand sinophobia. In part this reflected the different nature of ethnic relations in the two countries. Maori were much more involved in the public sphere than Aboriginals, and indeed were partially exempt from a dominant form of racism in New Zealand at this time. The theory of a European origin for Maori, the so-called Aryan Maori thesis, was widely disseminated and persisted well into the twentieth century. Belich has argued that *Pakeha* (European) co-option of Maori culture at the turn of the century was a means of negotiating a colonial identity crisis brought on by economic stagnation, a changing relationship with Great Britain, and the prospect of Australian Federation.[101] In Australia at this time the need to establish a distinctive identity was based on the idea of a white nation, which meant the exclusion of Aboriginals as well as the Chinese and other coloured immigrant groups. In New Zealand, however, a whitened Maori was incorporated, though never on equal terms, into an emergent national identity. Maori, therefore, fell on one side of a colour divide, the Chinese on the other. As Apirana Ngata, the leading Maori politician of the first part of the twentieth century, put it: 'Any integration between Maori and Chinese would bring racial contamination and moral degradation of the Maori people.'[102] Sinophobia in New Zealand, therefore, lacked the fear of miscegenation that compounded its intensity in Australia. In both countries, however, it was a constitutive element in the turn-of-century renegotiation of settler identity.

It was also believed that Maori had leprosy well before the arrival of Chinese immigrants. Arthur Thomson, a military surgeon and

---

[99] *Ibid.*, p. 229.   [100] *Ibid.*, p. 228.   [101] *Ibid.*, pp. 206–10.   [102] *Ibid.*, p. 231.

ethnographer who worked in New Zealand in the 1840s and 50s, had published a detailed account of a number of cases of *ngerengere* or leprosy *gangraenosa* among Maori in the *British and Foreign Medical-Chirurgical Review* in 1854. His observations were widely noted and found their way into much of the subsequent nineteenth-century writing on leprosy, including the 1867 College of Physicians' Report. Although it is unlikely that all the cases Thomson described were aetiologically similar, John Miles argues that leprosy had been introduced to New Zealand in the early days of European contact and persisted into the twentieth century. He concludes, for example, that five cases among North Island Maori reported by A. Ginders in 1890, and circulated in Britain by a medical press concerned to track the spread of the disease across the empire, were definitely leprosy.[103] Unlike Hawaii, however, there seems to have been little alarm that Maori would be infected by contact with other leprous groups. Arthur Mouritz, resident physician at Molokai from 1884-7, had regarded the native Hawaiian population as inherently susceptible to leprosy, 'the weak link in our chain of national health defence'.[104] In New Zealand, despite the contemporary belief in an indigenous form of the disease, there was no equivalent concern that a latent susceptibility within the Maori population might be activated by the presence of Chinese immigrants.

Compared with Hawaii the numbers involved were very small; in 1904 there were just five officially recorded cases of leprosy in New Zealand, four Maori and one Chinese.[105] But the fears prompted by leprosy were always disproportionate to their numbers and there was a growing feeling of the need for a permanent site for the isolation of sufferers. In 1906 a man admitted to Christchurch Hospital and found to have leprosy was isolated on Quail Island in Lyttelton harbour. More admissions followed and a small colony formed on the south side of the island. This remained until 1925 when the eight lepers at the colony were transferred to Makogai Island in Fiji, where they joined more than 400 other leprosy patients from around the Pacific.[106]

Quail Island had a long history as a place of quarantine. It had been established as an isolation island for immigrants in 1875 but was used primarily for New Zealand residents suffering from infectious diseases. In 1879 more than a hundred children from the Lyttelton Orphanage were

[103] See *British Medical Journal*, 2 (1890), 1094.
[104] Mouritz, *The Path of the Destroyer*, p. 22.
[105] John Miles, *Infectious Diseases: Colonising the Pacific* (Dunedin: University of Otago Press, 1997), pp. 41–51.
[106] P. J. Jackson, *Quail Island: A Link With the Past* (Christchurch: Department of Conservation, 1990), pp. 42–6, 52.

(a)

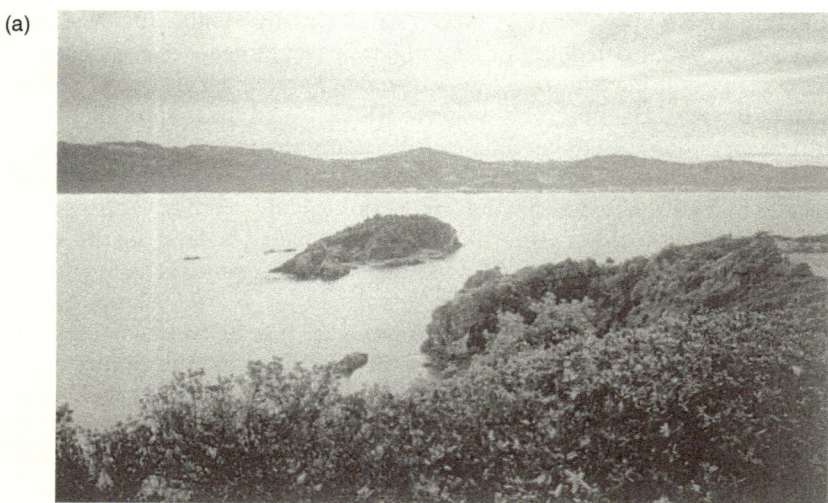

(b)

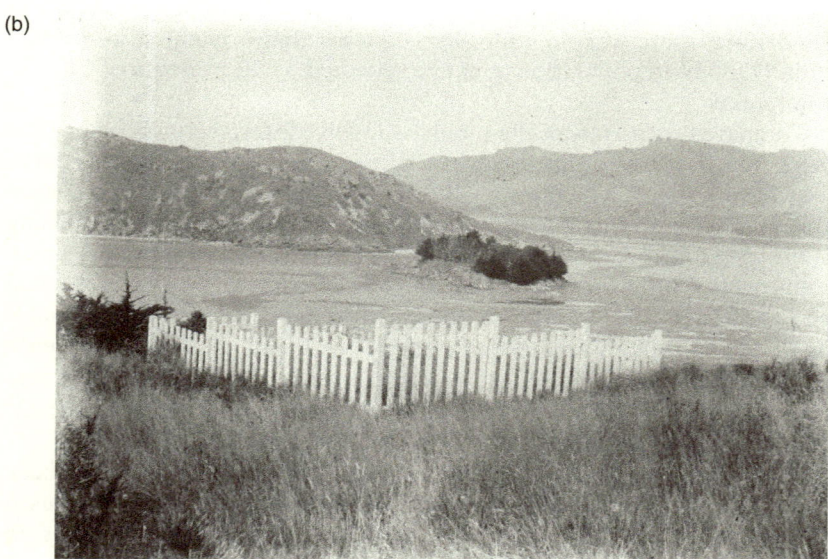

Figure 6. (a) Nga Mokopuna Island, off Somes/Matiu Island, Wellington harbour. Courtesy of Lynette Shum. (b) Leper grave of Ivan Skelton, Quail Island, Lyttelton harbour. The grave has been enclosed with a picket fence. W. A. Taylor collection, Canterbury Museum (Ref. 1968.213.123).

sent there following an outbreak of diphtheria. A smallpox patient was isolated there in 1910, and during the influenza epidemic at the end of the First World War it served as a convalescent sanatorium. In the early twentieth century Quail Island had been used as part of the corrective training for boys and girls sent to reform schools.[107] It also served as an animal quarantine station for imported livestock from England, including dogs and ponies used by Scott and Shackleton on their Antarctic expeditions.[108] And to complete this catalogue of isolation and rejection, from 1887 a bay on the western side of the island became a ships' graveyard for the dumping of vessels that had fallen into disuse. Skeletons of several of these ships can still be seen at low tide.[109]

The use of Quail Island as a leper colony was unpopular. Apart from the predictable disquiet of Lyttleton residents, its designation as an isolation site for lepers clashed with other actual or potential categories of exclusion. A plan to use it as a prison island for those with indeterminate sentences had to be abandoned, and it was objected that the colony would endanger the island's quarantine work.[110] Isolation of the leprosy patients was very strict. The first inhabitant, Will Vallane, was prohibited from going outside the fence round his hut, and his food was left on a small table by the fence. This practice of fencing-in even extended to the leper graveyard, which was enclosed by a prominent white picket fence. Regulations stipulated that no person should approach the lepers closer than six feet or enter their huts. Church services were outdoors and the vicar, suspicious of the regulations, kept 'some fifteen paces away'. A member of Holy Trinity Parish, Lyttelton, visiting the colony for a service in 1922, noted: 'We felt as though we were visiting some mission station in the New Hebrides and half expected to see a cannibal emerge from the shadows.'[111] The nativisation of the disease, and the contradictory attitude of Christianity towards it – the need to witness and tend combined with the fear of approaching – is well captured here.

The ethnic make-up of the colony was predominantly Polynesian, with two Chinese patients admitted in 1921. Local Maori interest in the colony is demonstrated by the photo of a large community group from Rapaki visiting the colony in 1924.[112] From the evidence of names and two extant photos of some of the inhabitants it is likely that Will Vallane and George Philips were Pakeha. Philips, admitted in 1916, was said to have contracted the disease from sleeping in a hut in Samoa while serving with the New Zealand Army. Ivan Skelton, who died at the colony in 1923, had been born in Samoa.[113] Life on Quail Island was austere but probably better

---

[107] *Ibid.*, pp. 40–1, 54–5.   [108] *Ibid.*, pp. 59–76.   [109] *Ibid.*, pp. 81–8.
[110] *Ibid.*, p. 42.   [111] *Ibid.*, pp. 43–50.   [112] *Ibid.*, p. 52.   [113] *Ibid.*, pp. 46, 50.

provisioned than many colonies elsewhere in the empire. Nevertheless, in 1911 there was a confrontation between a new patient and the caretaker's wife over the quality and quantity of food. This resulted in Mrs Thomas defending herself with a clothes-prop and a police constable being called.[114] A letter from residents at the colony was sent to the *Lyttelton Times* in 1924 complaining about the lack of space and recreation amenities. In 1925 George Philips escaped and, in a nice touch, was last seen heading for Christchurch dressed as a clergyman.[115] With the removal of the remaining patients to Makogai two years later New Zealand effectively rid itself of 'the leper problem'.

Summary

Foucault, in *Discipline and Punish*, selected the traditional casting out of the leper as his example of the practice of 'exile-enclosure'. He contrasted this act of total rejection with the historically later response to plague, in which the sick were closed off within the town rather than sent 'without the camp'. Unlike the leper who 'was left to his doom in a mass among which it was useless to differentiate', 'those sick of the plague were caught up in a meticulous tactical partitioning' in which every aspect of their life was subject to the closest scrutiny, regulation and record-keeping. Foucault understood this contrast as representing two distinct ways of exercising power, of controlling personal and social relations and 'of separating out the dangerous mixtures'.[116]

At one extreme, the discipline-blockade, the enclosed institution, established on the edges of society, turned inwards towards negative functions: arresting evil, breaking communications, suspending time. At the other extreme ... is the discipline-mechanism: a functional mechanism that must improve the exercise of power by making it lighter, more rapid, more effective, a design of subtle coercion for a society to come.[117]

Foucault also understood this contrast as representing different historical epochs. He describes the movement 'from a schema of exceptional discipline to one of generalised surveillance' as occurring during the seventeenth and eighteenth centuries, and spreading through the social body to form the modern disciplinary society.[118]

Within this schema, the leper colonies I have been discussing would represent the persistence of vestigial forms of 'exile-enclosure' into a

---

[114] *Ibid.*, p. 46.   [115] *Ibid.*, pp. 51–2.
[116] Michel Foucault, *Discipline and Punish: The Birth of the Prison* (London: Penguin, 1991), pp. 195–9.
[117] *Ibid.*, p. 209.   [118] *Ibid.*

modern world in which power elsewhere functions more subtly. Indeed Alison Bashford sees Australia's island leper colonies in precisely this way, contrasting them with leper colonies elsewhere in the British empire which were being remodelled along more therapeutic and corrective lines.[119] Elsewhere in *Discipline and Punish*, however, Foucault suggests that the relation of exile-enclosure to the therapeutic-corrective institution is one of overlap as much as succession. Although different projects, they were not incompatible ones:

We see them coming slowly together, and it is the peculiarity of the nineteenth century that it applied to the space of exclusion of which the leper was the symbolic inhabitant (beggars, vagabonds, madmen and the disorderly formed the real population) the technique of power proper to disciplinary partitioning. Treat 'lepers' as 'plague victims' [for Foucault the leper has become merely figurative by the nineteenth century], project the subtle segmentations of discipline onto the confused space of internment, combine it with the methods of analytical distribution proper to power, individualize the excluded, but use procedures of individualization to mark exclusion – this is what was operated regularly by disciplinary power from the beginning of the nineteenth century in the psychiatric asylum, the penitentiary, the reformatory, the approved school and, to some extent, the hospital.[120]

Foucault is here suggesting that rather than one phase following another, pre-modern forms of coercion somehow merge with modern techniques of observation, the inducement to conform with the production of consent. According to this, Australian 'exceptionalism', as Bashford has it, is less an anachronism than an enduring practice still waiting to be modified by therapeutic correction. Elsewhere, in fact, Bashford complicates the sharp contrast that Foucault's schema can encourage and acknowledges that in Australia, too, segregation and differential management could co-exist within the repertoire of leprosy control.[121]

There is no doubt that some aspects of Molokai, and even Robben Island by the turn of the century, can be made to fit Foucault's category of the modern institution. But the fit is never more than loose, and it leaves many features of these and other leper colonies of the time unexplained. This, in turn, raises a larger question about the appropriateness of Foucault's schema for colonial settings. Ann Laura Stoler has pointed out that Foucault's account of the cultivation of the bourgeois self in the nineteenth century ignores the constitutive role played in this process by

---

[119] Bashford, *Imperial Hygiene*, pp. 82, 90.
[120] Foucault, *Discipline and Punish*, p. 199.
[121] Bashford, *Imperial Hygiene*, p. 109.

imperial racial configurations.[122] Her question as to why, in Foucault's work, colonial bodies never figure as a site for the articulation of nineteenth-century European sexuality has wider application.[123] The attempt to use Foucault's sequence of 'exile-enclosure to therapeutic-corrective' is greatly complicated when cast in an imperial rather than a metropolitan context. Foucault's account of the emergence of modernity, whether it be the sexual body of the bourgeois self or the institutional structures through which distinctively modern forms of power were being fashioned, can never be more than half the story, ignoring as it does both the colonial project itself and its 'return effect', that is the role that colonialism played in ordering social relations at home.[124]

In regard to leprosy, there is a complex asynchronicity between metropolitan and colonial centres. We have already seen how mid-nineteenth-century metropolitan medicine regarded the idea that leprosy was contagious as a mark of colonial ignorance and superstition, only to be pulled in that direction itself by the discovery of the leprosy bacillus and a feared increase in the incidence of leprosy across the imperial world. Bashford argues that it was important for colonial management to differentiate just and modern British treatment of lepers from medieval practices and unjust indigenous exclusions.[125] This was certainly the case for Milroy and some others in the 1860s and 70s, but by the closing decades of the century metropolitan medicine was just as likely to be complaining about the harmful indifference of indigenes to leprosy, and urging stricter, even compulsory, segregation for its victims.

It is also difficult to accommodate the high level of missionary involvement with leper colonies at this period in Foucault's model. Even in Australia, as we have seen, members of religious orders stepped in to palliate the worst effects of a crude and harsh quarantine response to the disease. The example of Damien on Molokai is the ideal type of this form of intervention, which has a very long history quite distinct from both punitive dumping and therapeutic correction. Megan Vaughan's analysis of missionary-run African leper colonies discussed earlier suggests some superficial similarities with a modern productive disciplinary institution

---

[122] Ann Laura Stoler, *Race and the Education of Desire: Foucault's History of Sexuality and the Colonial Order of Things* (Durham, N.C., and London: Duke University Press, 1995), p. 8. Megan Vaughan had earlier pointed out the differences between the colonial power/knowledge regime and that described by Foucault; see *Curing their Ills*, pp. 8–12. Her emphasis, however, is on the incommensurability of metropolitan and colonial worlds, whereas I am concerned with their intersections.

[123] Stoler, *Race and the Education of Desire*, p. vi.

[124] *Ibid.*, p. 75, acknowledges that Foucault's 1976 Collège de France lectures on race are a partial exception to this.

[125] Bashford, *Imperial Hygiene*, pp. 81–2.

such as the sanatorium, but mission leper colonies had a different orientation. If the emphasis of the sanatorium was on hygienic discipline as a preparation for re-entering social life, isolation as a prelude to reintegration as it were, in the mission colony lepers were educated to accept their life-sentence, abandon all other identities and wait for better things in the afterlife. And even within emergent public health forms of leprosy management in the early decades of the twentieth century, the orientation of the sanatorium towards education and reintegration could not become a serious option for the leper colony while the disease remained incurable and belief in its contagious nature persisted.

A further difficulty with applying Foucault's schema to the history I am tracing is its top-down nature. The typological shifts and differences he describes would have meant little to the inhabitants of Robben Island. This is not to pit some unproblematised notion of 'experience' against the work that cultural theory and history can perform, but to insist nevertheless on the importance of those scattered accounts of the actual residents of leper colonies that we possess. That is why I have included passages of narrative in the discussion of particular colonies, intending these as a kind of check and control on the abstractions of 'exile-enclosure', 'therapeutic corrective' and such like. These narratives also alert us to differences between leper colonies in different colonial settings, and help us to see micro-change through shorter periods as well as macro-change over epochs. Bashford and Strange theorise this well when they point out that for Foucault the leper and the lunatic were always 'other', by definition excluded from the cultivation and techniques of the self that he analyses. We have seen above how Foucault's leper has become entirely figurative by the nineteenth century. Bashford and Strange, however, remind us that 'spaces of isolation are not simply made from above, by legislators, architects, doctors and overseers: they are constantly reshaped by those whom they aim to reform, cure or expel'.[126] We have already seen this to be the case in leper colonies, and it is an emphasis to be kept in mind as we now move on to look at further examples of colonisation and enclosure.

---

[126] Alison Bashford and Carolyn Strange, 'Isolation and Exclusion in the Modern World', in Carolyn Strange and Alison Bashford (eds.), *Isolation: Places and Practices of Exclusion* (London and New York: Routledge, 2003), pp. 13–14, 19 n48.

5 Concentrating and isolating racialised others, the diseased and the deviant: the idea of the colony in the later nineteenth and early twentieth centuries

The colony

As European empires spread across the world in the nineteenth century, the meanings and applications of the word 'colony' multiplied. Etymologically colony was an agricultural metaphor, from the Latin *colere* to till, and *colonus* a husbandman. Thus *colonia*, a colony, meant an estate in the country or a rural settlement. It was then applied to the new cities that settlers came to from Rome, and the imperial associations of this usage were extended in Greek where the word also had the sense of civilising barbarous people. There is an implicit contrast here between the colonist and the townsperson, or *civis*, from which the word civilisation derives. A *civis*, unlike a colonist, is someone whose home does not move. In the early modern period colonies were made by sending people to settle and plant; thus in Hobbes's *Leviathan*, colonies are sent from England to plant Virginia.[1] Swift, in *Gulliver's Travels*, offers perhaps the first post-colonial usage of the word:

Ships are sent ... the natives driven out or destroyed ... a free licence given to all acts of inhumanity and lust, the earth reeking with the blood of its inhabitants: and this execrable crew of butchers employed in so pious an expedition, is a *modern colony* sent to convert and civilise an idolatrous and barbarous people.[2]

The connection between a parent state and a new settlement is integral to all these usages, and it is the settler who establishes and maintains this relation. In the early modern period the settlers themselves were the colony, but once the settlement was firmly established the colony came to be seen more as the territory. Although these two senses remain inter-dependent, the word 'colonist' (1701 is the first recorded usage in the *Oxford English Dictionary*), and later 'colonial' as a noun (first recorded

---

[1] All references to the meanings of 'colony' derive from the *Oxford English Dictionary* unless otherwise stated.

[2] Jonathan Swift, *Gulliver's Travels* (Harmondsworth: Penguin, 1977), pp. 343–4.

usage 1865) reflect the process whereby the meaning of 'colony' shifted from people to territory. By the mid-nineteenth century, therefore, Herman Merivale would define a 'colony' as 'a territory of which the soil is entirely or principally owned by settlers from the mother country'.[3] The relation with the mother country, however, remained central. As Seeley expressed it in *The Expansion of England* (1883): 'By a colony we understand a community which is not merely derivative, but which remains politically connected in a relation of dependence with the parent community.'

The centrality of this relation with a parent state meant that two main kinds of colony came to be distinguished from each other during the nineteenth century. There were the white settler colonies that were moving towards some form of self-government, and there were the predominantly black crown colonies that were military outposts or providers of staples for the metropole.[4] In terms of the trope of family that was so often applied to the British empire during the nineteenth century, settler colonies were like children and crown colonies like servants. This distinction between colonies that were increasingly free of restriction and those that were to remain under control is to be found within other applications of the word as these proliferated during the nineteenth century.

The *Oxford English Dictionary* gives the 1880s as the first use of 'colony' to mean the people of a particular nationality residing in a quarter or district of a foreign city or country, or as people of the same occupation inhabiting a particular locality. Here the word is being applied to any group or concentration of people living in some way separate from the rest of society, even within metropolitan society itself. In this usage there was a clear difference between colonies that were established by official authorities and agencies for the purposes of containment and segregation, and those that were voluntary and self-concentrated for the purpose of social or artistic experiment or freedom. Examples of the former kind would be the leper and penal colony, both closely related to nineteenth-century imperialism. The opposite, libertarian sense of the word had antecedents in Winstanley and the Diggers in the mid-seventeenth century but only became extensively used in the nineteenth. It was applied to Owenite and Fourierist communities, and to Feargus O'Connor's Chartist land settlements in the 1840s.[5] From the foundation of Ruskin's

---

[3] In Catherine Hall, *Civilising Subjects: Metropole and Colony in the English Imagination 1830–1867* (Cambridge: Polity, 2002), p. 213.

[4] *Ibid.*

[5] See Charles Gide, *Communist and Co-operative Colonies* (London: Harrap and Co., 1930); Dennis Hardy, *Alternative Communities in Nineteenth-Century England* (London and New York: Longman, 1979).

Totley Colony, near Sheffield, in 1876, such communitarian experiments were almost invariably described as colonies, and they increased rapidly in number towards the end of the century.[6] In naming themselves as 'colonies', these agrarian communities were drawing on the agricultural roots of the word while discarding the allied sense of connection to a parent society. They were conceived as independent alternatives to the dominant culture rather than adjuncts to it; the artists' colony becoming common at this time was another version of this model. These internal colonies, socialist or artistic islands in a capitalist or philistine society, were small worlds that had retreated in order to be productive, whether agriculturally, artistically or politically. Some also harboured the utopian aim of providing a model that society at large would come to imitate. The colonies of empire, on the other hand, were settlements to be exploited for the benefit of those living elsewhere in metropolitan centres. Leper and penal colonies were places of forcible exile in which any productive activity was always compulsory.

Other, more ambiguous forms of internal colony developed in the nineteenth century. As Felix Driver points out, over the last two centuries 'the regeneration of society, the cultivation of citizenship and the reclamation of character have often been said to require the colonisation of whole neighbourhoods within the city, and the planting of new colonies elsewhere – including labour colonies, model communities, new towns or indeed overseas settlements'.[7] A classic example of this was the agrarian colonies for the residential re-education of delinquent adolescents established in Germany, France and the Netherlands in the 1840s and which spread to other west European countries. Their prototype was the Mettray colony near Tours; the Philanthropic Society's farm school at Redhill in Surrey, set up in 1848, was a British version.[8] Foucault chose the date of the official opening of Mettray in 1840 to mark the completion of what he

---

[6] Hardy, *Alternative Communities in Nineteenth-Century England*, has a national map of such communities (p. 15), a map of colonies in Essex where they were particularly concentrated (p. 187), and a complete list of alternative communities in the Appendix.

[7] Felix Driver, 'Colonies', in Stephan Harrison, Steve Pile and Nigel Thrift (eds.), *Patterned Ground: Entanglements of Nature and Culture* (London: Reaktion Books, 2004), p. 93.

[8] See Jeroen J. H. Dekker, 'Rituals and Re-education in the Nineteenth Century: Ritual and Moral Education in a Dutch Children's Home', *Continuity and Change*, 9: 1 (1994), 121–44; Jeroen J. H. Dekker, 'Transforming the Nation and the Child: Philanthropy in the Netherlands, Belgium, France and England, c.1780–c.1850', in Hugh Cunningham and Joanna Innes (eds.), *Charity, Philanthropy and Reform* (Basingstoke: Macmillan, 1998), pp. 136–43; Felix Driver, 'Discipline Without Frontiers? Representations of the Mettray Reformatory Colony in Britain, 1840–1880', *Journal of Historical Sociology*, 3: 3 (1990), 272–93; Felix Driver, 'Bodies in Space: Foucault's Account of Disciplinary Power', in Colin Jones and Roy Porter (eds.), *Reassessing Foucault: Power, Medicine and the Body* (London: Routledge, 1994). On Redhill see David Owen, *English Philanthropy 1660–1960* (Cambridge, Mass.: Harvard University Press, 1965), p. 153.

termed 'the carceral system', that is one in which all the modern 'coercive technologies of behaviour' were concentrated. The 'small, highly hierarchised groups' upon which Mettray was based combined the regulation of the family, the army, the workshop and the school.[9] Here we see that coming together of exclusion and regulation that was for Foucault the distinctive contribution of the nineteenth century to the modern interlocking of knowledge and power. This model of modern disciplinary power exemplified by Mettray was, as Felix Driver puts it, 'above all else, a colonising form of power; it cultivated new ways of seeing, calculating and ordering'.[10] Designed to isolate adolescents at risk from the dangers of city life and bring about their moral regeneration, it was organised around a meticulous 'pedagogical infrastructure' involving hard work, strict rules, and a total break between the adolescent and his home.[11] The wider intention was to raise the moral level of the poorer population and to avert public disorder through moral disinfection.

We have already seen there can be problems with Foucault's genealogy of institutional discipline, especially when placed in an imperial context. In respect of Mettray, Felix Driver has questioned whether the movement from punitive to reforming regimes was as clear-cut as Foucault's genealogy implies, and he notes the elision of intentions and outcomes in this schema.[12] Ann Laura Stoler's critique of Foucault's neglect of imperial discourses and landscapes in his account of the emergence of European modernity, and her insistence that his 'genealogy of bourgeois identity and its biopolitics should also be traced through imperial maps' offers a different context in which to consider 'the carceral system'.[13] Although Foucault's genealogy still remains useful in a broader imperial setting, the variety within the models he deploys, the complex entanglement of his two main institutional types, and the possibility of rather different models altogether need to be kept in mind. In exploring these matters I am concerned with the simultaneity of apparently different models across metropole and empire, the interaction and commonalities between these, the manner in which imperial colonies could, in some instances, serve as 'laboratories of modernity',[14] and yet at other times as a counterpoint to

---

[9] Michel Foucault, *Discipline and Punish: The Birth of the Prison* (London: Penguin, 1991), p. 293.

[10] Driver, 'Bodies in Space: Foucault's Account of Disciplinary Power', p. 127.

[11] Dekker, 'Rituals and Re-education in the Nineteenth Century: Ritual and Moral Education in a Dutch Children's Home', 132.

[12] Driver, 'Bodies in Space', pp. 119–20.

[13] Ann Laura Stoler, *Race and the Education of Desire: Foucault's History of Sexuality and the Colonial Order of Things* (Durham, N.C., and London: Duke University Press, 1995), p. 16.

[14] *Ibid.*, p. 15.

the liberal modernity of Europe. Reforming colonies of the Mettray kind, being markedly different from conventional penal institutions, could provide a contrast with penal and corrective practices in colonial territories where the nature of the inhabitants was thought to require a different kind of regime. There was also, however, an increasing tendency through the nineteenth century to compare the metropolitan underclass, and other marginalised groups at home, with 'uncivilised' colonial subjects. In other words, there was a profound ambivalence at the heart of liberal reform and philanthropy that found expression in the control and coercion of reforming institutions. This becomes clearer when colonies at home and across the empire are brought into the same frame.

Broadly speaking, colonies such as Mettray were of an intermediate kind between the commune and the prison. Philanthropically inspired, the help they provided was compulsorily administered. Common to all these new nineteenth-century applications of the term, however, was the idea of concentrations of people cut off, whether voluntarily or forcibly, from the world in which they had lived. And there has emerged within the word a tension between connection – that of colony and parent state, and separation – enforced isolation for the good health and order of that parent state.

By the eighteenth century 'colony' was also being used in natural history to describe groups or swarms of animals or insects that were conspicuously co-operative. Analogies between human and insect empires became frequent in the works of natural philosophers, political economists, novelists and settlers. European colonisers in West Africa and the Caribbean were fascinated with how colonies of termites made castles of mud from which to make raids beyond their walls.[15] Natural and scientific applications of the word ramified during the nineteenth century. 'Colony' was used to describe a group of fossil forms that were temporally out of place. The word was also applied to aggregates of individual animals or plants, such as coral-polyps, that formed a physiologically connected structure. In an interesting extension of its imperial usage that simultaneously involves a return to the roots of the word in agriculture, an animal or plant that established itself in a place where it was not indigenous was also being termed a 'colonist' by the later nineteenth century.

Most significantly for my purposes, as the germ theory of disease was elaborated in the 1870s and 80s, the term 'colony' was applied to groups of micro-organisms, those minute clusters of life that could be seen only through a microscope. When producing or culturing such a colony in a

---

[15] Driver, 'Colonies', p. 94.

laboratory the main fear was of contamination – how to protect the purity of the culture. And so plate culture technique was developed to allow bacteriologists to grow a given species of micro-organism in isolation from all others and thereby guarantee the purity of the culture. There is an interesting collocation of metaphor here. Isolation is essential if the purity of the culture or colony is to be secured. Contamination is the worry. Bacterial and imperial colonies are homologous.[16]

Camp-thinking

Paul Gilroy has explored the process by which the nation-state in the era of high imperialism redefined itself in terms of 'biocultural kinship'. Those who fell outside the boundaries of this 'official community were despised, reviled and subjected to entirely different political and juridicial procedures'. Gilroy calls the resulting national and governmental formations 'camps'.[17] He might equally well call them colonies. Gilroy argues that the 'antinomies of modernity' were first produced in the social order of the colony, which was sharply distinguished from that of the metropole in terms of culture, language, biology and 'race'. This 'camp-thinking', articulated in terms of race, is for Gilroy the defining element of the distinctive European nationalism produced by colonial expansion.[18] He also follows Césaire and Fanon in seeing this model of inclusion and exclusion eventually brought home to Europe in the form of Nazi genocide.[19] I want to refine this argument and suggest that the antinomies of modernity Gilroy sees at the colonial margin were simultaneously present, in muted and less extreme forms, in the metropole. Camp-thinking was already part of the structure of thought and practice of European governments at home in the later nineteenth century, with a discourse of health and disease central to the construction of boundaries within the metropole as well as across the empire. At home the forms of exclusion and

---

[16] Plate culture technique was developed by the German bacteriologist Robert Koch, whose state-based forays into Africa were consciously figured in terms of the imperial emissary rooting out pathogenic bacteria as Germany extended its colonial empire (the microbiologist as small-game hunter). Imperial and bacterial language frequently borrowed from each other. A new culture of bacilli was described in the French press as 'new French colonies'; see Laura Otis, *Membranes: Metaphors of Invasion in Nineteenth-Century Literature, Science, and Politics* (Baltimore and London: Johns Hopkins University Press, 1999), pp. 30–6.

[17] Paul Gilroy, *Between Camps: Race, Identity and Nationalism at the End of the Colour Line* (London: Allen Lane/Penguin, 2000). In the United States this book is titled *Against Race: Imagining Political Culture Beyond the Colour Line* (Cambridge, Mass.: Harvard University Press, 2000).

[18] *Ibid.*, p. 82.   [19] *Ibid.*, pp. 71, 81.

containment were based more on class and gender than race, although the language used to describe these three categories of difference was frequently interchangeable and a health/disease dichotomy as a marker of difference was common to all. Without disputing the connection between the coercive systems for treating colonial subjects and the genocide of the Holocaust, I am suggesting a different kind of linkage in which the camp-thinking that produced often extreme suffering in the colonies of overseas empires can be understood in relation to analogous, if normally less acute, discomfort produced by a similar structure of thought and practice in the nineteenth-century metropole. In other words, embryonic or less conspicuously malign versions of camp-thinking were apparent in Europe as well as its empires at this time, and were already being turned on marginalised groups within metropolitan culture.

Camp mentalities, Gilroy argues, have a 'biopolitical potency' that derives from an appeal to national and ethnic purity. The veneration of homogeneity and purity raises, in turn, questions of 'prophylaxis and hygiene', with the regulation of fertility and the bodies of women at the centre of this concern.[20] Extending Gilroy's argument, I want to show how disease, infection and contamination were closely associated aspects of this camp mentality. The imperative to fortify the nation was an inevitable concomitant of camp-thinking, and was characteristically expressed in terms of containing and excluding disease. This was both metaphoric and literal. Figuratively the body of the nation could be represented as threatened with infection from the impurity of outsiders, by cultural germs. More literally, there was the fear of specific diseases that those coming from unsanitary tropical zones would bring with them. This resulted in the need for a cordon sanitaire, quarantine and other methods of isolation and exclusion. Camp-thinking produced camp-practice.

Camp-practice was a political technology producing institutions of 'useless suffering and modern misery'.[21] In the following pages I shall consider the origins of the concentration camp in the South African war, and the establishment of native reservations in the United States and Australia, as examples of this method of containing and extinguishing indigenous cultures. I shall then consider lock hospitals, tuberculosis sanatoria and other forms of disease-based encampment in Britain at this period, including the setting up of a leper colony in south-east England in 1914, as examples of camp-thinking at home. In the process I shall try and make clear the overlapping between camp-thinking in metropole and colony.

---

[20] *Ibid.*, pp. 83–4.   [21] *Ibid.*, p. 85.

There are difficulties with this. If the linkages made by Gilroy might seem to undermine the supposed uniqueness of the Nazi genocide, the various historical examples of encampment that I am bringing together could be said to occlude significant differences, and to suggest an equivalence between metropolitan discomfort and colonial wretchedness that minimises the extent of the latter. The comparative evaluation of degrees of suffering across different cultural contexts is impossible. Gilroy argues that 'a condition of social death is common to camp inmates in regimes of unfreedom, coercion, and systematic brutality'.[22] All the different kinds of forced encampment I shall be considering involve, to widely varying extents, the experience of 'social death'. These range from temporary isolation, to long-term segregation, to the life-long incarceration of the leper colony; the kinds of 'social death' involved range from the temporary loss of the 'home world' that confirms one's sense of self,[23] to the death-in-life condition of the incarcerated leper. I am not suggesting an equivalence of suffering, but rather the recurrence of underlying structures of thought and practice whose intentions could vary from the severe to the inhuman, and whose effects range from short-term discomfort to abjection and death. In doing so, I am arguing that in this respect, at least, metropole and colony need to be understood as simultaneously the condition and effect of the other. During the nineteenth century Britain itself became a colonial construction, although this is not to deny that many aspects of national life were wholly or relatively untouched by colonial expansion (which was itself a contested project).

Whether we call forced concentrations of targeted and pariah groups camps or colonies, they were produced within the fortified nation as well as across the imperial world. 'Encamped ethnicity' was, of course, palpable among colonisers in many territories; the greater the European's sense of vulnerability, the more the need for protective encirclement. The hill station, the club, the administrative compound and the military barracks were among many such forms of self-protective encampment established by the colonisers. Karen Blixen records that, in Kenya, the outbreak of the First World War resulted in a plan for 'a concentration camp for the white women of the country . . . [who] were believed to be exposed to danger from the Natives'.[24] The focus of this chapter, however, is on imposed rather than self-imposed forms of ethnic encampment. Gilroy argues that camp-thinking deprives in-between locations, that is alternative spaces within

[22] *Ibid.*, p. 88.
[23] Erving Goffman, *Asylums: Essays on the Social Situation of Mental Patients and Other Inmates* (Harmondsworth: Penguin, 1975), p. 23.
[24] Karen Blixen, *Out of Africa* (Harmondsworth: Penguin, 1984), p. 228.

which non-polarised collectivities might be conceived and inaugurated, of any significance.[25] However, camp-thinking simultaneously produces a concern with this very possibility. When sharply polarised camps are established, the space falling between them becomes crucial. This becomes imagined as a no-man's-land, a moat or a channel, a cordon sanitaire safeguarding the health and integrity of the coloniser's camp but which is constantly under threat.

The camp life of an imperial nation at home is not always as tense as this. Nevertheless, when the health of the metropole itself is thought to be threatened the drawbridge is likely to be pulled up. This was the case at the end of the nineteenth century. Selecting almost at random, the period-ical *The Nineteenth Century* in 1888 included articles titled 'The Swarming of Men', on population explosion; 'The Invasion of Pauper Foreigners', on the immigration of Jewish people from eastern Europe; 'The Chinese in Australia', criticising the imperial government for obstructing the attempt of several Australian colonies to end Chinese immigration; and 'The Defencelessness of London', about the vulnerability of the capital to foreign invasion.[26] This was the climate in which leprosy and other so-called tropical diseases took on heightened significance. Unlike a Russian Jew from Odessa, disease was invisible, a secret agent impossible to intercept. Threats from without readily become threats from within, and then cultural paranoia is prone to turn on itself. The forms of internal camp or colony I shall be discussing were all disease-based, though not necessarily aimed at tropical diseases. They are evidence, however, of a felt need to isolate various kinds of contaminant that were believed to threaten the health of the nation. Isolation was not a new idea but it was only in this period that it took on such strict and rigorous institutional definition. One reason for this was the emergence of the germ theory of disease. Another was the camp-thinking that accompanied the spread of overseas empire. It is in these terms that I argue for a close affiliation between the practice of ethnic encampment in colonised territories and the segregation of so-called risk groups at home.

Gilroy places the rise of camp-thinking in the context of 'that fateful shift from species to ethnos and the transformed understanding of human-ity and its limits' that followed. 'The Jew' and 'The Negro', he argues, were reconfigured by the interplay of raciology, modernity, selfhood and alter-ity during the nineteenth century.[27] We can also find variants of ethnos at work within the metropole itself: other figures of particularity, defined more by class and gender than race, that were being isolated at home.

---

[25] Gilroy, *Between Camps*, p. 84.   [26] *The Nineteenth Century*, 1 (1888).

[27] Gilroy, *Between Camps*, p. 94.

The prostitute and the tuberculosis patient are two that I have selected because of their direct association with disease. But the mental patient and the conscientious objector would be further examples of this process. And the shape-shifting figure of the leper, found in both colony and metropole, forever an outcast and forever threatening to return, is a particularly vivid example of the instability of such figures and the anxieties that accumulated around them. This racialised figure constantly threatened to deracialise, to become European as well as African, Oriental or Polynesian; in Gilroy's terminology, to replace ethnos with species. This, however, would have been a dangerous and tainted species, a diseased thing.

There is, finally, another sense in which the leper and the leper colony can be seen as an extreme type of camp-thinking. The leper embodies the instability of selfhood and alterity, and therefore the impossibility of securing difference. In like manner the leper colony demonstrates the impossibility of camps. The supposedly native and tropical disease of leprosy had a long European history, was a danger to Europeans in colonial settings, and threatened to return to the centres of empire. The strictly segregated leper colony was a response to these fears but did not contain the disease. The example of Hawaii suggested that compulsory segregation did not work. Diagnosis was imprecise. Those who contracted the disease would often go into hiding. Camps were always leaky, places from which the fears they were designed to contain would always threaten to escape. Camps and those within them would not stay in place, while disease in general, and leprosy in particular, made a nonsense of inside/ outside, or membrane thinking; the higher the walls the greater the fears. Leprosy, the disease-condition above all others that permitted no in-between, became the locus of in-between fears.

The concentration camp

In the modern colonial period the threat of leprosy was met not by placing the leper 'without the camp', but rather by the construction of camps within which lepers could be concentrated. This, I would argue, was symptomatic of colonial ways of thinking in the nineteenth century and certainly not specific to leprosy. The diversifying applications of the term colony, especially in the later part of the century, indicate a cultural preoccupation with drawing lines, establishing boundaries, and constructing enclosures to separate different kinds of people from each other. This was in order to contain the dangers to social health and ordering that imperial expansion brought with it. The formalising of the leper colony at the end of the century, for example, coincided in time and intention with the development of the concentration camp by the British Army during the South African war. These two forms of containment had much in common.

The concentration camp was partly a consequence of Kitchener's scorched-earth and population-clearance policies that resulted in the displacement of thousands of rural inhabitants, black and white. These were, however, camps of concentration rather than refugee camps. The families of fighting burghers, their black servants, 'undesirable' women and other suspect elements of the population were driven into the camps to create controlled enclaves and deny information and sustenance to the republican commandos.[28] Boer women were the especial targets of this policy. Kitchener hoped that by isolating them the Boer men would be forced to return to their families. The camps therefore were partly intended as 'hostage sites'.[29] They were also death camps. Concentrations of people meant concentrations of disease, and infection spread rapidly in the unsanitary conditions that were created by herding almost 120,000 people into fifty camps within a few months. Measles, dysentery, pneumonia and whooping cough devastated the internees, children especially; an estimated 26,000 women and children died in the white camps.[30]

It is often pointed out that the Spanish in Cuba had adopted a similar policy of large-scale concentration several years earlier. This might well have been the first military example of such practice but the idea of the forced displacement and concentration of populations was becoming widespread in colonial thinking and policy at this time. The fact that in the case of leper colonies or native reservations it was applied almost exclusively to indigenous populations has perhaps obscured its significance as part of the apparatus of colonialism in the South African war. This was, as Paula Krebs has shown, a singular imperial war, fought for the control of a non-European land by a European power against a European-descended people.[31] Officially, at least, the indigenous population had no part in it, although they suffered the highest mortality rates of all. In many ways, however, the Boer population in South Africa substituted for native subjects in other colonial territories.

Kitchener described the back-veld Boers as 'uncivilised Afrikaner savages with a thin white veneer'. In thus nativising the Boers he focused

[28] Bill Nasson, *The South African War 1899–1902* (London: Arnold, 1999), pp. 220–1; S. B. Spires, 'Women and the War', in Peter Warwick (ed.), *The South African War: The Anglo-Boer War 1899–1902* (Harlow: Longman, 1980), pp. 167–8.
[29] Nasson, *The South African War*, p. 221.
[30] Warwick, *The South African War: The Anglo-Boer War*, p. 61; Byron Farwell, *The Great Boer War* (London: Allen Lane, 1977), pp. 397–9.
[31] Paula M. Krebs, *Gender, Race, and the Writing of Empire* (Cambridge: Cambridge University Press, 1999), pp. 35–6.

especially on the women: 'The Boer woman in the refugee camps who slaps her great protruding belly at you and shouts, "When all our men are gone these little khakis will fight you", is a type of the savage produced by generations of wild lonely life.'[32] Though extreme, this was not unrepresentative. The Boers were regarded by Britain and its dominion allies as backward, congenitally unclean and unsanitary.[33] This emphasis on dirt was pronounced. The Boer's imputed 'sanitation malaise'[34] was also used to explain and excuse the appalling mortality rates in the camps that prompted concern and opposition to the war in Britain. Although Millicent Fawcett's report on the camps for the War Office was frank about the dreadful conditions she had observed, it also made much of the backwardness of Boer women and their 'filthy habits': 'the Boer woman has a horror of ventilation; any cranny through which fresh air could enter is carefully stuffed up, and the tent becomes a hot-bed for the breeding of disease germs'. In 'the pestilential atmosphere of these tents', Fawcett concluded, 'It is ... no wonder that measles ... had raged through the camps and caused many deaths; because the children are enervated by the foul air their mothers compel them to breathe and fall more easy victims to disease than would be the case if the tents were fairly ventilated.'[35]

Outside the camps the nativised Boer woman transmitted information to the enemy. Inside the camps she was the source of the dirt and diseases that killed her own children, and was making the war unpopular in Britain. Either way she was represented as contagious. Concentrating her within the camps produced a new set of problems, however, and not solely in relation to infant mortality. Sexual relations with British soldiers became a problem and punishment enclosures were constructed within the camps for those who transgressed.[36] It is the logic of concentration that successively smaller enclosures will need to be created within the larger structure. The coffin is the last stage in this process.

Paula Krebs has demonstrated the complexity of the representation of Boer women, and I am emphasising only one aspect of this. Emily Hobhouse's famous campaign against the camps involved a very different image of the noble Boer mother starving with her doomed children.[37] Hobhouse was recuperating the Boer woman as a suffering European in her efforts to bring the real state of the camps to public attention. But the

---

[32] In Farwell, *The Great Boer War*, p. 400.   [33] Nasson, *The South African War*, pp. 243–4.
[34] *Ibid.*, p. 244.
[35] Millicent Fawcett, *Report on the Concentration Camps*, 1902, in Krebs, *Gender, Race, and the Writing of Empire*, p. 74.
[36] Farwell, *The Great Boer War*, p. 414.
[37] Krebs, *Gender, Race, and the Writing of Empire*, pp. 70–1 also makes plain the conservatism and ambiguities of Hobhouse's representation.

dominant representation of the Boer woman as native subject shows how a war fought against a European-descended people could be translated into a more familiar colonial conflict. The easily recognised tropes of colonial discourse were being applied to a different kind of colonial subject, thereby explaining and justifying the herding of fellow whites into camps.

There were also concentration camps for natives. These had a stronger refugee element because the displacement of blacks was often a by-product of the conflict between the main antagonists: 'collateral damage' in the sanitising vocabulary of our own time. Many black servants and labourers, however, were at first concentrated with the white families they worked for, and then re-concentrated as the camps were divided along colour lines.[38] By the middle of 1902 more than 115,000 Africans had been placed in over sixty camps. There were 14,000 recorded deaths, mainly of children, and many more went unrecorded because of official and philanthropic indifference to the suffering of Africans. Record keeping in the black camps was irregular, and neither Emily Hobhouse nor Millicent Fawcett visited these camps. Insofar as black mortality rates were discussed at all, they were normally put down to traditional African lifeways and a failure to adapt to new conditions. According to the head of the Native Refugee Department in the Transvaal: 'natives do not thrive under abnormal conditions and sudden changes; if transplanted to new conditions, water, soil, food, etc. they appear to require time to become acclimatized'.[39] This redirected version of acclimatisation theory supplemented the idea that those Africans who died in the camps were victims of their own culture.

In many ways it is the black concentration camps that bear the closer resemblance to leper colonies. Their relative invisibility made them to the white camps what leper colonies were to the colonial infirmary: an easily forgotten dumping ground. Like leper colonies, and unlike the white camps, black concentration camps were intended to be self-sufficient; inmates were to erect their own huts and grow their own crops rather than depend on provided rations.[40] Whereas there was always some unease at the relocation and imprisonment of Boers (for example, Milner, Governor of the Cape, was never in favour of the plan), there were no qualms about this policy being applied to Africans. A report on black camps by the Society of Friends in 1902 found conditions to be satisfactory

---

[38] This short section derives from Peter Warwick, *Black People and the South African War* (Cambridge: Cambridge University Press, 1983), pp. 145–54; also Spiers, 'Women and the War', p. 172.

[39] In Warwick, *Black People and the South African War*, p. 152.

[40] Warwick, *The South African War: The Anglo-Boer War*, p. 172; Warwick, *Black People and the South African War*, p. 149.

and in several respects an improvement on their usual mode of living. Requiring the people to grow crops and to send their children to school to learn English was, the report concluded, beneficial: 'It seems possible that this experience may have far-reaching effects on the natives.'[41] African colonial subjects did not really know what was best for them; within the concentration camp and the leper colony they could be taught. Both forms of enclosure provided a setting within which native peoples could be more effectively colonised. Both were intended to control through segregation and by rendering the inmates dependent on the authorities that regulated their lives. These micro-colonies, the result of disease and war, could then be represented as an ideal type of the colony, a model for other natives who were yet to be brought to heel.

The Native American reservation

The black concentration camp of the South African war had antecedents in the Native American reservation and the Australian Aboriginal reserve, both of which involved the forced relocation and concentration of large numbers of indigenous people, and are further evidence of a colonial discourse and practice of segregation and enclosure that was being fashioned at this time. As empires and colonised territories expanded, indigenous populations were being penned in. This form of confinement was fundamentally different from punishment by incarceration and other kinds of judicial retribution. The policy of concentration was applied to whole groups rather than deviant individuals, and was not because of any alleged criminality. Indeed it was often represented as protective rather than punitive, to rescue native subjects from themselves or even from the lawlessness of the white man at the frontier. Large groups of people could never simply be locked up. Instead, boundaries were established: cordons sanitaires with the economic, social and hygienic purpose of keeping the native out of the way of the European.

In the case of the Native Americans, removal policies of the 1830s and 40s under which some 100,000 people were pushed across the Mississippi had given way to a reservation policy based on confinement by the later decades of the century.[42] This was because of the settler desire for land west of the Mississippi, and the belief of Eastern liberals that Native Americans

---

[41] In Warwick, *Black People and the South African War*, p. 146.
[42] This short section derives from Maldwyn A. Jones, *The Limits of Liberty: American History 1607–1980* (Oxford: Oxford University Press, 1983), and James S. Olson and Raymond Wilson, *Native Americans in the Twentieth Century* (Urbana and Chicago: University of Illinois Press, 1986).

needed to be detribalised if they were ever to assimilate to white civilisation. The establishment of bounded reservations, therefore, involved the concentration of hitherto territorially distinct Native Americans with the intention of freeing land for settlers and breaking down tribal structures. The Navajos, for example, after defeat in 1864 'were herded to a bleak reservation (more like a concentration camp) at Bosque Redondo in eastern New Mexico to live with Mescalero Apaches who had also been forcibly removed there in 1863'. A smallpox epidemic soon killed more than a quarter of the 800 people detained there.[43]

By the 1880s the Native American people had been confined to reservations – 'ghettos in the wilderness'[44] – which left them economically dependent on the federal government and undermined by diseases such as smallpox, measles, cholera and syphilis. Their population had been reduced from one million to less than 300,000. The protective and educative intentions of Eastern liberals had misfired as the often heavy-handed and culturally insensitive attempts by missionaries and government agents to introduce European values were resisted. And the railroad companies, ranchers and other economic interests regarded the reservations as obstructions to expansion and development. The idea of the reservation itself came under attack, and a scissors movement between reformers and developers resulted in the further break-up of land into allotments for Native American families. Reformers had come to believe that the reservations were perpetuating tribal values and economic dependence. Children became the new focus of their attempt to destroy tribal affiliation, and a federal system of boarding schools well away from reservations was set up.[45] Once more the initial stage of mass concentration is followed by further removals involving ever-smaller forms of concentration. The boarding schools scheme for Native American children in some ways resembles the European agricultural colonies for delinquent adolescents discussed earlier. The creation of individual and family allotments under the Dawes Act of 1887, rather than producing a class of yeoman farmers, pauperised the Native American and facilitated further land grabbing by whites. The last two decades of the century saw rapid reductions in the amount of land under Native American control and the enclosure of the native population within ever-narrower boundaries.[46]

[43] Olson and Wilson, *Native Americans in the Twentieth Century*, p. 43.
[44] *Ibid.*, p. 50.   [45] *Ibid.*, pp. 56–62.
[46] Jones, *The Limits of Liberty*, p. 285; Frederick E. Hoxie, 'The Reservation Period, 1880–1960', in Bruce G. Trigger and Wilcomb E. Washburn (eds.), *The Cambridge History of the Native Peoples of the Americas*, 3 vols., *North America*, vol. I, part 2 (Cambridge: Cambridge University Press, 1996), p. 187.

All these intensifying forms of concentration that Native Americans were subjected to in the second half of the nineteenth century involved the attempt to create borders between them and so-called civilisation, even as attempts were being made to civilise them. The European desire for land was overriding, but the belief in some quarters that Native Americans needed to be prepared for entry into the white world was genuinely held, though misapplied. Cultural and political frontiers were established to manage this process, and the boundaries within which Native Americans could live contracted further under the pressure of economic development. Native lifeways came under intense pressure, and in spite of the tenacity of tribal cultures, considerable autonomy and freedom of movement were lost.[47] Attempts to mitigate the worst effects of this process characteristically involved new kinds of displacement and re-concentration that further atomised Native American social organisation. The United States government that implemented these policies in the 1880s and 90s was at the same time pressing the Hawaiian government for ever-stricter segregation of lepers at the Kaulapapa colony on Molokai. In both cases the construction of a cordon sanitaire had seriously damaging cultural consequences, while conspicuously failing to produce the kind of impermeability that was intended.

The Aboriginal reserve

Reserves were also being established for Aboriginal Australians in the later nineteenth century. This had first been tried in Tasmania much earlier in the century when the 1828 Demarcation Proclamation removed the indigenous population from white settlement districts, initially to a remote part of Tasmania itself, and then to confinement on Flinders Island. Although justified on the grounds of protecting Aboriginal people from white settlers, it was designed to clear the colony for those settlers. This rationale of 'displacement for protection' was to inform policy towards the Aboriginal people for more than a hundred years.[48] Concentration policies removed Aboriginal Australians from valuable land assets and enabled missionaries and state governments to control their lifeways through cultural conversion or neglect.

---

[47] Hoxie, 'The Reservation Period, 1880–1960', p. 185; Olson and Wilson, *Native Americans in the Twentieth Century*, p. 56.

[48] C. D. Rowley, *The Destruction of Aboriginal Society* (Canberra: Australian National University Press, 1970), pp. 46–7; Richard Broome, *Aboriginal Australians: Black Response to White Dominance 1788–1980* (Sydney: Allen and Unwin, 1992), p. 48.

Across the middle and later years of the century there was a variety of attempts to establish reserves. Some were sponsored by state governments, with missionaries usually undertaking the management; some were at the request of the Aboriginal population itself; still others were initiatives by mission groups or individual European settlers. Although there were variations across the different states, there was also a shared pattern with similarities to the history of the Native American reservations. Those who were removed to reserves lacked freehold or security of tenure, and were often relocated when white settlers wanted the land for grazing. The Poonindie reserve, for example, which had been successfully self-supporting from the 1860s, was dismantled by the South Australian government in 1894 to open up land for European settlers. The Aboriginal population was then left with the poorest land and the reserves became ration depots rather than farms.[49] The balance between protection and control, uncertain from the beginning, had shifted decisively towards control by the later part of the century, and the management of the reserves became increasingly authoritarian. In 1897 an Act in Queensland, 'to make provision for the better Protection and Care of the Aboriginal and Half-Caste Inhabitants of the Colony, and to make more effectual Provision for Restricting the Sale and Distribution of Opium', provided the model for similar legislation in other states. Many of its provisions, however, were already widely in practice. As C. D. Rowley puts it, the Aboriginal had stepped 'into the convict's shoes'.[50]

This and subsequent legislation meant all Aboriginal people, including 'half-castes', were liable to be moved to reserves. Once corralled on a reserve, obedience to the superintendent was compulsory. Reserve managers had powers of search, confiscation, confinement and expulsion to other reserves. Medical inspection was compulsory and Aboriginal cultural practices were prohibited. Inhabitants of a reserve were liable for up to thirty-two hours of unpaid work per week. Sexual relations with Europeans were prohibited but European names and clothing were imposed on the inhabitants.[51] Any idea of protection disappeared in this draconian and racially based legal restriction that provided the basis for the institutional and separate management of Aboriginal people in Australia until after the Second World War.[52]

The reserves had an important role within the colonial labour market. They were 'enclaves where the Aboriginal family produced in safety the

---

[49] Broome, *Aboriginal Australians*, pp. 80, 85.
[50] Rowley, *The Destruction of Aboriginal Society*, pp. 173, 182.
[51] Broome, *Aboriginal Australians*, pp. 98–9.
[52] Rowley, *The Destruction of Aboriginal Society*, p. 183.

labourers of the future. From here they were to go into rural employment, and here they were to return when not required ... The system could thus operate as a subsidy to the pastoral and other industries.'[53] This persisted well into the twentieth century; for example in New South Wales in the 1930s many Aboriginal people living in towns and cities were pushed back into the reserves to save dole payments during the Depression.[54] But although the creation of a disposable labour supply was important, the main purpose of the reserves was racial separation. At first this simply meant removing the Aboriginal Australians from the path of the white settlers. Soon, however, the reserve policy was complicated by a concern to distinguish 'full bloods' from 'half-castes'. The former, it was assumed, would wither away on the reserves, a people doomed to extinction. The latter were to be assimilated to the European population until the taint of their Aboriginal origins was bred out of them. Legislation in Western Australia (1905), the Northern Territory (1911), and a Children's Act in Queensland (1911) made the Chief Protector of Aborigines in these states the legal guardian of all Aboriginal and 'half-caste' children. This gave him the right to remove children from their parents and place them in an institution or with a foster family, something that became general practice with light-skinned children.[55] Cecil Cook, chief medical and quarantine officer, and chief protector of Aborigines in the Northern Territory between 1927 and 1939 wanted to give the half-caste an 'opportunity to evolve into a white man'.[56] As with the Native Americans, we can see an alternation between concentration and dispersal that results from the intricate process of trying to prevent social relations between different groups of people, and, in the case of Australia, of attempting to distinguish between them according to some theory of racial make-up.

The arithmetic upon which different categories of race and age were based became increasingly bizarre. The Victoria Aborigines Act 1886 ruled that only 'full bloods' and 'half-castes' over the age of thirty-four could remain on reserves. Younger 'half-castes' were to begin the process of being blended to whiteness through assimilation.[57] However, the category of 'half-caste' was itself unstable, and legislation struggled to distinguish between those with Aboriginal mothers or fathers, parents or grandparents, those with Aboriginal or non-Aboriginal spouses, and so on.[58] The more precise the arithmetic, the more tortuous became the distinction. J. W. Bleakley, Chief Protector of Aborigines in Queensland from 1913 to

---

[53] *Ibid.*, p. 221.   [54] *Ibid.*, p. 143.   [55] Broome, *Aboriginal Australians*, p. 134.
[56] Warwick Anderson, *The Cultivation of Whiteness: Science, Health and Racial Destiny in Australia* (New York: Basic Books, 2003), p. 244.
[57] *Ibid.*, p. 82.   [58] Rowley, *The Destruction of Aboriginal Society*, p. 231.

1940, refined his measurement down to the category of 'octoroon' (one eighth Aboriginal 'blood') in his attempt to control the growth of a mixed-race population. The Aboriginal woman became the particular focus of these miscegenation fears and there were even moves for sterilisation.[59] Cecil Cook was particularly concerned to absorb half-caste women into white society, partly to ensure they did not become a 'native reservoir' of disease.[60] Different categories required different kinds of concentration. In Darwin, between the wars, Aboriginal Australians with jobs in the town were required to return each night to a compound two miles outside the town boundary where they lived in a collection of huts with earth or concrete floors and no beds. Young Aboriginal people of mixed descent were crammed into a small house within the town limits, known as 'Halfcaste House'.[61]

Metropolitan colonies

Comparable forms of enclosure and segregation were practised in Britain in the later nineteenth and early twentieth century. Although these were usually medically based, some involved the control or attempted re-education of groups of people who were marked as much by their class, gender or way of life as by the stigma of disease. The Mettray colony for the residential re-education of delinquent adolescents has already been touched upon. This 'colony without walls' practising a 'discipline without frontiers' acquired many admirers among reformers and policy makers in Britain. The idea of bodily discipline within a circumscribed location as a means of moral training had especial appeal, and versions of it were found in the reformatory schools that were established in the 1850s and the pauper schools of the 1870s. Even at the turn of the century, movements for the rural regeneration of the urban poor through agricultural colonies were citing Mettray as the model to emulate. Mettray had, by then, come to be regarded as appropriate for dependent children, paupers and the morally endangered, as well as the actually criminal or deviant.[62]

One of the factors contributing to the spread of Mettray-type institutions was the emerging construction of juveniles as a distinct category with an under-developed moral sense and therefore a disturbing potential for criminal or anti-social behaviour. This concept of the half-formed juvenile had close analogies with some of the more optimistic constructions of the

---

[59] Broome, *Aboriginal Australians*, pp. 160–2.
[60] Anderson, *The Cultivation of Whiteness*, p. 244.   [61] *Ibid.*, p. 123.
[62] Driver, 'Discipline Without Frontiers?' 280–4; 'Bodies in Space', pp. 125–6; personal communication with Felix Driver, 30 July 2004.

colonial subject at this time. As the narrator of Robert Louis Stevenson's novella 'The Beach of Falesa' (1892) has it: 'it's easy to find out what kanakas think. Just go back to yourself anyway round from ten to fifteen years old, and there's an average kanaka.'[63] Ann Laura Stoler has written of the discursive connection between the 'savage as child' and the 'child as savage', both constructs of a civilising, custodial mission and a growing anxiety about degeneracy.[64] Intersecting concerns about individual development and social degeneration were affecting the definition and treatment of groups both at home and in the colonies that it was felt should be isolated, at least as much for the protection of nation and empire as for their own good.

A vivid example of this in Britain was a new category, the feeble-minded, one of a growing number of target groups being segregated in colonies around the turn of the twentieth century. Hitherto regarded as a mild form of mental deficiency, a borderland between imbecility and normality, this was now reconceptualised as pathological, more dangerous than more severe and visible forms of mental retardation, and hence in particular need of attention.[65] Mark Jackson has shown how concern with a 'residuum of educationally inept and socially dangerous defectives' in the later 1890s became caught up with wider concerns about degeneration and declining imperial strength.[66] The remedy for this, vigorously proselytised by Mary Dendy in Manchester, was a system of permanent segregation and care in purpose-built working colonies.[67] The first of these, Sandlebridge Boarding Schools and Colony, opened in 1902 'in the sylvan glades of sunny Cheshire', as a contemporary description put it. This was for boys, but a separate house for girls opened soon after, and was followed by separate establishments for adult women and men as well.[68]

Sandlebridge, in its spatial and temporal organisation, resembled Mettray and other such institutions. Clusters of small houses facilitated strict gender and age segregation, creating a familial structure in which all the children addressed the matrons as 'mother', and enabling the continual observation and supervision of inmates. The day was carefully structured with mornings devoted to 'head work' and afternoons to 'hand work' – gardening, farming and workshop tasks for the boys, laundry, sewing and kitchen work for the girls.[69] The feeble-minded were often explained as

[63] Robert Louis Stevenson, 'The Beach of Falesa', in Roslyn Jolly (ed.), *Robert Louis Stevenson: South Sea Tales* (Oxford and New York: World's Classics, 1996), p. 55.
[64] Stoler, *Race and the Education of Desire*, p. 141.
[65] Mark Jackson, *The Borderland of Imbecility: Medicine, Society and the Fabrication of the Feeble Mind in Late Victorian and Edwardian England* (Manchester and New York: Manchester University Press, 2000), pp. 1–13.
[66] *Ibid.*, pp. 62–3.   [67] *Ibid.*, pp. 66–7.   [68] *Ibid.*, p. 70.   [69] *Ibid.*, pp. 70, 176–9.

examples of racial damage, even racial degeneration, although unlike so-called 'Mongols' they were not conflated with a specific ethnic group. They were, however, understood as associated with the pauper and criminal classes.[70] Jackson is clear that they were removed to colonies because they were regarded as contaminants. Segregation was not primarily a 'humanitarian endeavour validated by medical science ... but [an] overtly political enterprise designed to subdue and control'.[71] It was one of a number of such boundaries being configured at this time intended to draw a clear line between a healthy imperial nation and internal contaminants threatening to infect or undermine it. Jackson compares colonies for the feeble-minded with contemporary examples of racial segregation in colonial societies in British West and South Africa. He also notes the choice of the term 'colony' to describe these settlements for the feeble-minded, and the way it echoed a discriminatory politics of punishment as well as reclamation operating in both metropole and empire at this time.[72]

This association of colonies at home with those of empire was made quite explicit in William Booth's *In Darkest England and the Way Out* (1890). By deliberately echoing the title of Henry Morton Stanley's *In Darkest Africa*, published a few months earlier, Booth found a powerful trope for the condition of Britain's urban poor: 'Darkest England, like Darkest Africa, reeks with malaria. The foul and fetid breath of our slums is almost as poisonous as that of the African swamp. Fever is almost as chronic there as on the Equator.'[73] If England's cities are like an untamed jungle, the answer lies in colonisation. Booth advocates a three-stage process of colonisation. The first of these is the City Colony, 'harbours of refuge' for all those 'shipwrecked' in 'the ocean of misery'. After 'a course of regeneration by moral and religious influences', those without employment or suitable homes to return to would pass on to the Farm Colony, reversing the damaging flow of population from city to country. Here the 'reformation of character' begun in the City Colony would be extended to include 'those forms of labour and that knowledge of agriculture which ... will qualify [the Colonist] for pursuing his fortunes under more favourable circumstances in some other land'. While some in the Farm Colony might settle in cottages or on Co-operative Farms, 'the great bulk, after trial and training, would be passed on to the Foreign Settlement ... The Over-Sea Colony'. This would be established in some 'empty space' in South Africa, Canada, Western Australia or elsewhere and settled with 'a prepared people'. This step-by-step progress would culminate in 'laying the foundations ... of another Empire to swell to vast

---

[70] *Ibid.*, pp. 129–30, 133.   [71] *Ibid.*, p. 131.   [72] *Ibid.*, pp. 149–50.
[73] William Booth, *In Darkest England and the Way Out* (London: Charles Knight, 1970), p. 14.

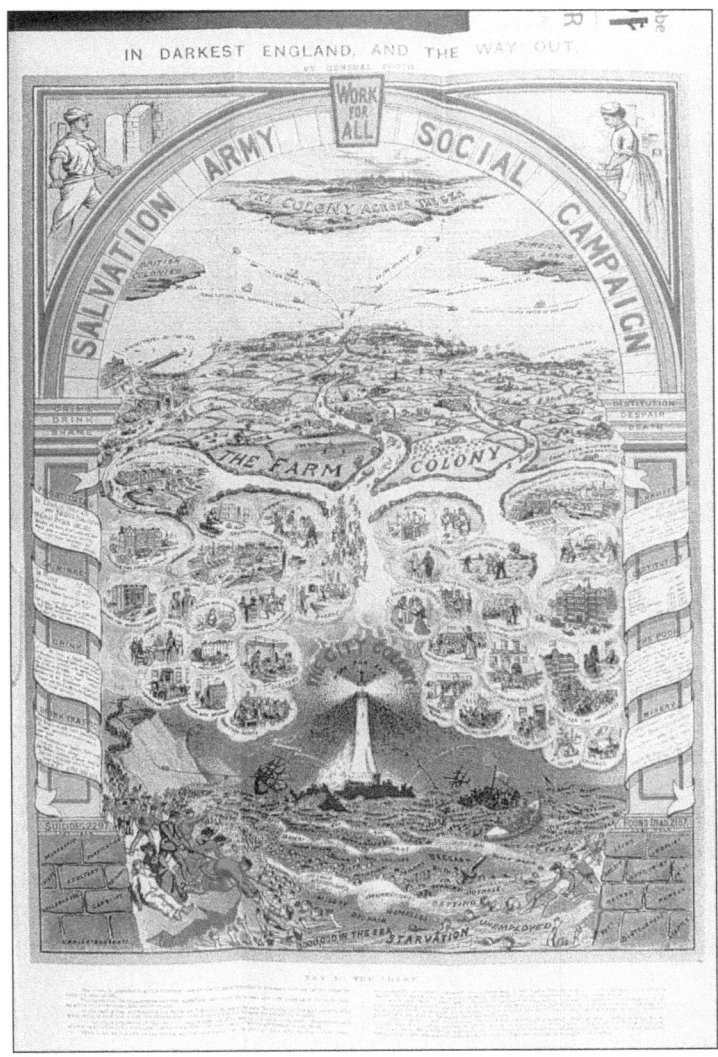

Figure 7. Frontispiece to William Booth's *In Darkest England and the Way Out* (1890).

proportions in later times'.[74] *In Darkest England* has an elaborate frontispiece, with the lighthouse of the Salvation Army as a haven for those rescued from the sea of beggary and ruin at the bottom, and the City Colony, Farm Colony and the Colony Across the Sea spreading up the

[74] *Ibid.*, pp. 92–3.

page as the city is left behind for farms and allotments, with the distant prospect of a utopian Colony Over-Sea at the top.

In devising this scheme Booth was obviously drawing upon the long nineteenth-century tradition of the domestic colony I have already touched on. As with other end-of-the-century versions of this idea, Booth's scheme is inflected by contemporary theories of urban degeneration, and based upon a conviction that the problem of poverty could be addressed by moral training. His idea of the colony as reformatory could be applied to children, the morally unfit and other sub-categories of the residuum at home, as well as to natives abroad.[75] The third phase of Booth's grand plan, the Colony Over-Sea, failed to win much support, although Driver notes that it was revived during the early twentieth-century debate over physical deterioration and national efficiency.[76] The Colony Over-Sea was a notion rather than a programme, although it was an interesting attempt to graft much earlier schemes of planned colonisation, such as Edward Gibbon Wakefield's in the 1830 and 40s, on to an end-of-the-century concern about urban and national degeneration. The Farm Colony, however, was more practical and very much in tune with the moment. By 1892 the Salvation Army had established one at Hadleigh, in Suffolk, where several hundred colonists were employed in market gardening, animal husbandry and brick-making.[77]

Other disease-specific forms of enclosure and segregation were multiplying in the second half of the nineteenth century. Of course there was nothing new about isolating those suffering infectious diseases, nor about the conflict between the regulation of public health and the rights of individuals and groups. The creation of a cordon sanitaire was a long-established method of preventing the spread of disease. Dorothy Porter gives the example of the British Plague Act (1604) by which plague-sufferers were put under house arrest, infected houses were marked with an insignia, and militia could be posted outside to prevent exit and entrance.[78] Such measures, however, had normally been an immediate response to a suddenly perceived danger. The public health measures of the later nineteenth century were far more elaborate and systematic in their application and in the range and kind of control they imposed. The new understanding of the role of bacteria in causing disease was one reason for this. Bacteriology highlighted the significance of individual habits and behaviour in the spread of infection, with the result that preventive environmental medicine

[75] Felix Driver, *Geography Militant: Cultures of Exploration and Empire* (Oxford: Blackwell, 2001), pp. 193–4.
[76] *Ibid.*, pp. 189–90.   [77] *Ibid.*, p. 192.
[78] Dorothy Porter, 'Public Health', in W. F. Bynum and Roy Porter (eds.), *Companion Encyclopedia of the History of Medicine*, 2 vols. (London: Routledge, 1993), vol. I, p. 1233.

increasingly brought social behaviour as well as the social environment within its purview. This involved the identification of risk groups as well as the education and policing of domestic hygiene.[79] But even more significant than the emergence of bacteriology was a cast of mind that saw segregation as an essential means of protecting nation and empire from many different kinds of threat, real and imagined, internal and external, physiological and ideological. Segregation as ideology and technology was reconfiguring both colonial outposts and the cities of Britain at this period.

Lock hospitals

The Contagious Diseases Acts designed to check the spread of venereal disease through the confinement of prostitutes believed to be so infected were more than just a response to a specific medical problem; they provide a telling example of the way in which disease models and social anxieties were mutually reinforcing in the second half of the nineteenth century. Furthermore, as a measure common to Britain and virtually every British colony between the 1860s and 1880s, this legislation provides an interesting example of metropole and empire as a single but differentiated site.

From their beginnings in eighteenth-century Britain as hospitals with separate venereal wards, lock hospitals had by the mid-Victorian period acquired moral and disciplinary functions as well.[80] The origin of the term is disputed. A nineteenth-century explanation by William Acton was that it derived from the French *une loque*, meaning the rags, bandages or lints in which lepers bound their sores, because the original lock hospital at Southwark had been founded on the site of a medieval leper house. Philippa Levine gives this some credence, noting the practice from the sixteenth century of leper hospitals taking patients with venereal disease, but also suggests *un loquet* (latch), as another possible origin.[81] Admission to lock hospitals was voluntary until a series of Contagious Diseases Act in 1864, 1866 and 1869. These began as an exceptional measure to control the spread of venereal disease in garrison towns and ports, but evolved into a method of enforcing social discipline on an unruly section of the non-respectable poor. This involved two closely related forms of concentration: the detention of prostitutes with venereal diseases in lock hospitals until

---

[79] *Ibid.*, p. 1256.

[80] This short section derives from Judith R. Walkowitz, *Prostitution and Victorian Society: Women, Class and the State* (Cambridge: Cambridge University Press, 1980); Paul McHugh, *Prostitution and Victorian Social Reform* (London: Croom Helm, 1980); Frank Mort, *Dangerous Sexualities: Medico-Moral Politics in England since 1830* (London and New York: Routledge, 2000).

[81] Philippa Levine, *Prostitution, Race and Politics: Policing Veneral Disease in the British Empire* (New York and London: Routledge, 2003), pp. 70–1.

they were no longer infectious, and the establishing of strict geographical limits within which non-infected prostitutes could work. Arguments justifying this legislation were increasingly in terms of its moral benefits rather than any social amelioration it might offer.[82]

Under the Contagious Diseases Acts, hospital authorities engaged in what Judith Walkowitz describes as 'a colonising effort'.[83] Inmates were subjected to strict routines of time and labour, prayers and laundry work punctuated their day, and a total regimen designed to teach the women deference and subordination was imposed. Particular emphasis was placed on domestic training in the hope that many of the women would return to the public sphere as domestic servants.[84] Resistance to the rigorous discipline of confinement resulted in a further tightening of the system to ensure stricter enclosure and, where necessary, isolation. Walls were made higher, internal segregation wards were set up to isolate disruptive inmates, and hardened long-stay patients were kept apart from new arrivals.[85] The structures of confinement and discipline multiplied in the attempt to control and educate through hygiene and segregation. Nothing, however, was less amenable to control and concentration than prostitution. A major reason for extending the first Contagious Diseases Act had been the ability of prostitutes to slip out of the districts covered by the Act when threatened with hospital internment.[86] Confinement prompted resistance, and further confinement in the interests of good order could never be more than a temporary expedient. And with the diagnosis of venereal disease so imprecise, there could be no confidence about when it was safe to release the cured and reclaimed prostitute back into the world.

The earliest contagious disease legislation in the empire occurred in Hong Kong in 1857, anticipating Britain's domestic measures, but the bulk of colonial legislation was enacted in the late 1860s: for example, Jamaica in 1867, Barbados, Trinidad, Cape Colony, India and Queensland in 1868, New Zealand in 1869.[87] Although colonial and domestic laws both used the registration of prostitutes as a means to compulsory examination, and required compulsory in-patient treatment for all infected women, there were significant differences between them as well. British legislation was limited to specified garrison and port towns, but colonial laws applied colony-wide. In the colonies the registered brothel was the focus of attention, whereas in Britain brothels were never recognised. And the emphasis on reclamation through work training and moral instruction was much

[82] Walkowitz, *Prostitution and Victorian Society*, p. 78.   [83] *Ibid.*, p. 220.
[84] *Ibid.*, pp. 220–3.   [85] *Ibid.*, pp. 224, 226–7.   [86] *Ibid.*, p. 78.
[87] Levine, *Prostitution, Race and Politics*, pp. 40–1.

less pronounced in colonial lock hospitals, which were more overtly prison-like than their British counterparts.[88]

Contagious disease laws were disliked and resisted both at home and in the empire, but the focus of opposition differed. Most hospital provision in the empire was outpatient, and so colonial lock hospitals were markedly different from the norm and resented as such by native subjects.[89] In Britain, the class and gender-specific nature of the measures was the main point of resistance. The legislation of the 1860s coincided with and encouraged middle-class feminism, and anti-contagious disease campaigners made resentful comparisons, often heavily saturated with imperial racial assumptions, between their inferior status and that of non-white colonised female subjects.[90] One prominent member of the campaigning Ladies' National Association also likened lock hospitals to the horrors of the lazar house.[91]

Although contagious disease legislation in metropole and colony differed, it shared a fundamental commonality in which working-class women at home and native women across the empire were identified as threats to social purity and national identity. The boundaries between the included and excluded within nineteenth-century national and colonial societies were unlikely to be identical but, both at home and across the empire, medical discourse on the dangers of infection and contagion through prostitution readily became a discourse on cultural and moral contamination.[92] Ann Laura Stoler, in her critique of Foucault's 'tunnel vision of the West', argues that nineteenth-century discourses of sexuality were inseparable from those of race, nation and empire.[93] More particularly, she asks if any of Foucault's four target figures of sexual discourse – the hysterical woman, the masturbating child, the Malthusian couple and the perverse adult – existed 'without a racially erotic counterpoint, without reference to the libidinal energies of the savage, the primitive, the colonised'.[94] The figure of the prostitute, at home threatening the good health of the armed forces and the boundaries of class upon which the social order depended, and in the empire the health of the barracks and the boundaries of race upon which national and imperial identity depended, is a telling

---

[88] *Ibid.*, pp. 40, 74.   [89] *Ibid.*, p. 70.   [90] *Ibid.*, p. 7.

[91] Walkowitz, *Prostitution and Victorian Society*, p. 130.

[92] Ann Laura Stoler and Frederick Cooper, 'Between Metropole and Colony: Rethinking a Research Agenda', in Frederick Cooper and Ann Laura Stoler (eds.), *Tensions of Empire: Colonial Cultures in a Bourgeois World* (Berkeley, Los Angeles and London: University of California Press, 1997), pp. 24–6.

[93] Stoler, *Race and the Education of Desire*, pp. 11, 133–4.

[94] *Ibid.*, pp. 6–7. On Foucault's four target figures of sexual discourse, see Michel Foucault, *The History of Sexuality*, vol. I (London: Allen Lane, 1978), p. 105.

witness for Stoler's case. Prostitution was one of those mobile discourses of empire that, in this case, resulted in forms of confinement marking and defending the interior frontiers upon which the health and order of both metropolitan and colonial society depended.

Contagious disease legislation was, of course, repealed in Britain in 1886, and in its colonies several years later. But this was after an unprecedented and sustained campaign by middle-class feminists in which the particular issue of segregation as a form of defending social health became entangled in other questions of gender and alternative notions of social purity. Speculum examination, for example, a particular focus of the campaign in Britain, was denounced as a degrading and voyeuristic intrusion into the womb, which as one campaigner put it, had been planted by God deep within the body for shelter and protection.[95] Such arguments were limited to the Contagious Diseases Acts at home, and colonial legislation only became a matter of serious concern after repeal had been won in Britain. All the cases of confinement and segregation being considered in this section were debated and sometimes opposed. All would eventually disappear, though we are currently finding new forms of detention and concentration to meet the felt or imagined imperatives of our own time. Compulsory detention in lock hospitals was relatively short-lived, and ended because of concerted opposition that the confinement of leper patients, Australian Aboriginals or the feeble-minded never attracted. It nevertheless marked an intensive and empire-wide project of defending men from the medical consequences of sexual encounter across the borders of class and race.

Smallpox isolation

Other historians have noted the spread of institutions for confinement and isolation around the turn of the twentieth century.[96] Each of the social or medical conditions it was felt necessary to segregate had its own specificity, but there was an underlying cultural reflex common to these various forms of exclusion that resulted in similar techniques and palliatives. Most striking was the habit of medicalising and then moralising a range of different kinds of condition, whether physiological, psychological, social or imagined. Smallpox would seem a rather poor example of this broad cultural

---

[95] Walkowitz, *Prostitution and Victorian Society*, p. 130.
[96] Linda Bryder, *Below the Magic Mountain: A Social History of Tuberculosis in Twentieth-Century Britain* (Oxford: Clarendon Press, 1988), p. 29; Alison Bashford, *Imperial Hygiene: A Critical History of Colonialism, Nationalism and Public Health* (Basingstoke: Palgrave Macmillan, 2004), pp. 61–2.

tendency, and indeed the short-term isolation of smallpox sufferers is in many ways much closer to the traditional practice of isolation as an immediate response to a sudden outbreak of disease than to the more long-term and morally driven forms I am discussing. Even so, there are parallels between later nineteenth-century responses to smallpox and these other forms of isolation. In the first place, isolation arrangements were considerably tightened at this time. Before the severe smallpox epidemic of 1870–2, isolation arrangements were haphazard. There was a smallpox hospital at Highgate, but when this was full patients would be received into the workhouse or parish infirmary where they might or might not be isolated.[97] The 1870–2 epidemic caused a rapid extension of isolation facilities, including the use of Thames hospital ships that provided a floating island on which the infected could be temporarily marooned.[98]

On-shore isolation hospitals established in the aftermath of this epidemic were often regarded as nests from which infection might spread, and some of London's medical officers supported local residents who campaigned against their siting.[99] A smallpox outbreak in 1880 led to a canvas camp being set up near Dartford in Kent, and two warships being chartered from the Admiralty and moored off Greenwich. By now regarded as a port disease, smallpox also raised those boundary anxieties common to other diseases and foreign bodies at this time. In the 1880s the London port sanitary authorities (set up in 1872 to prevent the introduction of infectious diseases) introduced more stringent regulation of smallpox, and following a commission into the siting of smallpox hospitals in the metropolis, three hospital ships were anchored at Long Reach, between Dartford and Purfleet in Essex, seventeen miles below London Bridge.[100] As always, however, removal and concentration shifted the problem without removing the fear. The Thames was narrow, and around Purfleet where the hospital ships were within a few hundred yards of the village, they were regarded as a source of contagion.[101]

Attitudes to confinement also had a marked class bias, as a report on isolation hospitals to the Medical Department of the Local Government Board in 1912 reveals. Accommodation, it recommended, should be basic, anything better being 'quite out of place, especially in view of the class of

---

[97] Anne Hardy, *The Epidemic Streets: Infectious Diseases and the Rise of Preventive Medicine, 1856–1900* (Oxford: Clarendon Press, 1993), p. 123.

[98] G. C. Cook, *From the Greenwich Hulks to Old St. Pancras: A History of Tropical Disease in London* (London: Athlone Press, 1992), pp. 51–4.

[99] Hardy, *The Epidemic Streets*, pp. 137–9.

[100] *Ibid.*, p. 142; J. R. Smith, *The Speckled Monster: Smallpox in England 1670–1970, with Particular Reference to Essex* (Chelmsford: Essex Record Office, 1987), p. 161.

[101] Smith, *The Speckled Monster*, p. 167.

people from whom the majority of small-pox patients come'. The report recommended that as smallpox patients were 'often of the vagrant class', on-shore isolation hospitals should be surrounded by a fence 6 feet 6 inches high to prevent escape.[102] In this report smallpox convalescence has become a form of internment, justified by the class origin and peripatetic life-style of those who were its main victims. In fact, with smallpox clearly in decline, compulsory vaccination had been relaxed several years earlier, and this report seems as much concerned with social regulation as with the disease itself.

Tuberculosis sanatoria

Linda Bryder has argued that the expansion of tuberculosis sanatoria in the early twentieth century should be seen in the wider context of the growth of institutions in general: 'The decades between 1860 and the First World War saw the proliferation of institutions on a scale rarely known before ... There appeared to be a new faith in the medical and social value of institutions; by 1900 ... they had become a universal panacea.'[103] Underlying this faith in institutional solutions was the cultural imperative of separating those who were physically and morally healthy from those who were not. Different kinds of quarantine were being set up to protect the fit from the threat of infection or contamination. Although many of these new or intensified forms of concentration and enclosure had a medical basis, the characteristic elision of physical and moral disease ensured that they were also forms of social isolation and exclusion.

Tuberculosis and leprosy were often linked at this time. Robert Koch's Nobel Lecture in 1905 made this connection in calling for the strict isolation of these two chronic contagious diseases.[104] Others compared the tuberculosis sanatorium with the leper house. Dr Mercier, in his Fitzpatrick Lectures to the Royal College of Physicians in 1916, argued that in modern Europe tuberculosis had replaced leprosy as the most serious of chronic infective diseases, and declared: 'the ancient leper house has not only its modern representative, but also its lineal descendant, in the modern sanatorium for consumption'.[105]

The sanatorium movement that developed in Britain at the turn of the twentieth century was aimed at the working and lower-middle classes.[106]

---

[102] *Ibid.*, p. 168.   [103] Bryder, *Below the Magic Mountain*, p. 20.
[104] Bashford, *Imperial Hygiene*, pp. 88, 209 n.32.
[105] *British Medical Journal*, 1 (1916), 54–5.   [106] Bryder, *Below the Magic Mountain*, p. 27.

Alison Bashford's genealogy of Australian sanatoria is also applicable to Britain. Turn-of-the-century treatment of consumptives in both countries, and elsewhere in the settler colonies, drew upon a mixture of penal, charitable, preventive, educative, therapeutic and restorative traditions of quarantine.[107] The prototype of sanatorium treatment for tuberculosis had been developed at Dr Otto Walther's sanatorium at Nordrach in the Black Forest, which had opened in 1889. This involved an open-air therapy that, together with its 'authoritarian management and high-minded austerity', proved congenial to doctors and philanthropists involved in the sanatorium movement in Britain and elsewhere.[108] Rather like the Mettray colonies, sanatoria using the Nordrach brand-name spread to other parts of Europe and Britain. Although Britain lacked the extensive pinewoods that gave Walther's sanatorium its distinctive therapeutic character, a rural setting was considered an essential part of the treatment. Sanatoria were typically converted smallpox hospitals or country houses with added 'shelters' or 'chalets'. Fear of infection often prompted opposition from those living in their neighbourhood, and in 1914 the Royal College of Physicians felt it necessary to issue a statement that such fears were 'exaggerated', and that 'no risk is incurred in living in the immediate neighbourhood of institutions for the treatment of tuberculosis which are properly conducted'.[109]

One particular model of a 'properly conducted' institution was the Frimley Sanatorium in Surrey under Dr Marcus Paterson, its medical superintendent from 1905 to 1912. F. B. Smith describes Paterson's regime as 'absolutist', based on a determination to prevent the 'work-shirking' and 'moral deterioration' that residence in sanatoria was thought liable to induce.[110] Again we see the grim logic of concentration whereby isolation produces problems that can only be countered by ever-stricter forms of regulation and segregation. The whole day at Frimley was mapped from rising at 6.50 until lights-out at 9.15. Work was the heart of the system, and the 'Frimley method' involved a graded scale of labour from 1 to 6 that patients were expected to ascend in the climb towards recovery.[111] Behind this lay the theory of 'auto-inoculation', according to which increasing levels of work caused an inoculation of the patients by their own bacterial

---

[107] Bashford, *Imperial Hygiene*, p. 62.
[108] F. B. Smith, *The Retreat of Tuberculosis 1850–1950* (London: Croom Helm, 1988), pp. 98, 103. Also Thomas Dormandy, *The White Death: A History of Tuberculosis* (London and Rio Grande: Hambledon Press, 1999), p. 152; Dormandy relies more heavily on Smith than his referencing would suggest.
[109] Bryder, *Below the Magic Mountain*, p. 49.
[110] Smith, *The Retreat of Tuberculosis*, p. 116.
[111] Bryder, *Below the Magic Mountain*, p. 58.

products. Paterson explained this phenomenon in terms of a military metaphor:

The aim of the physician is to keep the blood well garrisoned and well armed, swarming with its protective sentinels the anti-bodies so that all invading forces may be overcome at once . . . if we allow our patient to exert himself, we make him liberate a certain amount of . . . toxin, to overcome which the body immediately re-acts and produces anti-toxin, which at once neutralises or kills the tuberculosis poison . . . Exercise or work, in graduated amounts is therefore, in every sense of the term, scientific treatment.[112]

Male and female patients at Frimley were strictly segregated, with walks for men marked with red stakes and those for women with green. Visitors were prohibited and letters were censored to protect the patient from anything likely to cause mental agitation.[113] Paterson's methods were widely admired. Frimley was co-winner of the sanatorium prize at the International Tuberculosis Congress in 1908, and Paterson's techniques were applied in the United States to the treatment of 'certain classes of criminals, dipsomaniacs ... [and] those exhibiting degenerate symptoms'. This was exactly the time at which open-air labour was becoming routine in colonies established for the unemployed, mental defectives, epileptics and other targeted groups.[114]

Sanatoria accommodation and therapies mirrored the class structure.[115] Frimley was the model for the treatment of working and lower-middle-class patients; luxury, it was said, would be 'wasteful' and 'confusing'.[116] Tuberculosis was by now accepted to be a bacterial infection that flourished in conditions of dirt and poverty, and those who contracted it were to be re-educated as well as cured. Work therapy had its own fallacious medical justification but was equally a form of moral reclamation. Upper-class patients, however, escaped the stigmatisation of dirt and ignorance that attached to the mass of tuberculosis patients. Many would be attended at home, and for those in need of institutional care a different kind of sanatorium was established, yet another form of cordon sanitaire ensuring that upper-class patients were clearly distinguishable from others. These institutions were less common and more select. Exercise rather than work was the rule, and one even included a golf course.[117] Most sanatoria, however, were of the Frimley type in which the patients lived according to

---

[112] *Ibid.*, p. 57.   [113] *Ibid.*, p. 58; Smith, *The Retreat of Tuberculosis*, p. 119.
[114] Bryder, *Below the Magic Mountain*, p. 61.
[115] Smith, *The Retreat of Tuberculosis*, p. 104.
[116] Bryder, *Below the Magic Mountain*, p. 52.
[117] Dormandy, *The White Death*, p. 172.

the gospel of work and hygiene. T. N. Kelynack, physician to a sanatorium in Middlesex, wrote in 1904 of the benefits to patients from receiving regular lectures on the conduct of a healthy life: 'they become enthusiastic missionaries in the cause of hygienic righteousness'.[118] Home missions for the semi-civilised indigenes of Edwardian Britain echoed missionary and other colonising activity in remoter parts of its empire. Alison Bashford's description of Australian sanatoria is equally applicable to the metropolitan centre: the aim was to produce reformed and safe consumptive subjects: embodiments of hygienic citizenship.[119]

Robert Philip, a prominent figure in anti-tuberculosis work in the early twentieth century, described his ideal sanatorium in these terms: 'My idea of a sanatorium for the working class is that of a busy hive, where patients, subject to doctors' directions, contribute . . . by their own regulated efforts to the upkeep and beauty of the place – a kind of working colony.'[120] This captures the overlap between sanatoria for tuberculosis patients and other contemporaneous forms of collective isolation aimed at protecting the social order from deviancy and disease, and providing, where possible, a rigorous education for return to the community. Philip established such a farm colony attached to a hospital just out of Edinburgh in 1910. One of his prototypes was the Salvation Army Colony for the unemployed that had been established in Suffolk in the early 1890s. In fact the unemployed and the tubercular were often linked at this time.[121] Both were urban risk groups to be targeted, isolated and decontaminated. Tuberculosis had powerful social resonance, and unemployment was a social disease with disturbing implications for social order. Poverty and unemployment were significant causes of tuberculosis, and the disease itself was a frequent cause of pauperisation.[122]

Although there was an obvious practical impulse behind the establishment of sanatoria and farm colonies, in both cases the emphasis was as much on moral instruction as on treatment. As with lock hospitals, the targeting and isolation of a group perceived as representing a specific social or medical threat was the prelude to a more radical attempt at transforming the whole way of life of a social group deemed to be in need of correction. Social defence through segregation and correction became the prime aim.

[118] Bryder, *Below the Magic Mountain*, p. 67.   [119] Bashford, *Imperial Hygiene*, pp. 79–80.
[120] Bryder, *Below the Magic Mountain*, p. 56.   [121] *Ibid.*, p. 65.
[122] Smith, *The Retreat of Tuberculosis*, p. 105.

The Essex leper colony

Special provision for the isolation of leprosy sufferers in Britain had been mooted since the time of Damien's death and the alarm created by the story of the leper in the London meat market. Calls for such provision recurred from time to time over the next two decades, usually prompted by some event that brought leprosy back to public attention. The Berlin Conference in October 1897, which had recommended stricter enforcement of the isolation of lepers, was followed at the beginning of 1898 with another 'startling discovery' of a case of leprosy in London. In response the *British Medical Journal* described the lack of provision and highlighted the need for a dedicated institution: '[U]nless their friends are well off and able to provide the poor creatures with proper care and nursing, they must either remain more or less neglected, as objects of disgust and alarm to all around, or perhaps they may drift into the Poor-law infirmaries, where also they are not always welcome.'[123] Such reports were concerned to warn but anxious not to alarm. Although this case was 'startling', the *British Medical Journal* also insisted there was 'nothing so very alarming or remarkable' in finding a leper in London. It repeated Abraham's reassurance following the Berlin Conference that although the imperial connection with India and the colonies meant there were always cases of leprosy in Britain, the disease did not spread in this country. Nevertheless, the article concluded, the present case in which a leper 'lies in a private house in one of the busiest parts of the town' demonstrated at the very least the need for a separate annex for lepers at a hospital for diseases of the skin. The spectre of lepers in the streets of London continued to disturb.

The matter of dedicated provision was revived after the Second International Leprosy Conference in Bergen in 1909. The conference had reaffirmed the contagious nature of the disease, and declared: 'Every country of whatever latitude ... is within the range of possible infection by it.'[124] The British delegation at Bergen had endorsed this, and now called for the disease to be made subject to compulsory notification. This was a new element in the leprosy debate. Leprosy had not been included in either the Infectious Diseases (Notification) Act 1889, or the extension of this legislation from London to the rest of the country in 1899. Nor for that matter had tuberculosis, although voluntary notification had been

---

[123] *British Medical Journal*, 1 (1898), 392.
[124] John Bhoyroo, 'The British Leper: A Study of Leprosy in Britain 1867–1951' (unpublished dissertation, Wellcome Institute for the History of Medicine, London, 1997), p. 55.

introduced in 1899, with compulsory notification following in 1913. Syphilis was brought under this legislation at the same time.[125]

In 1912 the *British Medical Journal* rebuked St Pancras Borough Council for applying to have leprosy added to the list of contagious diseases, accusing it of causing unnecessary alarm. This provoked a response from Dr H. Bayou, a former superintendent of the Robben Island leper colony and a member of the British delegation to the Bergen Conference. Bayou supported the call by St Pancras and disputed the *British Medical Journal*'s claim that there had been no recorded case of leprosy originating in Britain in the last two hundred years, citing Hawtrey Benson's Dublin case and one currently being treated by Abraham.[126] This, in turn, elicited letters from Hutchinson and Abraham; the leading figures in the world of leprosy in Britain had not changed much over several decades. For Hutchinson, who now believed that leprosy was 'a dietetic modification of tuberculosis', registration and isolation were 'unjust' and 'cruel': 'The word "leprosy" carries with it, in the popular imagination, such a frightful amount of exaggeration that it is much to be desired that it should be entirely disused.'[127] Abraham argued that even if several cases of leprosy had developed in Britain over many years, the disease had never spread. The 'occasional stray leper' was not a serious danger to others:

When the carriers of such easily communicable diseases as tuberculosis and syphilis are allowed to go freely about and to engage in any or every occupation, it would appear ... somewhat redundant to unnecessarily penalise the poor sufferers who are afflicted with leprosy. The official stamp of danger which notification would imply would doubtless further enhance the popular fear of its contagion, and render the burden of the unfortunate leper still more hard to bear.[128]

Old debates persisted even as their context changed.

There were also new takes on old debates. A reply to Hutchinson and Abraham by 'A Leper' argued in favour of notification and isolation. This anonymous correspondent had worked in a leper asylum for seven years and become infected. It was precisely because there were so few lepers in Britain, he argued, that measures should be taken to prevent contagion. Prevention could only be enforced when the number of lepers was few. In endemic areas like India segregation was impossible. Only through notification and investigation would it be possible to learn how the disease was communicated. This idea of Britain itself as a suitable laboratory for studying leprosy reversed the usual metropolitan habit of seeing remote

---

[125] *Ibid.*, p. 52.   [126] *British Medical Journal*, 1 (1912), 703–4.   [127] *Ibid.*, 757–8.
[128] *Ibid.*, 757–8.

tropical colonies as the best site for such investigation. The letter also turned inside out the argument that isolating lepers was an act of cruelty. The writer insisted that those infected with the disease wished to take every precaution to prevent its spread. Furthermore, the leper asylum offered the patient a secure and known world where they would not be shunned.[129]

The debate about notification was loaded with contradiction. The obvious reasons for excluding leprosy from the Infectious Diseases acts were the small number of actual cases in Britain, the continuing medical disagreement about whether it really was infectious, and the cost of providing dedicated shelter. But there was also the problem that to make the disease notifiable would increase the anxiety it caused and the stigma it carried. For doctors such as Abraham and Hutchinson, who represented a strand of thinking that stretched back to Milroy and the 1867 Report, this was of great concern. Paradoxically, therefore, public apprehension of the disease helped keep it off the list of notifiable diseases. If there had been less fear it might have been added much sooner than 1951 when it finally became a notifiable disease under the Public Health (Leprosy) Regulations. Although the main reason for this in 1951 was concern that leprosy might spread in the post-war world of returning servicemen and Indian independence, it was also the case that with the disease by then treatable, much of the fear surrounding it had vanished. It was therefore safe enough to be added.

Similar contradictions informed debate over the provision of shelter for lepers in Britain. There had long been concern that a leper asylum in Britain would exacerbate public fears and attract lepers from around the empire, and although segregation across the empire was supported in Britain there had been no matching response in the metropolis. The Bergen conference and the debate over notification created a new climate for the question of a leper asylum at home to be revived. There were other immediate reasons as well. In 1911 the President of the Local Government Board, John Burns, received a letter from a former government official in India describing himself as being in an advanced state of leprosy, unable to care for himself but unable to find a London hospital that would admit him. Inquiry revealed a handful of similar cases in London, and the Senior Medical Inspector for Poor Law purposes, Sir Arthur Downes, confirmed another twenty-five such cases across the country, although he suspected the actual number to be twice that.[130]

[129] *Ibid.*, 925–6.
[130] Tony Gould, *Don't Fence Me In: Leprosy in Modern Times* (London: Bloomsbury, 2005), pp. 283–4.

The founding of the St Giles leper asylum outside the village of East Hanningfield, in the parish of Woodham Ferrers and Bicknacre, near Maldon in Essex in 1914 was the result of concern at the refusal of London hospitals and Poor Law institutions to admit leprosy sufferers.[131] As well as Burns's concern and inquiries, Father William of the Anglican Franciscan Order the Society of the Divine Compassion, while visiting among the poor of London, had come across a man with leprosy and his wife, who were under notice to leave their lodgings because of the man's condition and had nowhere to go.[132] This seems a different case from the one that Burns's attention had originally been drawn to, and together they contributed to the process of getting St Giles established.

Impetus also came from a couple of lectures by Dr Bayou delivered to the Royal Society of Medicine in 1913. Bayou argued that strict segregation of lepers prevented spread of the disease. In the Philippines, where the United States administration had implemented a rigorous segregation policy, new cases had been reduced by 90 per cent. In southern Africa, where only half the leper population had been segregated, the incidence of the disease had remained constant. Bayou ignored the example of Hawaii where strict segregation had not brought any comparable reduction in the disease. Hawaii, previously a stumbling block for the anti-contagionists, was now a difficult example for the segregationists. Even though the death of Damien had inaugurated much of the contemporary debate about leprosy, the example of Hawaii was still often left out of the discussion because it was such a difficult case from which to draw a conclusion. Bayou conceded that segregation in India would have to remain voluntary, but argued that in other colonies where the scale of the disease was less overwhelming there should be compulsory segregation in well-conducted asylums with properly trained staff.[133] The *British Medical Journal* endorsed Bayou's argument: 'it is a matter of history that the abandonment of segregation which followed the report of the London College of Physicians in 1867, in which the theory of contagion was rejected, was followed by a great increase in the number of lepers in our tropical and subtropical colonies'.[134] This argument had become a commonplace, but

---

[131] This section on the founding of St Giles derives from M. J. Turner's privately printed and distributed pamphlet, 'The Hospital and Home of St Giles: A History of an Old English Farmhouse that became a Hospital for Leprosy, visited by Royalty', n.d. A shorter version of this appears in the same author's privately printed book, *A Short History of Woodham Ferrers and Bicknacre*, n.d., pp. 97–102. See also Bhoyroo, 'The British Leper', pp. 42–4; Gould, *Don't Fence Me In*, pp. 285–7.

[132] Geoffrey Curtis, *William of Glasshampton: Friar, Monk, Solitary 1862–1937* (London: Society for Promoting Christian Knowledge, 1947), pp. 37–8.

[133] *British Medical Journal*, 2 (1913), 1420–23.   [134] *Ibid.*, 1449.

was now being extended to include the case for a leper colony in the temperate zone of Essex.

Bayou's second lecture was about the Robben Island leper colony he had formerly managed. On this occasion the leprosy specialist Sir Malcolm Morris also spoke about the pitiable position of lepers in London, and proposed an institution where they could be 'segregated and properly looked after'. This plan, Morris argued, should be kept secret to prevent the influx of lepers from the colonies of the empire. Abraham supported the idea of an institution but thought it should deal with all disfiguring diseases of the skin. Familiar disagreements, based on different ideas of the contagion of leprosy, resurfaced. The *British Medical Journal* dismissed the proposal for a mixed institution as 'a standing negation of the idea of contagion on which the case for segregation rests':

Disfiguring skin diseases do not cause the same horror as leprosy, which is 'a name of fear' . . . it is doubtful whether sufferers from skin affections would accept shelter under the same roof with lepers. And if they did, it cannot be denied that there would . . . be some risk of their acquiring leprosy, and as they could not be compelled to stay in the home, it is conceivable that they might spread the disease outside.[135]

Abraham's position was too close to that of the supposedly discredited 1867 Report and he lost the argument; a farmhouse with twenty-seven acres of land was purchased for £1,500 outside East Hanningfield. An appeal for a building programme was launched 'privately and very discreetly, so as not to cause any public alarm'.[136] Lord Strathcona, a personal friend of John Burns, donated £5,400 and died the following day. The colony presumably took its name of St Giles, the patron saint of the crippled and afflicted, from that of the medieval leper hospital founded near Maldon in the reign of Henry II 'for the relief of such burgesses of this town as should have the leprosy'.[137] Father William's Order, the Society of the Divine Compassion, took responsibility for the running of the colony, and by the middle of 1914 two sisters from Guy's Hospital and two Franciscan monks had taken up residence in the farmhouse, 'Moor House'.[138] Once the purpose of the settlement became known there were letters of protest in the local paper, and a parish meeting in July 1914 expressed 'detestation and alarm'. When the first lepers arrived later that

---

[135] *Ibid.*   [136] Bhoyroo, 'The British Leper', p. 41.

[137] Stephen P. Nunn, *St. Giles' Leper Hospital, Maldon* (Maldon Archaeological Group, 1983), p. 1.

[138] Turner, 'The Hospital and Home of St Giles' (alternative version in my possession) records that the chaplain of Robben Island, also a member of the Society of Divine Compassion, had been raising funds for a leper refuge in Britain since 1912.

month they were brought from Woodham Ferrers railway station under cover of night to avoid creating alarm in the neighbourhood.[139] At first only one local tradesman would sell provisions to the settlement and he lost business because local residents were afraid of contracting the disease if they purchased from his store.[140] Later that year Father William came to live at the colony as its first chaplain.

The first two residents of St Giles were Charles Clemsen, a seventy-three-year-old retired Indian police officer, and George Giraud, a thirty-four-year-old Mauritian who was accompanied by his wife. Clemsen, who was virtually blind, died in 1918. Giraud was an astonomer who had worked at the Greenwich Observatory and had been brought to St Giles after being turned out of his lodging house in Greenwich. It seems very likely this was the case Father William had discovered; he died in 1922.[141] At first the lepers lived in Moor House with the sisters, while the brothers slept in the cowsheds, but after the war ten bungalows were built for patients.

The example of a resident named Bax (forename unrecorded) is an interesting case study of a St Giles patient. His brother had been born in British Guiana and died of leprosy. Bax himself was born in Manchester and had never been abroad. At the age of eleven he had developed symptoms of leprosy and been withdrawn from school and isolated at home without medical treatment. He was admitted to St Giles in 1920, at the age of fifteen, where he died seven months later.[142] Bhoyroo's analysis of the ethnic origin of the fifty-four patients housed at St Giles between 1914 and 1950 shows that thirty-two were white British, ten were non-white British, one was Belgian, and eleven were unrecorded; only nine of the fifty-four were women but this was partly because women patients, as distinct from women who accompanied their infected husbands, were not admitted until 1925.[143] The incomplete records of the country of origin of these patients show that twenty-six were from the Indian sub-continent, between five and ten were from Africa, South America, the West Indies and South-East Asia, with less than five from Palestine, Malta and Britain.[144] Incomplete as these records are, they indicate that by far the largest group of patients at St Giles comprised white British men who had been born and lived abroad, mainly in the Indian sub-continent. The numbers were small, the evidence of infection negligible, but the pattern

---

[139] Bhoyroo, 'The British Leper', p. 42.
[140] Turner, 'The Hospital and Home of St Giles', p. 99.
[141] Bhoyroo, 'The British Leper', p. 42 and Appendix C; Gould, *Don't Fence Me In*, pp. 283, 286.
[142] Bhoyroo, 'The British Leper', p. 87.   [143] Gould, *Don't Fence Me In*, p. 287.
[144] Bhoyroo, 'The British Leper', p. 82.

of the disease as one of return conformed to the exaggerated fears of end-of-the-century commentators.

Sister Clare, one of the first two nurses at St Giles, wrote of how the settlement was at first 'boycotted by the neighbourhood', but the war soon gave local residents more urgent concern. She described Zeppelins fighting above them, searchlights and shrapnel in the skies, and how young soldiers in the nearby training camp would attend Father William's Vespers before leaving for the front, spending Sunday afternoons resting on the lawns at St Giles.[145] With time, the colony seems to have become accepted, although there are glimpses of persisting fear and isolation, as for example in an exchange of letters between Sister Isabella at Moor House and Essex County Council in 1949. Sister Isabella had written to the Chief Education Officer inquiring about a correspondence course for a thirteen-year-old patient. Her letter was referred to the County Health Department, which wrote to the doctor in Maldon who attended the patients at St Giles. As well as requesting more information about the boy's condition, the Health Department also sought the doctor's opinion 'as regards the question of conveyance of infection by books or papers used in a correspondence course'. In reply the doctor ventured his 'personal opinion ... that the risk of conveying infection via papers used in a correspondence course is negligible'.[146] When leprosy patients were invited to local people's homes, they would bring their own cups, plates and cutlery.[147]

The colony, as it was termed by the *British Medical Journal*,[148] was administered by the Society of the Divine Compassion, with a management committee including prominent doctors in the field of leprosy, until in 1936 patient care and day-to-day management was taken over by another Anglican order, the Community of the Sacred Passion. The Mother House of this Community was based in (then) Tanganyika where it worked among leprosy sufferers, and St Giles also became a rest house for sisters coming home to recuperate. Following the Second World War and the founding of the National Health Service, state provision for leprosy patients was finally established. The opening of the Jordan Hospital at Redhill, near Reigate, in 1951 also met strong local opposition at first. At the same time leprosy was finally made subject to notification, although in recognition of the enduring public fear of the disease the Ministry of Health rather than local medical officers were to be notified, in order to maintain 'strict secrecy'.[149] The Jordan Hospital closed in 1967

---

[145] Curtis, *William of Glasshampton*, pp. 43–4.
[146] Bhoyroo, 'The British Leper', Appendix C.
[147] Turner, 'The Hospital and Homes of St Giles', p. 115.
[148] *British Medical Journal*, 1 (1924), 246.   [149] Gould, *Don't Fence Me In*, pp. 298–9.

by which time the combination of successful drug control and outpatient clinics had made long-term isolation redundant. Some patients were transferred to St Giles, which once again became the only dedicated provision in the country. In 1969 the word 'Hospital' was added to its title 'The Homes of St Giles', and in 1986 St Giles was taken over by the Springboard Charitable Trust, a Christian housing association providing residential care for people with mental health and learning disabilities. The nine remaining leprosy patients stayed on under the new arrangements, and in 2004 there were still four in residence.

Conclusion

At the point in Henry James's *The Turn of the Screw* (1898) where the unnamed governess is becoming aware of her beleaguered position, she refers to the household at Bly as 'our small colony'.[150] The term is well chosen. Cloistered in a country house, yet another colony in Essex, enjoined never to trouble her employer but to look after his enigmatic young charges, the governess finds herself caught between several different worlds, not least that of the living and the dead. The colony of Bly is a place of exile and retreat, cut off from the fashionable West End world of her employer that the governess has so tantalisingly glimpsed, inhabited by two rejected children and the disturbingly named Mrs Grose, and haunted by the spectral presences of Quint and Miss Jessel. It is both a sanatorium and a prison, and like other such colonies is less secure than intended. It is also unlikely that James would have chosen the word 'colony' to describe such a community half a century earlier.

This is, no doubt, the most strained of all the comparisons I have been pursuing between colonies of empire and colonies at home. But my argument has been that behind all these proliferating uses of 'colony' in the later nineteenth century was the same need to enclose and isolate the primitive, the diseased and the backward: different kinds of 'risk group' that could not be assimilated and must therefore be rejected or refashioned. In the case of leprosy, disease itself was the reason for isolation. In other cases disease was mapped on to the 'risk group'. But the distinction between isolating the pathological and pathologising the isolated was always blurred; one reinforced the other. Disease thinking in some shape or form was common to all the different types of isolation I have been discussing.

[150] Henry James, *The Turn of the Screw and Other Stories* (Harmondsworth: Penguin, 1983), p. 40

In trying better to understand this process I have brought together Foucault's argument about the constitutive role of biopolitics in the emergence of Western modernity, and Gilroy's insistence that imperialism provided the defining context for the emergence of 'biocultural kinship' as the central element of the modern nation-state. Foucault's neglect of empire in his account of European modernity has already been rehearsed. Giorgio Agamben's implied criticism that Foucault failed to carry his argument forward to the exemplary places of modern biopolitics, the concentration camp and the totalitarian state, also repeats this neglect. Only at the very end of *Homer Sacer* does Agamben extend his gaze beyond Europe and suggest that 'the entire population of the Third World' has today been transformed into 'bare life'.[151] This belated recognition is not only cursory, but entirely undifferentiated. And to read Foucault back through the worst atrocities of the twentieth century runs the risk of sensationalising his arguments. Encamped ethnicity and its metropolitan variants became embedded in everyday life during the nineteenth century. The quotidian nature of colony formation and its resultant 'bare life' can be obscured by Agamben's insistence that the historical culmination of Foucault's *grand renfermement* is the Holocaust.

In a different way this is also true of Gilroy's argument. His emphasis on 'camp-practice' as an instrument of empire neglects Europe itself as a site of the production of that biopolitics upon which empire rested. And his emphasis on the Holocaust and its colonial antecedents and parallels can also obscure the point that the exemplary places of modern biopolitics are also to be found in the everyday. In trying to draw these different emphases together, the work of new imperial historians such as Ann Laura Stoler and Catherine Hall, that understands metrople and colony as simultaneously cause and effect of each other, has been of great assistance. My own study has been concerned with the role of one particular disease within the far wider context of modern imperial biopolitics. In pursuing this I have examined leprosy itself, changing disease constructions during the period, and the disease-based institutions that were being fashioned at home and away to assist in the process of defining, explaining and protecting nation and empire. In comparing these institutions I have tried to keep in mind the specificities of each particular instance, and also the differences within the same example across metropole and empire. I must also concede the vast differences of scale between, say, the native reservation and the tuberculosis sanatorium. Nevertheless, all the examples I have discussed were part of the dialectic of dilation and contraction that was at the heart of

---

[151] Giorgio Agamben, *Homo Sacer: Sovereign Power and Bare Life* (Stanford, Calif.: Stanford University Press, 1988), p. 180.

modern colonialism. As European empires expanded, the need for ever-more carefully calibrated forms of enclosure and segregation increased.

In the context of nineteenth- and early twentieth-century culture, there-fore, it becomes more readily understandable that the leper should have become an especially powerful type of the other, the unclean, of 'bare life', Agamben's 'state of exception'. Disease became a particular focus of concern, and an especially powerful trope for figuring other kinds of concern, because it expressed so readily the dangers of spreading and mixing that were the underside of the power and confidence of modern empires. A disease such as leprosy whose primary symptoms were expressed on the skin captured these kinds of anxiety perfectly. The resurgence of a belief in the infectious character of leprosy, a persisting and now intensifying fear that it was communicated by touch, made it an exemplary disease for an era in which contact – both literal and cultural – marked and defined European expansion across the globe. Many new kinds of stigmatisation were being elaborated, especially that of race; and leprosy was, par excellence, the disease of stigma.

6   Writers visiting leper colonies: Charles
     Warren Stoddard, Robert Louis Stevenson,
     Jack London, Graham Greene and Paul
     Theroux

Crossing the boundary

Leper colonies attracted visitors. As the spread of European empires
improved communications and made ocean voyaging easier, a new kind
of traveller-writer was drawn to the more remote and hazardous outposts
of the imperial world. Damien's colony on Molokai became part of the
itinerary for those embarking on Pacific voyages from the eastern sea-
board of the United States: Charles Warren Stoddard, Robert Louis
Stevenson, Jack London and Charmian Kittredge all visited and wrote
about the experience. The pull of the leper colony continued well into the
twentieth century. Graham Greene became its most famous cicerone, and
Paul Theroux provides a further example later in the century. These writers
will be the focus of my concluding chapter.

The draw of the leper colony was another consequence of the revived
fear of leprosy and the more rigorous confinement of its victims in the later
nineteenth century. Unlike those who wished to be protected from the
sight and danger of the leper, these traveller-writers – most of them critical
of imperial power – were tempted to transgress the boundaries placed
around the leper and enter the camp. They had different individual reasons
for making this journey but as each of them passed over to the other side
they inevitably became entangled in the complex Judeo-Christian tradition
of abjuring and cherishing the leper.

There were financial rewards for penetrating the camps, colonies and
dark places of the earth. The economics of contemporary publishing
enabled Stevenson and London to finance their Pacific cruising by selling
their reports and stories to the expanding newspaper and periodical
market. Stevenson's leprosy story 'The Bottle Imp' was published serially
in both New York and London in 1891 several years before its volume
publication in *Island Nights' Entertainments* (1893). Also in 1891, his wife
Fanny Stevenson published a leprosy story 'The Half-White' in *Scribner's
Magazine*. Stevenson's account of the week he spent at the colony on

Molokai was serialised in the New York *Sun* in the same year. When Jack London went foot-stepping after Stoddard and Stevenson in 1906, the account of his visit to Molokai first appeared as a commissioned series of articles in *Harper's* before later being included in his travel book *The Cruise of the Snark* (1911). And like Stoddard and Stevenson before him, London also wrote several leper stories, again for magazines that paid well for short fiction that would appeal to their readers.

There was clearly a market for writing about braving the hazards of the leper colony. Like most modern travel writing, such work offered the frisson of apprehension and risk from the safety of the armchair. A prototype of this particular kind of writing was Richard Burton's *Personal Narrative of a Pilgrimage to Al Madinah and Meccah* (1855), in which the author narrated his furtive pilgrimage to Mecca disguised as an Arab pilgrim. In Burton, as in the writers I am to discuss, the main interest derives from a confrontation with the feared or forbidden rather than the unknown. The extremity of the experience lay in what was already known to be dangerous or discomfiting rather than in what was yet to be discovered.

There was a further dimension to this. Since at least the eighteenth century the body, travel and health had been discursively entangled. As the body was increasingly medicalised, travel came to be seen as both a therapy and a source of pathology.[1] The confrontation between these traveller-writers and the extreme medical condition of leprosy frequently involved their own precarious health. Stevenson went to the Pacific in search of health and in fear of imminent death, and this gave both edge and compassion to his observations of lepers, and more generally of what he believed at first were the dying cultures of Oceania. London's Pacific cruise was ended by the eruption of his skin with a condition that resembled leprosy and was probably psoriasis. Having visited Molokai his body began to mimic the condition of the leper. In Greene's novel *A Burnt-Out Case* (1960) the spiritual health of the main protagonist Querry is at stake, and leprosy becomes a correlative for ennui and spiritual drought. In Paul Theroux's autobiographical essay 'The Lepers of Moyo' (1994), the author's understanding of leprosy as a form of 'bare life' is partly won through his own experience of severe illness. In each of these cases, though in very different ways, a kind of sympathy is established between the colonised leper and the Western visitor that seems to remove the barriers that imperialism had erected.

---

[1] Richard Wrigley and George Revill (eds.), *Pathologies of Travel* (Amsterdam and Atlanta, Ga.: Rodopi, 2000), pp. 10–12.

Charles Warren Stoddard

Stoddard was an important link between a number of writers who travelled in the Pacific and were fascinated by Molokai. He was friendly with Mark Twain, and met both Stevenson and London in California before they embarked on their Pacific voyages. He also introduced Stevenson to Melville's writing, something that won him a guest appearance in Stevenson's novel *The Wrecker* (1893) as 'a certain San Francisco character ... known to many lovers of good English',[2] and resulted in on-going correspondence between the two. Stoddard was the earliest of these writers to visit Molokai, making his first call in 1869 several years before Damien's arrival at the colony. This resulted in a short fiction 'Joe of Lahaina' published in Stoddard's collection *Summer Cruising in the South Seas* (1873), titled *South Sea Idylls* in the United States. He returned to Molokai in 1884 and wrote *Lepers of Molokai* (1885), the first book on the colony and one that was influential in bringing Damien's work and example to an international audience. Stoddard also kept a diary of this visit that appeared in an expurgated edition in 1933, and he published a further book about the colony, *Father Damien: the Martyr of Molokai* early in the twentieth century.

Stoddard's writing is best described as 'camp', in almost every sense of that word: high, gay and encircled. He was one of the earliest writers to make explicit the homosexual allure of the Pacific. His style, however, is simultaneously so arch and so sentimental that 'explicit' is not, perhaps, the right word. It is unlikely but just possible that an innocent reader beguiled by Stoddard's account of the Pacific as a scattering of Tennysonian 'happy isles' might have missed the nature of the narrator's relationship with the beautiful native boy Kana-ana, in his story 'Chumming with a Savage':

Again and again [Kana-ana] would come with a delicious banana to the bed where I was lying, and insist upon my gorging myself, when I had but barely recovered from a late orgie [sic] of fruit, flesh, or fowl. He would mesmerize me into a most refreshing sleep with a prolonged but pleasing manipulation.[3]

Stoddard's leprosy story 'Joe of Lahaina' also uses Stoddard's favourite narrative of the European male deliciously enslaved by an enchanting Polynesian boy. The opening section gives an idyllic account of the

---

[2] Robert Louis Stevenson, *The Wrecker* (London: Heinemann, 1928), pp. 118–19.
[3] Charles Warren Stoddard, 'Chumming with a Savage', in *Summer Cruising in the South Seas* (London: Chatto and Windus, 1873), pp. 41–2. For an informative and witty discussion of this collection see Nigel Rigby, 'A Sea of Islands: Tropes of Travel and Adventure in the Pacific 1846–1894' (unpublished PhD thesis, University of Kent, 1995), pp. 209–18.

domestic felicity shared by the narrator and Joe in which the trope of 'housekeeping' is an unlikely substitute for bananas. The concluding section, set months after the amicable break-up of this blissful arrangement, has the narrator landing on Molokai. He tours the island, revelling in its beautiful desolation and exquisitely mourning 'the ruins of a nation', before reaching 'the brink of a great precipice, three thousand feet in the air' from where he looks down upon the leper colony. The descent, predictably, is an entry into 'the valley of death, and the very mouth of hell', though embroidered by 'floral avenues'. At the colony he sees 'Gorgonlike faces ... listen[s] in vain for the voices that have been hushed for ever by decay; breathe[s] the tainted atmosphere'. While the lepers 'hover about ... forbidden to touch you, yet longing to clasp once more a hand that is perfect and pure', the visitor is threatened by the possibility that 'the insidious seeds of the malady may be generating in your vitals'.[4]

The narrator is approached by one of the inhabitants who turns out to be Joe, now deformed beyond recognition. They talk separated by a latticed fence, which an accompanying illustration represents as if it were a prison gate, with the cloaked figure of death at Joe's shoulder. Their plangent reminiscences are punctuated by Joe singing, echoed by a faint chorus from the whole community. Even the sea joins in, 'breathing its long breath under the hollow cones of lava, with a noise like a giant leper in his asthmatic agony'. At this operatic climax Joe looks beseechingly at the narrator: 'The desolated beauty of his face pleaded for measureless pity, and I gave it, out of my prodigality, yet felt that I could not begin to give sufficient.'[5] The tragic focus has shifted from Joe to narrator, lavish even wasteful in his sympathy, but powerless to help and thus equally to be pitied.

After this melodramatic tosh, Joe is finally reconfigured as a snake, 'his pitiful face growing gradually as dreadful as a cobra's, and almost as fascinating in its hideousness'.[6] More than just a simile for Joe's repellent skin, this renders the once beautiful boy as phallic tempter. The narrator has recalled that Joe was 'naturally bad' and how little effect the attempt to instil precepts ever had. At this point the narrator himself is implicated. A particularly beguiling evening is coyly remembered, in which we are told: 'He forgot my precepts then, and I'm afraid I forgot them myself.'[7] Nigel Rigby has neatly described how in this story 'the language of sentiment packages the horror of disease'.[8] This is so, but the figuring of Joe as a cobra also distances the narrator from this rapidly degenerating figure.

---

[4] Stoddard, 'Joe of Lahaina', in *Summer Cruising in the South Seas*, pp. 109–11.
[5] *Ibid.*, p. 115.   [6] *Ibid.*, p. 116.   [7] *Ibid.*, p. 114.   [8] Rigby, 'A Sea of Islands', p. 223.

The association between Joe's promiscuous homosexuality and the disease he suffers is all but explicit; the narrator's role in this, and his relation to it, anything but.

If the suggestion that leprosy can be caused by homosexuality is displaced wholly on to the native, other threats to the clean European body from the leprous Polynesian one cannot be so easily allayed. The touch and breath of the diseased indigene are threats to the visitor, and this ever-present sense of danger sustains both *The Lepers of Molokai* and Stoddard's diary. This is heightened by the impression that Stoddard stayed at the colony much longer than he actually did. Damien is the other focus of this fear of infection, becoming a kind of alter ego for the author. Shortly after Stoddard's 1884 visit it was confirmed Damien had contracted leprosy. In *The Lepers of Molokai* Damien's escape from being infected thus far is described as 'almost miraculous'. The thin line between clean and unclean is highlighted in the description of a mass, 'at which all save the priest and I were lepers'. The courage and anxiety of the visitor, rather than the suffering of the visited, has become the main concern of the text.

Robert Louis Stevenson

Stevenson himself confessed: 'The ideas of deformity and living decay have been burdensome to my imagination since the nightmares of childhood.'[9] A particular horror of leprosy is signalled in *The Black Arrow* (serialised 1883, volume publication 1888), written some years before his visit to Molokai. Two young characters, Dick Shelton and John Matcham, are confronted and pursued by a blind leper. His clanking bell, tapping stick, and the eyeless white hood veiling his face so terrifies them that one turns 'dead-white ... as if by the mere sight he might become infected'. Worse, the leper holds the clapper of his bell so his approach cannot be heard. As Matcham exclaims: 'Who ever heard the like, that a leper, out of mere malice, should pursue unfortunates? Hath he not his bell to that very end, that people may avoid him?'[10] Eventually the leper breaks cover and hurls himself on the boys, only to be revealed as the disguised Sir Daniel Brackley, guardian of Dick Shelton. This narrative in which the horror of leprosy is exploited only to be allayed recalls Doyle's 'The Blanched Soldier'.

[9] Robert Louis Stevenson, 'The Eight Islands', in A. Grove Day (ed.), *Travels in Hawaii: Robert Louis Stevenson* (Honolulu: University of Hawaii Press, 1973), p. 64.
[10] Robert Louis Stevenson, *The Black Arrow* (London and Glasgow: Collins, n.d.), pp. 79–81.

After finishing *The Master of Ballantrae* in Honolulu in April 1889, Stevenson took himself off to the Kona Coast of Big Island where he stayed at Ho'okena, ten miles south of Kealakekua Bay where Captain Cook had been killed. It was here that Stevenson first saw leprosy. On 1 May he watched a young leprous girl being deported to Molokai accompanied by her mother. His account of this departure opens with a defence of the Hawaiian government's policy of segregation, which he compares favourably with Chinese, English and French indifference to the problem of leprosy in their tropical possessions. This policy, however, he describes as incomprehensible to 'the native mind'. Stevenson is outside a wooden house standing isolated in a field of broken lava. This is a holding station for lepers waiting to be taken to Molokai, one of whom has just escaped by cutting through the floor and taking refuge with a friend and fellow sufferer in the mountains. Stevenson blames the shelter commonly given to such escapees on Hawaiian family affection, which he describes as 'luxuriously self-indulgent, circumscribed within the passing moment', and in which the 'presence and approval of the loved one, it matters not how purchased, is the single demand'. This is the rock on which the law of segregation founders. Stevenson reinforces his account of the unthinking nature of Hawaiian family affection by describing how leprous parents of clean children born on Molokai resist having their children removed from the island and offered 'life and health and liberty'. At Ho'okena he notes with 'grief' the unrestrained physical contact between the young girl and those around her.[11]

This frames the painful scene he is now to describe of the girl's departure for Molokai. 'Sympathy may flow freely for the leper girl; it may flow for her mother with reserve; it must not betray us into injustice for the government whose laws they had attempted to evade.' The girl, when first seen, crouches motionless, swathed in a black shawl, concealing her face. Her mother sings of her grief. Stevenson emphasises the theatre of the occasion. The actual departure scene is 'a grief perhaps – a performance certainly'. The girl is now decked out in a red dress with a fine red feather in her hat, although she crouches apart from the company on the rocks. Her mother, however, moves with 'swaggering gait . . . swinging her hat, rolling her eyes and shoulders, visibly working herself up'. She is centre-stage and Stevenson is slightly vexed by this and by the theatricality of her performance. The mother, after all, can return; her daughter 'took leave forever'. Standing on those same rocks and watching the performance of departure, Stevenson decides he must follow them to their 'place of exile'.[12]

---

[11] Stevenson, 'The Eight Islands', pp. 39–40.   [12] *Ibid.*, pp. 41, 43–5.

It is thought that Stevenson's story 'The Bottle Imp' was written on the Kona coast of Big Island around the time that he watched the leprous girl and her mother departing for Molokai. If so it was written very quickly because by 3 May, a week after arriving on Big Island, he was back in Honolulu and making arrangements to visit Molokai himself. Whatever the precise date of its composition, 'The Bottle Imp' was certainly written during Stevenson's first visit to Honolulu and his encounter with its leprosy problem.[13] Stevenson's acknowledged source for his story was an early nineteenth-century melodrama by Richard Brinsley Peake, itself based upon a German folktale. With its Hawaiian setting, and Stevenson's professed aim of designing and writing the tale for a Polynesian audience, it also had its generic origins in Pacific storytelling.[14]

A young Hawaiian man, Keawe, visiting San Francisco, purchases a magical bottle, 'white like milk', within which 'something obscurely moved, like a shadow and a fire'. The imp in the bottle will give its owner anything they wish, but to die before selling the bottle is to be damned. Further, the bottle must always be sold for less than it was purchased, otherwise it returns 'like a homing pigeon' to its owner. The bottle has by now become dangerously cheap. Keawe uses it to build a wonderful modern house on the Kona coast. When the house is completed, Keawe and his friend Lopaka who has agreed to purchase the bottle ask that the imp should reveal itself to them. The sight of the imp leaves them as if turned to stone. Lopaka departs with the bottle, and in time Keawe meets and falls in love with a young woman, Kokua (her name being the word used to describe those who accompanied leprous companions to Molokai). Before they can marry, Keawe discovers a patch on his skin resembling a 'lichen on a rock', and realises he has contracted 'the Chinese Evil', leprosy. He therefore sets out to recover the bottle to cure him of his disease and allow him to marry Kokua. By the time he catches up with it the price has slumped to one cent. He buys back the bottle and cures himself of leprosy but to sell it again must travel to Tahiti where French currency, with its smaller denominations, operates. After much difficulty the bottle is finally sold to 'an old brutal *Haole*' (European) and the obstacle to Keawe and Kokua's love is removed.

---

[13] 'The Bottle Imp' was published serially in the New York *Herald*, February–March 1891, in England in *Black and White*, March–April 1891, and was translated into Samoan and published in a missionary magazine *O Le Sulu Samoa*, May–December 1891. It was collected in Stevenson's volume *Island Nights' Entertainments* (1893).

[14] In a prefatory note to the story Stevenson described it as 'designed and written for a Polynesian audience'; see Roslyn Jolly (ed.), *Robert Louis Stevenson: South Sea Tales* (Oxford and New York: World's Classics, 1996), p. 72.

This story also had origins in near-contemporary Hawaiian history. William P. (Billy) Ragsdale was a *hapa-haole* (mixed Hawaiian and European ethnicity) lawyer who was official interpreter in Hawaii's bilingual legislature during the 1860s. In 1873 he was diagnosed as having leprosy and sent to Molokai. He is said to have discovered that he had the disease when one day he picked up an overheated oil lamp, burned himself but felt nothing. Fanny Stevenson's leprosy story, 'The Half-White' uses this episode but transfers it to a priest, thereby creating an amalgam of Ragsdale and Damien.[15] Mark Twain gave Ragsdale's story another twist that seems to have found its way into 'The Bottle Imp'. In this version, Ragsdale discovered his infection just as he was about to marry a beautiful 'half-caste' girl but refused to deceive her and surrendered himself to the authorities.[16] The story of his self-surrender is accurate. Ragsdale, who according to Daws was known for his sense of theatre, made a very public departure for Molokai. He came down to the boat with his Bible and lawbooks, wearing a gardenia *lei*, and was seen off by hundreds to the accompaniment of a Hawaiian glee club.[17] There seems to be an echo of this in Stevenson's account of the departure of the mother and daughter from Ho'okena. Ragsdale's history also appears to have influenced several of Jack London's stories, 'Good-By, Jack' which combines a cross-cultural love story with another departure-for-Molokai scene, and 'The Sheriff of Kona', in which a prominent *haole* citizen is exposed as suffering from the disease and voluntarily departs for Molokai.

All these different versions of Ragsdale's story, with the exception of Stevenson's, highlight the significance of mixed ethnicity in leprosy narratives. It was widely believed that such people were particularly susceptible to the disease and were also a bridge for its transmission from the Hawaiian to the European. Stevenson makes no such use of the 'mixed-race' figure. Nevertheless, and for all his approval of the segregation policy, he shapes a disease narrative that enables his hero to avoid the fate of being sent to Molokai. Keawe is saved from repeating Ragsdale's self-sacrifice by the agency of the bottle imp, which also rescues him from losing Kokua. The imp in the bottle is also a figure for the disease itself and the destruction it causes. Throughout the story the bottle is like a virus, and the uncorking scene described above hastens the infection it spreads it around Honolulu. Once Lopaka has purchased his schooner he sells the

---

[15] 'The Half-White' was published in *Scribner's Magazine*, March 1881.

[16] Mark Twain, *Following the Equator: A Journey Around the World*, 2 vols. (New York and London: Harper and Brothers, n.d.), vol. I, pp. 41–2.

[17] Gavan Daws, *Holy Man: Father Damien of Molokai* (Honolulu: University of Hawaii Press, 1973), p. 89.

bottle as quickly as he can, and so on through the city, its price falling all the while.

As Keawe walks the streets of Honolulu in his search to retrieve the bottle he follows a trail of wealth, secrets and misery. When the current owner of the bottle is eventually tracked down he is showing physical symptoms that suggest leprosy: 'here was a young man, white as a corpse, and black about the eyes, the hair shedding from his head, and such a look in his countenance as a man may have when he is waiting for the gallows'. Keawe purchases the bottle, declares his wish to be a 'clean man', and is restored: 'his flesh was whole like an infant's'.[18] But there is a complex relation between the bottle and infection; it is simultaneously cure and curse. Although now cured of leprosy Keawe will be damned for eternity unless he can sell the bottle. When he and Kokua try to sell it in Tahiti they are shunned as if they were lepers: 'children ran away from them screaming ... Catholics crossed themselves as they went by; and all persons began with one accord to disengage themselves from their advances.'[19] The bottle, which signifies material greed, is also itself leprous. When Kokua persuades an old man to buy it from Keawe, so she herself can buy it back and rescue her husband from its curse, she can hardly bear to touch it: 'my hand resists, my flesh shrinks back from the accursed thing'. The bottle has become an object of 'unutterable fear and ... loathing'.[20] Finally, the greed and the disease it signifies are returned to their source. Originally purchased from a rich Californian with a fabulous house overlooking the Pacific, Keawe eventually sells it back to another white man, 'an old brutal *Haole*' and some-time Pacific adventurer, now wrecked and beached in Tahiti. Already in his own mind condemned to hell, the man is guaranteed a never-ending supply of rum for the term of his natural life. For Keawe and Kokua, his helper, the cork is at last back in the bottle.

Returning to Honolulu in early May, Stevenson made plans for his own crossing to Molokai. In a letter to the Board of Health requesting permission to visit the leper settlement he explained that he wished to include an account of it in his projected work on the Polynesian Islands. And he added that he wanted 'to see with my own eyes how the sufferers are disposed; as I have already had occasion to see something of the horrors and dangers of the disease in other islands less considerately managed'. He was also concerned to correct any misapprehension that he might be a mere newspaper correspondent: 'I trust that you will

[18] 'The Bottle Imp', in *Robert Louis Stevenson: South Sea Tales*, pp. 88, 89.
[19] *Ibid.*, p. 93.   [20] *Ibid.*, pp. 96, 98.

consider that I scarcely belong to the same class, and that I visit the
settlement with no design to make capital.'[21]

Landing scenes in island narratives are always significant, and as
Stevenson made the short voyage to Molokai he worried about the
moment of his arrival. As he wrote to Fanny: 'Every hand was offered;
I had gloves, but I had made up my mind on the ... voyage *not* to give my
hand, that seemed less offensive than gloves.'[22] He also had the uncomfortable sense that his identity as a writer made him an intruder and
'a spy'.[23] From the moment he landed, his understanding of the relation
between the leper and the world was turned inside out. The first leper he
speaks with, a young woman, is 'comely in face and person', 'infinitely
engaging and (in the old phrase) towardly'.[24] She assumes Stevenson is a
new patient and is disappointed to discover he is not. In view of his own
horror of the disease and trepidation at his visit, Stevenson finds her
reaction difficult to comprehend.

During his stay, however, he comes to understand that: 'Within the
precinct to be leprous is the rule.' Out riding one afternoon, Stevenson
comes upon a party of young men and women decked out in their best
clothes, garlanded with flowers, singing and laughing: 'They made from a
distance an engaging picture: I had near forgotten in what distressful
country my road lay.' Coming up to them he sees that several of the
company are 'unhumanly defaced'. Among them he recognises the young
woman recently removed from Big Island. The only one of the group not
showing signs of facial disfigurement, she is also the only one to keep her
head lowered. In time, however, her face will be lifted even as it deforms.
Molokai, Stevenson reflects, 'confounds the expectation of the visitor ...
another norm arises'.[25] Stevenson was especially drawn to the Bishop
Home for Girls at Kalaupapa. He presented the Home with a croquet set
and spent several days teaching the game to the children; after his return to
Oahu he sent them a piano.[26] His admiration for the courage of the girls
and the Catholic sisters who taught and tended them found complicated
expression: 'As for the girls in the Bishop Home, of the many beautiful
things I have been privileged to see in life, they, and what has been done for
them, are not the least beautiful.' The litotic construction captures
Stevenson's hesitant though profound admiration as language strains

---

[21] Bradford A. Booth and Ernest Mehew (eds.), *The Letters of Robert Louis Stevenson*, 8 vols.
(New Haven, Conn., and London: Yale University Press, 1994–5), vol. VI, p. 298.
[22] *Ibid.*, vol. VI, p. 306.   [23] Stevenson, 'The Eight Islands', p. 64.
[24] Booth and Mehew, *The Letters of Robert Louis Stevenson*, vol. VI, p. 306.
[25] Stevenson, 'The Eight Islands', pp. 67–8.
[26] Nicholas Rankin, *Dead Man's Chest: Travels After Robert Louis Stevenson* (London:
Phoenix Press, 2001), pp. 282–4.

against the difficulty of expressing his perception of 'the brief gaiety of these afflicted'.[27]

Nevertheless, the boundary between health and disease, 'clean' and 'unclean', structures Stevenson's narrative. As he describes, the visitor to the colony is isolated from everything around him: 'No patient is suffered to approach his place of residence. His room is tidied out by a clean helper during the day and while he is abroad. He returns at night to solitary walls.'[28] The free and clean man in this place of detention and disease finds himself in solitary confinement. Walking by the shore – 'along the brink' – he finds that in this 'tainted place the thought of the cleanness of the antiseptic ocean is welcome to the mind'.[29] On the day of his departure his 'heart panted for deliverance', and he was alarmed to discover that he had mistakenly been issued with a one-way pass. But this was sorted out and soon Stevenson was 'eating untainted food, drinking clean sea air'.[30]

The next section of 'The Eight Islands' is titled 'The Free Island', and celebrates Stevenson's release from the captivity of the peninsula and his exploration of the rest of the island, its untainted hinterland, as he comes ashore further down the coast. The spectacular scenery he now rides through is a relief after the human extremity of the colony, yet he becomes increasingly conscious of the emptiness of this landscape. He asks his guide, 'Where are the people?' and is told; 'Pau kanaka make' (the people are dead). Stevenson's first response to this is to muse that 'The place of the dead is clean; there is a poetry in empty lands.' But then he guiltily recalls Kalaupapa and the girls of the Bishop Home. Like the bereaved Wordsworth in his sonnet about his daughter's death, 'Surprised by joy', he wonders how he could have forgotten 'the shadow, the sorrow, and the obligation' so quickly.[31] Eventually the ride comes almost full circle, to the top of the *pali* where the narrator of 'Joe of Lahaina' had stood. Stevenson looks down from a safe altitude on to the peninsula below. From a distance it looks like any other coastal settlement, but the chapter ends by echoing the reply of the guide: 'Pau kanaka make'. The leper colony has become a synecdoche for the island, indeed for the dying cultures of the Pacific as Stevenson then saw them. It was almost a year later, in Sydney, that Stevenson read of the accusation that Damien had died of syphilis as a result of having sexual relations with female members of the colony, and wrote his blistering reply, 'An Open Letter to the Reverend Dr. Hyde of Honolulu'.

[27] Stevenson, 'The Eight Islands', pp. 69–70.   [28] *Ibid.*, p. 51.   [29] *Ibid.*, p. 49.
[30] Booth and Mehew, *The Letters of Robert Louis Stevenson*, vol. VI, p. 313.
[31] Stevenson, 'The Eight Islands', pp. 75–6.

Jack London

Jack London's account of his visit to Molokai and his subsequent leprosy fiction will be treated more briefly.[32] London's leprosy writing is in all respects more extreme than Stevenson's. The account of his visit in *The Cruise of the Snark* (1911), initially a series of articles commissioned by *Harper's*, is more upbeat than Stevenson's, while stories such as 'The Sheriff of Kona' and 'Koolau the Leper', collected in *The House of Pride and Other Tales of Hawaii* (1912), represent the disease as one of unmitigated horror.

Jack London and Charmian Kittredge were given permission by the Board of Health in Honolulu to visit Molokai in 1906 in the anticipation that they would endorse the segregation policy by giving a favourable picture of the colony. In their travel writing, at least, they both obliged. London's account in *The Cruise of the Snark* begins festively with a description of the sports and entertainments he witnessed on the Fourth of July, at which 'nearly a thousand lepers were laughing uproariously at the fun'. The settlement is a thriving community of churches, assembly halls, a bandstand, a race-track, a shooting range, an athletics club and two brass bands. Living conditions are better than those found in many cities of the United States or Britain: 'I have seen the Hawaiians living in the slums of Honolulu, and ... I can readily understand why the lepers, brought up from the Settlement for re-examination, shouted one and all, "Back to Molokai!"'[33] More than just a sanctuary for lepers, Molokai is a remnant of the traditional communities that once typified Hawaiian culture but which have otherwise been wiped out by white settlement of the islands. Segregation actually works to protect the diseased from the civilised. Charmian Kittredge's parallel account of the Fourth of July celebrations makes explicit this view of the colony as the flawed remnant of an indigenous culture:

The whole was a picture of old Hawaii not to be found elsewhere in the whole territory ... For no set reproduction of the bygone customs could equal this whole-souled exhibition, costumed from simple materials by older women who remembered days of the past, carried out in the natural order of life in one of the most beautiful spots in the islands.[34]

---

[32] For a detailed discussion of this see Rod Edmond, *Representing the South Pacific: Colonial Discourse from Cook to Gauguin* (Cambridge: Cambridge University Press, 1997), ch. 7; also chapter 1, p. 37 of this book.

[33] Jack London, *The Cruise of the* Snark: *A Pacific Voyage* (London and New York: KPI, 1986), pp. 99, 110.

[34] Charmian Kittredge London, *Jack London and Hawaii* (London: Mills and Boon, 1918), p. 123.

London's leprosy fiction, on the other hand, represents the disease and the colony very differently, and it was alleged to have damaged the Hawaiian tourist trade.[35] Several stories dramatise Western horror of the disease. In 'The Sheriff of Kona', the eponymous hero is exposed as having 'the mark of the beast' by a disreputable *hapa-haole* who has relatives on Molokai and can therefore recognise the signs. The sheriff is removed to the colony but his white friends cannot accept his segregation in an over-whelmingly Hawaiian and Chinese settlement, and they spring him from the island by night. This involves a bizarre struggle between one of the rescuers and a leper – 'noseless, lipless, with one ear swollen and distorted, hanging down to the shoulder' – who sinks his teeth into the rescuer's hand, leaving it looking 'as if it had been mangled by a dog'.[36] Seven years on, however, the man remains uninfected. This is another text that owes something to Billy Ragsdale's story, although in this case the *hapa-haole* is the accuser and implied bridge for the disease, rather than its target. It is the wholly white man who suffers. The story dramatises *haole* fears of leprosy and terror at its failure to discriminate between races. Equally it expresses the anxiety that uncertainty about the transmission of the disease caused. The source of the hero's infection is unknown, yet the vicious bite of a leper leaves his rescuer untouched by leprosy.

In 'Koolau the Leper', however, the angle is reversed. Based on an episode from recent Hawaiian history, this story is narrated from the indigenous point of view and leprosy becomes an image of the dismember-ing and putrefying effects of colonialism. In the real-life story, Koolau was refused permission to have his uninfected wife and child accompany him to Molokai. The three then took refuge in a remote valley on the island of Kauai and evaded capture for more than two years until both Koolau and his now leprous child died. Several attempts to capture Koolau resulted in the local sheriff and several soldiers being shot and killed.[37] In London's fictional version, a leper band makes its last stand against deportation to Molokai in the mountain passes of Kauai. Until the attempted capture this group has survived as a maimed community, planting gardens and culti-vating taro, melons and papaya. This fallen Eden, a kind of voluntary Molokai, is shelled and destroyed by the soldiers coming to deport the lepers. Most of the lepers surrender, but Koolau escapes and lives as a fugitive before eventually shooting himself. In this story the leper is a figure of the tragic but inevitable extinction of the culture of the colonised.

---

[35] *Ibid.*, p. 239.

[36] Jack London, *Tales of the Pacific* (Harmondsworth: Penguin, 1989), p. 133.

[37] *The True Story of Kaulaikoolau, as Told by his Wife, Piilani*, trans. Frances N. Frazier (Lihue, Hawaii: Kauai Historical Society, 2001).

Molokai has become a burial ground for the Hawaiians, a place to be feared and resisted rather than a vivid trace of a once vibrant people. The lines of division have also become starkly clear. There is no complicating *hapa-haole* element in this story; the lepers are all native Hawaiian and the force sent to capture them is led by 'a blue-eyed American'.

Graham Greene

There is nothing in *A Burnt-Out Case* (1960), nor the journal from which it grew, published as *Congo Journal* (1961), to suggest that Greene knew Stevenson's or London's leprosy writing. He had, though, once considered writing Damien's life, and the priest is mentioned in both Greene's texts as a possible type of the leprophil.[38] *Congo Journal* also has a luridly garbled version of Arning's inoculation experiment, but there is no invoking of literary predecessors who had crossed the leper boundary. Instead, the foundation text of Greene's leprosy writing is Conrad's *Heart of Darkness*.

At the end of January 1959 Greene had flown from Brussels to Leopoldville in the Belgian Congo with a novel taking shape in his mind. Its situation was to be 'a stranger who turns up in a remote leper-colony'.[39] From Leopoldville, Greene flew on to Coquilhatville, now Mbandaka, in Congo's Equator Province, from where he was taken to the leper colony of Yonda by its resident leprologist, Dr Michel Lechat. Lechat is the dedicatee of *A Burnt-Out Case*, and in his dedication Greene is at pains to make clear that neither the leprologist in the novel, Dr Colin, nor his *léproserie* are to be identified with Greene's host and the Yonda hospital. My Congo, the author insists, 'is a region of the mind'. From almost the beginning of his journal it is apparent that this region of his mind is being shared with Conrad. Shown the modern parts of Leopoldville – a university, the Stanley Memorial – Greene recalls the narrator of *Heart of Darkness*: ' "And this also, said Marlow suddenly, "has been one of the dark places of the earth." '[40] After a week at Yonda, Greene travels up-river stopping at several missions and *léproseries*, first Imbonga and then Lombo Lumba. These are stations on Greene's quest for a novel, and as he travels he is reading *Heart of Darkness*. He is also repeating part of the river journey that Conrad had made in 1890 as captain of the steamship *Roi des Belges*.[41] It is the first Conrad he has read for many years: 'I abandoned him about

---

[38] Norman Sherry, *The Life of Graham Greene*, vol. III: *1955–1991* (London: Jonathan Cape, 2004), p. 162; Graham Greene, *A Burnt-Out Case* (Harmondsworth: Penguin, 1975), p. 22; Graham Greene, 'Congo Journal', in *In Search of a Character* (Harmondworth: Penguin, 1968), p. 23.

[39] Greene, 'Congo Journal', p. 7.   [40] *Ibid.*, p. 15.

[41] Sherry, *The Life of Graham Greene*, vol. III, p. 154.

1932 because his influence on me was too great and too disastrous.' Now he is more critical; Conrad's language is 'too inflated for the situation. Kurtz never really comes alive.'[42] Nevertheless the pressure of Conrad's novella is inescapable, in the details as well as the settings of the river journey Greene recorded in his journal. For better or worse Greene found himself travelling in Marlow's wake. Whereas visiting a leper colony in the Pacific characteristically produces a 'horror in paradise' narrative, in Africa it becomes a 'heart of darkness' one.

Heart of Darkness echoes through the novel, *A Burnt-Out Case*, that resulted from this journey, affecting its shape and characterisation as well as the view of Africa as a dark and diseased continent that is common to both texts. *A Burnt-Out Case* opens with Querry, the stranger who is to turn up at the remote leper colony, journeying up-river towards his quarry. One evening he leaves the boat, which has anchored for the night, and follows a rough track 'towards what geographers might have called the centre of Africa'.[43] The scene recalls Marlow leaving his boat in search of the vanished Kurtz and cutting him off from the 'the gleam of fires, the throb of drums, the drone of weird incantations'.[44] In Querry's case, however, the village he finds is poor, the drums are old tins of sardines and Heinz beans, and the natives are mere pygmoids – 'bastard descendants of the true pygmies'.[45] The effect is reductive, but as so often with Greene the irony retains much of what it seems to undercut.

There is a broader pattern of influence from *Heart of Darkness* in Greene's novel. The journalist, Parkinson, who tracks Querry down in his leper hideaway and tells the world of this famous architect-become-reclusive-saint is a parody of Conrad's Marlow. Just as 'Kurtz discoursed . . . to the very last', becoming for Marlow entirely 'a voice',[46] so the normally taciturn Querry bursts into eloquence with the arrival of Parkinson. 'I have been waiting for you, Parkinson, or someone like you',[47] Querry tells the journalist, as if he can only explain himself to this wretched but exemplary representative of the world he has turned his back on. Marlow listens intently to Kurtz's flow: 'No eloquence could have been so withering to one's belief in mankind as his final burst of sincerity.' And Kurtz's final cry, 'The horror!' is glossed by Marlow as 'the expression of some sort of belief . . . the appalling face of a glimpsed truth'.[48] Parkinson, however, listens with neither interest nor understanding. Unlike Marlow, this hard-boiled cynical hack knows the story he will tell before he meets its subject.

[42] Greene, 'Congo Journal', pp. 42, 44.   [43] Greene, *A Burnt-Out Case*, p. 15.
[44] Joseph Conrad, *Heart of Darkness* (London: Dent, 1960), p. 144.
[45] Greene, *A Burnt-Out Case*, p. 15.   [46] Conrad, *Heart of Darkness*, p. 147.
[47] Greene, *A Burnt-Out Case*, p. 116.   [48] Conrad, *Heart of Darkness*, pp. 145, 151.

But he is like Marlow as well in that both men bring out lies from the heart of darkness. The readers of his journal, *The Post*, are as keen as Kurtz's Intended to have their illusions bolstered, as Greene takes pleasure in illustrating with an extract from Parkinson's write-up of Querry's story:

What is it that has induced the great Querry to abandon a career that brought him honour and riches to give up his life to serving the world's untouchables? I was in no position to ask him that when suddenly I found that my quest had ended. Unconscious and burning with fever, I was carried on shore from my pirogue, the frail bark in which I had penetrated what Joseph Conrad called the Heart of Darkness, by a few faithful natives who had followed me down the great river with the same fidelity their grandfathers had shown to Stanley.[49]

But whereas Marlow's lie has its partial justification – humankind can only bear so much reality and Kurtz's vision is incommunicable to the sepulchred cities of Europe – Parkinson's is flagrantly opportunist. It also contributes directly to Querry's death.

Querry is killed by Ryker, Greene's version of Conrad's Harlequin, the 'man of patches', 'admirer of Mr Kurtz' and another idealistic babbler.[50] Querry is murdered because his refusal to accept Ryker's need to worship him becomes entangled with Marie Ryker's marital servitude. For Marlow, 'the women ... are out of it – should be out of it. We must help them to stay in that beautiful world of their own, lest ours gets worse.'[51] For Greene, however, women are always somewhere at the heart of the matter. In fact Ryker's wife is an apparently bland but eventually poisonous amalgam of both of Kurtz's women, the savage and the Intended. Marie is the civilised girl in the jungle, and the casual misogyny of Marlow's remark is endorsed in Greene's text by the way that her lie about having sex with Querry leads to his death.

My point in tracing the patterns of this influence is to show that Conrad's novella provided Greene with a structure he could use and ironise. It also created some problems that I shall consider below. First, however, the heart of Greene's novel – the identification of Querry's plight with that of the leper – needs closer consideration. Early in *A Burnt-Out Case* Dr Colin describes 'the sweet gangrenous smell of certain leprous skins', and how this has for him become 'the smell of Africa'.[52] Greene's fascination with decay is always entangled with the possibility of salvation, and leprosy, which by this time was curable, is a powerful correlative for his most insistent concerns. Querry's emotional and spiritual numbness sends him from Europe to Africa to seek cure, solace or death in a leper

---

[49] Greene, *A Burnt-Out Case*, p. 133.   [50] Conrad, *Heart of Darkness*, pp. 131, 136.
[51] *Ibid.*, p. 115.   [52] Greene, *A Burnt-Out Case*, p. 18.

colony. The early sections of the novel emphasise the parallel between Querry's condition and that of the leper. Just as the young child examined by Dr Colin has patches on its back where 'the ... skin seemed to have grown an extra layer', so too the unnaturally thick-skinned Querry dreams of his inability to share the suffering of a girl 'he had once known and thought he loved'.[53] He excuses himself to the girl by explaining he can no longer feel, that he is a leper. And so on. He explains his avoidance of Marie Ryker when she visits the settlement by comparing himself with the leper who is afraid of striking his fingers because he knows they will not hurt any more.[54]

This equivalence is sustained by the identification of Querry with Deo Gratias, the actual burnt-out case who becomes Querry's double and secret sharer. Deo Gratias is the first leper Querry sees on disembarking at the riverside colony and he becomes the visitor's servant. When Deo Gratias disappears into the forest Querry discovers his injured servant and spends the night with him where he has fallen. As Querry tries to move Deo Gratias from the stream in which he is lying, the servant feels 'warm and wet like a hummock of soil'; sitting together in the darkness his fingerless hand 'felt as a rock might that has been eroded for years by the weather'.[55] Leprosy is a kind of bedrock, the condition of conditions, Agamben's 'bare life', and this links Deo Gratias's physical symptoms with Querry's emotional and spiritual ones. Once this identification has been established, however, Deo Gratias fades into the background. From the moment of Parkinson's arrival the novel is focused elsewhere.

The language used to describe Deo Gratias's disfigurement is consistently naturalising and objectifying. The stump of his arm is 'like a piece of wood which had been roughly carved into the beginning of a human hand'; when Deo Gratias brings Querry his morning water, the pail hangs on his wrist 'like a coat on a cloakroom-knob'. This truncated, rough-hewn, desensitised body provides the means by which Querry can make clear the nature of his own deformity. As he explains to the doctor: 'The palsied suffer, their nerves feel, but I am one of the mutilated.'[56] Thickening of the skin is a recurring trope. Dr Colin has ordered new apparatus from Europe that will enable him to anticipate the formation of leprous nodules and patches by measuring the varying temperature of the skin. There is, however, no such apparatus for measuring Querry's condition. Of course for Greene a simile is as irresistible as an adjective was to Conrad, but the objectifying and dehumanised language in which Deo

---

[53] *Ibid.*, pp. 27, 31.   [54] *Ibid.*, p. 75.   [55] *Ibid.*, pp. 56, 57.   [56] *Ibid.*, pp. 17, 25, 46.

Gratias is consistently described contributes to the recurring and uncomfortable implication that Querry's plight is worse than that of the lepers. This is not merely an aspect of Querry's self-pity, which Greene certainly dramatises, but it is a point of view reinforced by Dr Colin who repeatedly makes the Querry/leper analogy, and who suggests that the psychology of decay is more significant than its physical forms of expression.

This parallelism between Querry's aridity and the suffering of the leper is problematic in the way that Sylvia Plath's self-identification with Holocaust victims is also problematic. It threatens to reduce the leper colony to a necessary place of extremity in which Querry can recover his ability to feel and suffer, and it recalls Chinua Achebe's objection to the way in which Conrad's *Heart of Darkness* uses Africa as a mere backdrop for European angst: 'Can nobody see the preposterous and perverse arrogance in thus reducing Africa to the role of props for the break-up of one petty European mind?'[57] This criticism is, if anything, more pertinent to *A Burnt-Out Case*, where Greene seems much closer to Querry than Conrad ever is to Kurtz. Querry's death is tragic because it effaces the process of recovery that the novel has been tracing; Kurtz's death, on the other hand, is the end-point of his degeneration. Both are brilliant Europeans for whom Africa is a foil, but Greene's text works much harder to establish sympathy for Querry than Conrad's does for Kurtz. And the terms in which it does so are directly dependent on African suffering in a way that has no parallel in *Heart of Darkness*. Achebe has suggested that Greene avoided Conrad's appropriation of Africa and African people: 'He didn't want to explain Africans to the world. He made limited claims and wasn't attempting to be too profound.' Achebe's case against Conrad, first made in 1975, remains unchanged: 'you cannot compromise my humanity in order that you explore your own ambiguity ... My humanity is not ... to be used simply to illustrate European problems.'[58] But this seems precisely what Greene is doing in *A Burnt-Out Case*, and far less ambiguously than Conrad had half a century earlier.

This is not to suggest that *A Burnt-Out Case* has no interest in leprosy as such. Through the figure of Dr Colin, and especially in his conversations with Querry, a great deal of information about the understanding and treatment of the disease at the time is conveyed. The doctor represents the modern scientific approach to leprosy, in contradistinction to traditional religiously based attitudes. This is neatly illustrated in the scene where he and Querry sit on the steps of the hospital listening to the Superior saying

[57] Chinua Achebe, 'An Image of Africa: Racism in Conrad's *Heart of Darkness*', in *Hopes and Impediments: Selected Essays 1965–1987* (London: Heinemann, 1988), p. 8.
[58] Interview in *The Guardian*, 22 February 2003.

mass for a congregation of lepers in the open-sided church across the road. This deftly reverses the traditional arrangement whereby lepers were left on the outside looking in. As they listen to the sermon Querry asks the doctor if he feels like a Christian. His reply – ' "I'm not interested . . . I wish Christianity could reduce the price of cortisone, that's all" ' – is answered by Querry's retort that he hates simplifications. The doctor admits the reductionism of his position, acknowledging that whereas a negative skin test tells him if someone is cured there 'are no skin-tests for a good action'.[59] Querry is left somewhere between the religious and the scientific, a sceptic without a vocation. Later in the novel he begins to discover a vocation in the new hospital he plans and builds with Dr Colin, only to be killed by Ryker, the jealous Catholic zealot.

The medical science practised by Dr Colin is treated with sympathy and respect throughout. We see him ordering an Atlas of Leprosy, waiting for the apparatus that will warn of leprous patches, and planning to have wheel chairs for the worst cases. And Greene can make brilliant if mis-leading use of this material. The Atlas, with its 'gaudy page of swirling colour' illustrating bacilli swarming along the nerves, becomes an image of the contagion spread by Marie Ryker's lie that Querry is the father of her child.[60] Particularly interesting is the account of the side effects of DDS (diamino-diphenyl-sulphone) in which a patient is overcome by a kind of madness that renders him likely to kill his son.[61] There is still no simple cure. Too much from the patient's point of view, however, would threaten the Querry/leper analogy. Elsewhere we see Dr Colin reflecting on the psychological aspect of leprosy now that a cure was available for the physical disease. Touching his patients helped them to realise they were not untouchable.[62] Awareness of this psychological dimension, however, also facilitates the association of Querry's mind and soul with the leper's body.

The divide between modern scientific and traditional attitudes to lep-rosy goes back to the development of bacteriology in the late nineteenth century, exemplified by Arning's position in Hawaii in the mid-1880s. The new element in Greene's treatment of the disease is the idea of the lepro-phil. Dr Colin wonders at first if Querry is a leprophil, a type that he describes to the Superior at the colony:

Schweitzer seems to attract them. They would rather wash the feet with their hair like the woman in the gospel than clean them with something more antiseptic. Sometimes I wonder whether Damien was a leprophil. There was no need for him

[59] Greene, *A Burnt-Out Case*, pp. 81, 82.   [60] *Ibid.*, pp. 185–6.   [61] *Ibid.*, p. 104.
[62] *Ibid.*, p. 18.

to become a leper in order to serve them well. A few elementary precautions – I wouldn't be a better doctor without my fingers, would I?[63]

Later in the novel Dr Colin suggests that Damien had a death wish.[64] Cherishing the leper, once a mark of sainthood, has now become suspect; if Damien's sacrifice is ambiguous then Francis of Assisi was certainly a leprophil.

Saints were always problematic for Greene, but in *A Burnt-Out Case* the celebrity leprologist has become the model to avoid. Albert Schweitzer is the conspicuous example. Dr Colin is at first concerned that Querry might be a writer or photographer, an outrider of the world's press: 'There's no room for a writer here'[65] he tells Querry, a nice instance of Greene's self-reflexive irony. But the doctor has misidentified his guest. With Parkinson's arrival Querry himself becomes a version of Schweitzer, sacrificing fame for duty among the stricken of Africa. Although this unsought attention is most unwelcome to both Querry and the doctor, the acting Superior Father Thomas sees advantages in Parkinson's stories of 'the hermit of the Congo': 'Our leproserie may become famous – as famous as Schweitzer's hospital, and the British, one has heard, are a generous people.'[66] The funding of leper colonies, as well as the treatment of those suffering from the disease, has become secularised. Whereas in the nineteenth century metropolitan congregations raised money for missionaries and nurses, by the mid-twentieth century this funding has dwindled. The new kind of celebrity saint, though abhorrent to Querry and Doctor Colin, can bring in the money.

This transformation whereby the cult of the leprosy worker has encouraged the spread of leprophilia, with the world's press beating a track to Lamberene for Schweitzer to display his work, is a direct consequence of the curability of the disease. The danger has gone out of leprosy. Dr Colin comments on the previously high suicide rate among leprologists, explaining it as an inability to wait for the positive test they all expected. Post-DDS there are fewer 'vocations of doom', and therefore less 'unnecessary suffering'.[67] Rather than hearing from afar, the world can now see for itself, or at least be shown through the medium of mid-twentieth-century photo-journalism. For Querry this means there is no place to hide, and it threatens Dr Colin's ability to work in peace. Schweitzer is the modern version of the type of the leprophil, the latest impediment to a fully adequate scientific response to the disease. He was also a figure of scorn for Achebe:

---

[63] *Ibid.*, p. 22.   [64] *Ibid.*, p. 121.   [65] *Ibid.*, p. 28.   [66] *Ibid.*, pp. 134, 108.
[67] *Ibid.*, pp. 121–2.

In a comment which has often been quoted Schweitzer says: 'The African is indeed my brother but my junior brother.' And so he proceeded to build a hospital appropriate to the needs of junior brothers with standards of hygiene reminiscent of medical practice in the days before the germ theory of disease came into being. Naturally he became a sensation in Europe and America. Pilgrims flocked, and I believe still flock even after he has passed on, to witness the prodigious miracle in Lamberene, on the edge of the primeval forest.[68]

Querry can be seen as a reworking of the figure of Schweitzer. He too builds and designs a hospital, implicitly renouncing the famous churches he has built in Europe, exchanging the aesthetics of religion for the instrumentality of medicine. Querry's hospital, designed to meet the needs of a modern bacteriologist, while remaining hidden from the lepro-phils of the world, is the anti-type of Achebe's Lamberene.

The celebrity leprologist and the phenomenon of the leprophil has implications for Greene the writer who made his own journey to the Yonda leper colony, published an account of his experiences, and used them as the material for a novel which is dedicated to Dr Michel Lechat. Greene, like other traveller-writers at this time, can make his journey confident that in the unlikely event of his contracting leprosy it would be curable. The nature of the leper border has changed. Once the disease can be arrested, once it is recognised as having a very low contagion rate, crossing that border loses most of its danger, while still retaining some of its frisson. This helps explain the differences between Stevenson and London's fictional treatment of the disease, and Greene's. For the former writers, the distance between the leprous colonial subject and the clean Westerner is more uncertain, and this makes the disease a potent means of figuring both the ambiguities and the injuries of cultural contact and exchange. Greene's use of the disease is altogether more egocentric and Eurocentric. It becomes a correlative for the death-in-life state of mind of his European hero, for the burnt-out soul of the ex-Catholic, for the celebrity hiding from his success. No longer a death-sentence, leprosy can now be confidently appropriated as a metaphor and put to different kinds of use. Greene can run the parallel between Querry and Deo Gratias because there is no longer any fear of the European catching the disease, yet Querry's moral stature rests to a considerable extent on his apparent carelessness in braving the colony and getting his hands dirty. Those such as Ryker, who continue to worry about infection and are squeamish at the sight of a leper, are pictured as moral cowards. Greene draws on the boundary anxieties that leprosy has traditionally provoked, but has set his novel in a time when the medical reasons for fearing leprosy have

---

[68] Achebe, 'An Image of Africa', pp. 7–8.

disappeared. This sleight of hand enables him to exploit the danger and to appropriate the disease.[69]

Paul Theroux

My closing example of a traveller-writer who breached the cordon sanitaire of the leper colony is Paul Theroux. His autobiographical essay 'The Lepers of Moyo' was published in 1994 but looks back to his time as a young Peace Corps teacher in Malawi in the early 1960s. Theroux volunteers to spend a vacation teaching English to the inhabitants of a leper settlement and mission hospital at Moyo. The narrative begins with Paul's long train journey north from Blantyre, where he has been teaching in a school. Almost inevitably it is another 'heart of darkness' narrative. Paul wishes 'to know the inside of the continent – its secrets', to discover 'the Africa of my imagination'.[70] But his language class is a failure, and his other vain efforts to assist the colony are ended by a severe bout of fever.

The main focus of his narrative is on two women: one a young American nurse, Birdie, who frequently wears the habit of a nun; the other a young Malawi woman, Amina, inseparable companion of her conspicuously leprous and blind grandmother. A sexual encounter with the American nurse is comically unsuccessful. Paul turns to Amina and they make love in her hut under the sightless gaze of the leprous grandmother. Amina also has leprosy, although Paul had not realised this at first; her only visible symptom is a hard dry patch of skin on her arm. Immediately after his sexual encounter with Amina Paul leaves the colony and returns to Blantyre. This is not because of fear of infection but because he has 'violated a strict rule . . . created an area of disorder'.[71] Paul fears discovery by the priests with whom he has lived and leaves in confusion and shame.

The sexual theme is the most striking aspect of Theroux's narrative. In having sexual intercourse with a leper Paul crosses the final border. In a post-dapsone world the fear of catching the disease has almost entirely disappeared and this clears the way for his transgression of the last remaining prohibition. That said, it is worth noting that for all Greene's braving of the border in search of extremity, sex in his leprosy writing remains strictly without the camp. Marie Ryker, the only sexual focus of *A Burnt-Out Case*, lives well away from Yonda with a leprophobic husband.

---

[69] Dr Robert Cochrane, medical missionary and leprologist, wrote a highly critical review of *A Burnt-Out Case* in 1961, accusing Greene of having a medieval approach to leprosy and of sensationalising the disease. See Tony Gould, *Don't Fence Me In: Leprosy in Modern Times* (London: Bloomsbury, 2005), pp. 332–3.

[70] Paul Theroux, 'The Lepers of Moyo', *Granta*, 48 (1994), 131–2.   [71] *Ibid.*, 189.

Theroux brings sex inside the camp and uses it to breach the last physical boundary between the clean and the unclean. In doing so, of course, Theroux is drawing on the age-old tradition of sexualising the disease, and following in the footsteps of modern traveller-writers who have preceded him. Stoddard deployed the sexualisation of leprosy homoerotically; Stevenson had presented a gently eroticised encounter with a woman on Molokai as an important step in his coming to understand the world from the point of view of a leper, and had passionately defended Damien from the very charge that Theroux voluntarily confesses; London had vividly depicted the active sexuality of physically maimed sufferers of the disease. Indeed Greene's avoidance of the subject is almost as distinctive as the emphasis given it by Theroux.

The scene with Amina, played out against the background noise of celebrations from the leper village, is represented as mutually desired and satisfying. In stroking her arm Paul touches the leprous patch – 'the disc of dead skin' – but this is the only intimate reminder of the disease and it does not disturb him; 'I had been here long enough to know there was no danger to me.'[72] Even while dispelling the danger, however, we are still reminded of its lingering trace. And, more emphatically, their lovemaking is under the nose of Amina's unmistakably leprous grandmother whose repeated questions about the noises she is hearing makes the episode furtive and tense as well as erotically charged. The grandmother's obtrusive presence is a kind of displaced reminder of the horror that such a scene would formerly have provoked. The older and younger women are inseparable; the grandmother as well as the patch is forever on Amina's arm. In earlier narratives the constant presence of the older woman would have functioned proleptically to indicate the inevitable fate of the younger. In the post-dapsone world of Theroux's narrative this is no longer the case, but some of the former power of this kind of imaging persists. Nor is this entirely without foundation. Even though the disease has been arrested, while symptoms remain cure is something of a misnomer. As Birdie tells Paul, scarring means that very few of the lepers of Moyo will ever return to their own villages: 'A person with toes missing looks like he still has the disease.'[73] Nevertheless, for all the complexity of Theroux's narrative, it is not without a self-aggrandising note of having crossed over to the other side and returned to tell the tale.

The juxtaposition of the sexual encounters with Birdie and Amina draws out the healthy and affirming nature of the latter. The scene with Birdie in the convent, she in her habit, Paul in a cassock from performing altar duties, is wonderfully lowering, the porno-comedy undercutting the

[72] *Ibid.*, 187.   [73] *Ibid.*, 140.

transgression. That between Paul and Amina is made natural and passionate. Seen from a different angle, however, it is also the oldest colonial narrative we have, one in which the European male takes his pleasure and departs, abandoning the native woman to her fate. Amina is not tearfully waving farewell from the platform as the train pulls away, but her absence from the text once Paul has left her hut allows the narrative to bring sharply into focus the other main theme of the narrative, that of writing.

'The Lepers of Moyo' is Theroux's version of Wordsworth's *Prelude*, about the growth of a poet's mind. Writing is foregrounded from the opening paragraph where Paul waits for the train to leave Blantyre, *The Diaries of Franz Kafka* on his lap. As the train heads up-country Paul tells us that although he has not yet published any of his poems, 'this trip made me feel like a writer'. His yearning to know 'the inside of the continent' is an aspect of his desire to be a writer, to visit the dark places of the earth and to discover new forms of language. It is the sound of the word 'leprosarium' that has prompted him to write to the father superior and offer his services:

I had never heard this English word before and I was bewitched by it. Leprosy was a primitive and dark disease, like an ancient curse. It suggested the unclean and the forbidden. It called to mind outcasts. It was an aspect of old, unsubtle Africa. Leper, leper, leper. I was sick of metaphors. I wanted words to have unambiguous meanings: leper, wilderness, poverty, heat.[74]

Moyo, however, is strange in ways Paul finds difficult to understand. The words 'Leper, leper, leper' are repeated, but their meaning is changing. Observing the dressing and bandaging of leprous sores not only makes his plan to teach English seem irrelevant and frivolous, but also makes Kafka's *Diaries* sound like 'the whining of a highly-strung child'.[75]

The leper colony becomes a rebuke to writing, a negation of it. When the father superior picks up Paul's English textbook and Kafka's *Diaries* he looks at them 'as though the books were mute objects without any function, like worn-out shoes'. Paul, too, has come to think of them as 'dead weight'.[76] Opening his notebook and fashioning a simile that could have been penned by Graham Greene – 'the Africans looking as upright as exclamation marks' – he does not bother writing it down: 'Writing seemed irrelevant.'[77] He is repelled by his own poems and when he comes across a passage in the *Diaries* where Kafka describes his shortness of breath as making him 'feel like a leper', Paul digs a hole and buries the book, together with his own poems. In doing so he disturbs two lepers having sex. The woman runs away but the man hitches up his shorts and stares at Paul, who later reflects:

[74] *Ibid.*, 130.   [75] *Ibid.*, 139, 142.   [76] *Ibid.*, 143.   [77] *Ibid.*, 150.

This was a leper: guiltless, maimed, seeping into his bandages. He had just copu-
lated under a tree with a leper woman and was now staring me down. In many ways
he was healthy – certainly healthier than Franz Kafka. Reading meant nothing to
him; a book was a mute object. He was patient and contemptuous because he was
powerless and knew it. Nothing would change for him, nor would he change
anything. He had no illusions, and so he was fully alive every moment, looking
for food or water or shade or a woman.[78]

Paul falls seriously ill with fever, has lurid dreams of leprous and
sexually rampant women, and is convinced he is dying. Convalescing, he
understands for the first time 'the leprosarium's indifference to the world',
and that 'any effort here was pointless'. The experience of serious illness
has left him 'naked' like all the other inhabitants of the colony:

Naked ... was not a figure of speech ... Words here had definite meanings. There
were no metaphors, no symbols, nothing poetic or literary. Sick meant leprosy;
fever meant a week of suffering; hot meant this pitiless sun; dust, this sour powder
that covered the ground and was the grit in every mouthful of food. And desire ...
was a man kneeling against a woman in the dust, behind a blind of crackling
cornshucks at the edge of the village, pumping while she thrashed, and it was
brief and brutal.[79]

Paul's departure from Moyo is a return to 'the feebler and less secure
world of metaphors, where leper did not mean leper'. The father superior's
suggestion that he might write something about the colony merely height-
ens the impossibility of doing so. The narrative ends as it began, with Paul
sitting in the train waiting for it to depart. He no longer feels like a writer:
'I wanted to write something, but I felt as though I would never write
again, about Moyo or anything else.'[80] Dr Colin's remark to Querry –
'There's no room for a writer here' – seems to have been proved true.
In this sense 'The Lepers of Moyo' becomes an anti-*Prelude*, about the
death of a poet's mind. Leprosy, the most metaphorical of diseases, had
rendered all figurative language impossible and all but the most basic
emotions trivial. How to describe bedrock without sentimentality, embel-
lishment or evasion? How to bridge the worlds of 'the clean' and the
'unclean', even now that these ancient terms have lost any real medical-
scientific meaning? Is there any space for the writer between the horror that
rejects, the sympathy that appropriates, the detachment that naturalises?
Stevenson, having said of Molokai that, 'A horror of moral beauty broods
over the place', added: 'that's like bad Victor Hugo, but it is the only way
I can express the sense that lived with me all these days'. Theroux is
grappling eloquently with a different version of the same problem; as this
book, less eloquently, has also been attempting.

---

[78] *Ibid.*, 153.   [79] *Ibid.*, 160, 161, 162.   [80] *Ibid.*, 190, 191.

Postscript

This book is not a history of leprosy down to the present day. Its main focus has been the period 1840–1920, when fears of the revival and return of leprosy became entangled with the spread of Western imperialism across the globe. Nor is it a narrative of the progressive elimination of ignorance and superstition by modern medical science. As we have seen, a mid-nineteenth-century anti-contagionist like Milroy was mainly right, but for the wrong reasons, while micro-biologists were wrong about the nature of the bacillus they rightly identified as the agent of infection.

That is, of course, always assuming that leprosy really is caused by *M. leprae*. It was not until 1971 that the bacillus was successfully transmitted to an experimental animal, the nine-banded armadillo, and it has still not been cultivated *in vitro*. Leprosy's mode of transmission remains unknown, and this, together with its very low level of infection, long latency, uncertain onset and prolonged duration means that many of the debates reviewed in this book have endured or been revived. Several modern researchers have questioned whether the disease is caused by *M. leprae* after all, suggesting instead that it has a metabolic origin and even returning to Jonathan Hutchinson's fish theory. The discovery that the bacilli can survive outside the body for many weeks has also seen the resurrection of telluric theories of the disease.[1] And while old debates survive, the mapping of the genome of *M. leprae* has opened up an entirely new way of understanding the mycobacterium, while leaving unanswered those questions that have haunted discussions of the disease since the middle of the nineteenth century. Old uncertainties remain as new questions are opened up.[2] Confident mid-twentieth-century forecasts of dapsone's ability to eradicate leprosy have proved wrong. Leprosy bacilli

---

[1] Tony Gould, *Don't Fence Me In: Leprosy in Modern Times* (London: Bloomsbury, 2005), pp. 379, 381.

[2] Even the terminology of its classification has been reversed. Danielssen and Boeck's anaesthetic type of the disease is now called tuberculoid, and their tubercular type is termed lepromatous or anaesthetic; see Gould, *Don't Fence Me In*, pp. 41, 313.

resistant to dapsone appeared and so multi-drug therapy had to be developed. Leprologists have no idea how one of the three drugs currently used in multi-drug therapy, clofazimine (B663), actually works.[3]

In 2005, the World Health Organisation Year of Leprosy, an estimated 750,000 new cases were detected. Unlike the years of high imperialism, however, leprosy now hardly impinges on the consciousness of the Western world, except, that is, in cultural representation where it remains static and clichéd. Walter Salles' film *The Motorcycle Diaries* (2004) uses the episode of Che Guevara's sojourn at a leper colony on an island in the Amazon to presage his later role as a champion of the oppressed and the dispossessed. In doing so, it makes far more of his visit to the San Pablo leper colony than is justified by the few pages devoted to the episode in Che Guevara's text. It also traduces his account by representing the colony as governed by Catholic superstition and repression.[4] Rather like Greene's *A Burnt-Out Case*, this allows Salles to use the colony as a backdrop to highlight the distinctiveness of its hero, in this case Che's moral courage and his empathy, indeed his Christ-like qualities. As he departs the colony, grateful lepers line the banks to cheer him on to his destiny. He will journey on to try and change the world while theirs remains as it always was.

The idea of leprosy as an atonement for being evil, savage or different has faded without entirely disappearing, but Salles' film demonstrates that the disease can still figure powerfully as a means of redemption or apotheosis for those who mix with the unclean. Crossing the boundary allows the transgressor to return transformed. W. G. Sebald's rendering of Flaubert's version of the legend of St Julian illustrates this well. Sated by his compulsive slaughter of all animal life, and haunted by the ghosts of the animals he has killed, St Julian is rowed by a leper across the water to the end of the world:

On the opposite bank Julian must share the ferryman's bed, and then, as he embraces the man's fissured and ulcerated flesh, partly hard and gnarled, partly deliquescent, spending the night breast to breast and mouth to mouth with that most repellent of all human beings, he is released from his torment and may rise into the blue expanses of the firmament.[5]

The Motorcycle Diaries begins as a road movie but is transformed by its hero's Damascene experience at the leper colony, the anagnorisis which redeems Che by putting him on the road of revolutionary politics. Having crossed over to the other side, Che can return cleansed and renewed.

---

[3] *Ibid.*, p. 16.
[4] Ernesto Che Guevara, *The Motorcycle Diaries: A Journey around South America*, trans. Ann Wright (London: Fourth Estate, 1996), pp. 131–8.
[5] W. G. Sebald, *Campo Santo* (London: Hamish Hamilton, 2005), p. 46.

The persistence of this narrative across many centuries is striking. Leprosy retains its traditional power of signification regardless of the state of medical knowledge, uncertainty or confusion. It would be difficult to find another time-lag so great than in the capacity of literature and related forms of cultural representation to retain and exploit forms of ignorance and superstition that would be scorned in other fields. Apart from the historical and cultural reasons for this that have been the burden of this study, there are others more intrinsic to modern cultural representation itself, particularly in the forms and conventions of psychological realism as they developed in the later eighteenth and into the nineteenth century. These rested on the idea that the outer reveals the inner, and that disfigurement is a symptom of malignity or corruption. The figure of the leper, therefore, could be recuperated as an emblem of our fallen state or, through its supposed condition of death-in-life, as anticipating our death and decay. When not a figure of horror, the leper has most commonly been one of sentimentalised pity. In this it shares something with the figure of the slave in abolitionist writing. As Marcus Wood has demonstrated, the suffering of the slave was often subordinated to the pain of abolitionist witnessing and testimony, with anti-slavery writing attesting to the sensitivity of the writer as much as to the enormity of enslavement.[6] Literature and its surrounding cultural discourses have continued to draw on a reservoir of stock images of disfigurement that should long ago have been discarded.

As I wrote this book the confinement of the leper in the modern imperial age came to seem exemplary of carceral reflexes that have persisted and are currently intensifying. The instinct to isolate and contain is, to some extent, cross-cultural and trans-historical, but not uniformly so. One of the defining characteristics of modernity has been the spatial definition of difference, in which increasing freedom of movement has as its necessary corollary the confinement of ethnic or social groups regarded as threatening or inimical. The parallels between medically based forms of segregation around the turn of the twentieth century and the construction of camps for undesired refugees, suspected terrorists and other aberrant groups became evermore apparent as I wrote. Elsewhere I have drawn a comparison between Australia's island solution to its leprosy problem at the end of the nineteenth century and its similar response to a perceived threat from refugees in 2001, when hundreds of such people were detained on Christmas Island before being distributed round the Pacific as their claims for asylum were very slowly investigated. Whereas lepers were

---

[6] Marcus Wood, *Slavery, Empathy and Pornography* (Oxford: Oxford University Press, 2002), *passim*.

formerly one of the pariah groups of the colonial world, refugees and asylum seekers had become their contemporary equivalent.[7] Such figures, as Hannah Arendt suggested, represent the limit of the idea of the rights of man, although in both cases this has been a contested limit.[8] This points to recurrent or enduring deep structures of thought, feeling and practice in the modern imperial world, epitomised by the penal colony at Guantanamo Bay, in which segregation and confinement persists even when the knowledge or evidence upon which it is based is demonstrably inadequate, or unlikely ever to be tested by due process.

[7] Rod Edmond, 'Abject Bodies/Abject Sites: Leper Islands in the High Imperial Era', in Rod Edmond and Vanessa Smith (eds.), *Islands in History and Representation* (London and New York: Routledge, 2003), p. 144.
[8] Hannah Arendt, *The Origins of Totalitarianism* (New York: Harcourt Brace Jovanovich, 1973), pp. 299–300.

Index

For EU product safety concerns, contact us at Calle de José Abascal, 56–1°,
28003 Madrid, Spain or eugpsr@cambridge.org.

www.ingramcontent.com/pod-product-compliance
Ingram Content Group UK Ltd.
Pitfield, Milton Keynes, MK11 3LW, UK
UKHW010854090126
466816UK00011B/228